D1260372

Issues in Palliative Care Research

ues in

lliative Care

Research

Edited by
RUSSELL K. PORTENOY, M.D.
EDUARDO BRUERA, M.D.

OXFORD
UNIVERSITY PRESS
2003

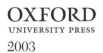

OXFORD
UNIVERSITY PRESS

Oxford   New York
Auckland   Bangkok   Buenos Aires   Cape Town   Chennai
Dar es Salaam   Delhi   Hong Kong   Istanbul   Karachi   Kolkata
Kuala Lumpur   Madrid   Melbourne   Mexico City   Mumbai
Nairobi   São Paulo   Shanghai   Taipei   Tokyo   Toronto

Library of Congress Cataloging-in-Publication Data
Portenoy, Russell K.
Issues in palliative care research/
by Russell K. Portenoy, Eduardo Bruera.
p. ; cm.   Includes bibliographical references and index.
ISBN 0-19-513065-0
1. Palliative treatment. 2. Terminal care—Research.
3. Terminally ill—Research.
I. Bruera, Eduardo. II. Title.
[DNLM: 1. Palliative Care. 2. Research.
WB 310 P843i 2003]   R726.8 .P665 2003
616'.029—dc21   2002070199

9 8 7 6 5 4 3 2 1

Printed in the United States of America
on acid-free paper

Preface

Palliative care is rapidly evolving, driven by the growing acknowledgment that the conventional medical care provided to those with life-threatening illness inadequately addresses the many sources of suffering and does little to prepare the patient and family for the process of dying. Given the complex, multidimensional, and dynamic nature of illness, palliative care is advancing as a therapeutic model that can address the physical, psychosocial, spiritual, and practical factors that may undermine quality of life from the time of diagnosis onward. When given appropriate emphasis, it intensifies as death approaches to reassure the patient and the family that decisions and values will be respected; physical, psychosocial, and spiritual needs will be managed; practical help will be provided; and opportunities for closure and growth will be supported.

This is work of extraordinary breadth. It includes a range of conventional medical interventions and a variety of concerns that traditionally have been at the fringes of the biomedical mainstream, such as ethics, communication, and the nature of suffering. In such a field, progress depends on many strategies.

In recent years, the need for improvements in the scientific foundation for palliative care has emerged as among the most important of these strategies. Without the science, the political and ethical rationale for improved care will be stymied, particularly in the setting of limited health-care resources. Verifiable evidence provides substance to the claim of benefits from one or more of the numerous interventions subsumed under the rubric of palliative care. Research may be able to chip away at the dogma that leads to thoughtless care, yield effective means for improving outcomes, and establish cost-benefit.

Not surprisingly, the types of research needed to advance palliative care are as broad as the field itself. With the exception of pain, there has been very little basic research into the nature of symptoms or disorders such as delirium. The promise of this type of work is profound but likely to be realized far in the future. More immediately, there is extraordinary promise from clinical epidemiology, treatment trials, psychosocial research, quality-of-life studies, and systems research.

This volume describes some of these efforts and is offered in the hope of spurring interest in palliative care research. The idea for such a book originated in a 1998 meeting focused on research that took place in Washington, D.C., at the National Institutes of Health. The meeting was designed to encourage a broad perspective on the research agenda for this field. It provided an opportunity for accomplished investigators to define the challenges inherent in the study of outcomes that are often subjective in populations with advanced illness. It recognized the fundamental importance of measurement to science and tried to clarify the types of methodology that could yield credible measurements of complex human occurrences and perceptions.

This volume includes updated proceedings of this meeting and additional chapters on selected topics. It is not intended to be an exhaustive review of the research agenda for palliative care or the methodological issues that must be addressed over time. Rather, it offers an overview of the most important research issues and aims at clarifying the range of relevant research concerns that should be addressed as palliative care advances as a therapeutic model.

We are grateful to all of the authors who contributed and then updated their work to maintain its topicality. They are the pioneers who are bringing the necessary scientific perspective to the fore. We also thank Ms. Marilyn Herleth, without whose efforts this book would not be published.

New York, New York   R.K.P.
Houston, Texas   E.B.

Contents

Part IX Research Issues in Special Populations

Contributors

MARILYN BOOKBINDER, PH.D., R.N.
Director of Nursing Education & Quality Improvement
Department of Pain Medicine and Palliative Care
Beth Israel Medical Center
New York, New York

WILLIAM BREITBART, M.D.
Chief, Psychiatry Service and Attending Psychiatrist
Department of Psychiatry and Behavioral Sciences
Memorial Sloan-Kettering Cancer Center
Professor of Clinical Psychiatry
Weill Medical College of Cornell University
New York, New York

ANNE BRUCE, R.N., PH.D.(C)
University of British Columbia, School of Nursing
Sessional Lecturer, School of Nursing
Lower Mainland Campus, University of Victoria
Victoria, British Columbia
Canada

EDUARDO BRUERA, M.D.
Professor and Chair
Department of Palliative Care and Rehabilitation Medicine
F.T. McGraw Chair in the Treatment of Cancer
The University of Texas M. D. Anderson Cancer Center
Houston, Texas

DAVID J. CASARETT, M.D.
Center for Health Equity Research and Promotion
Philadelphia Veterans Administration Medical Center
Assistant Professor, Division of Geriatrics
University of Pennsylvania
Philadelphia, Pennsylvania

DAVID CELLA, PH.D.
Professor, Department of Psychiatry and Behavioral Sciences
Northwestern University Medical School
Research Professor, Institute for Health Services Research and Policy Studies
Northwestern University
Director, Center on Outcomes, Research and Education
Evanston Northwestern Healthcare
Evanston, Illinois

HARVEY MAX CHOCHINOV, M.D.
Psychiatric Consultant
Manitoba Treatment & Research Center
Winnipeg, Manitoba
Canada

S. ROBIN COHEN, PH.D.
Research Director and Assistant Professor
Division of Palliative Care
Departments of Oncology and Medicine
McGill University
Medical Scientist, McGill University Health Center
Montreal, Quebec
Canada

JOHN J. COLLINS, M.B., B.S., PH.D.,
F.R.A.C.P.
Head, Pain and Palliative Care Service
The Children's Hospital at Westmead
Sydney, New South Wales
Australia

JESSICA CORNER, PH.D., B.SC.,
R.G.N.
Professor in Cancer and Palliative Care
School of Nursing and Midwifery
University of Southampton
Southampton, Hampshire
United Kingdom

NESSA COYLE, R.N., PH.D.(C)
Director, Supportive Care Program
Pain and Palliative Care Service
Department of Neurology
Memorial Sloan-Kettering Cancer Center
New York, New York

BETTY DAVIES, R.N., PH.D., F.A.A.N.
Professor and Chair, Department of
Family Health Care Nursing
University of California at San Francisco
School of Nursing
San Francisco, California

DEBORAH DUDGEON, M.D.,
F.R.C.P.C.
Director, Palliative Care Medicine
Associate Professor, Department of
Internal Medicine
Queen's University
Kingston, Ontario
Canada

LINDA L. EMANUEL, M.D., PH.D.
Buehler Professor of Geriatric Medicine
Director, The Buehler Center on Aging
Principal, The Education for Physicians
in End-of-Life Care Project
Northwestern's Feinberg School of
Medicine
Professor of Health Industry Management
Director, Health Section, The Ford
Center on Global Citizenship
The Kellog School of Management
Northwestern University
Chicago, Illinois

JOSEPH F. FOSS, M.D.
Director, Clinical Research and
Development
Adolor Corporation
Exton, Pennsylvania

ALICE INMAN, R.N., M.S.
Research Associate
Community Cancer Care, Inc.
Indianapolis, Indiana

PAUL B. JACOBSEN, PH.D.
Professor, Department of Psychology
University of South Florida
Program Leader, Psychosocial &
Palliative Care Program
Moffitt Cancer Center
Tampa, Florida

KRISTINA JONES, M.D.
Fellow, Psychiatry Service
Department of Psychiatry and Behavioral
Sciences
Memorial Sloan-Kettering Cancer Center
New York, New York

LINDA J. KRISTJANSON, R.N., B.N.,
M.N., PH.D.
Professor and Chair of Palliative Care
Faculty of Communications, Health &
Science
Edith Cowan University
Churchlands, Western Australia
Australia

CHARLES L. LOPRINZI, M.D.
Mayo Clinic and North Central Cancer
Treatment Group
Rochester, Minnesota

MITCHELL MAX, M.D.
Senior Investigator, Pain and
Neurosensory Mechanisms Branch
National Institute of Dental and
Craniofacial Research
National Institutes of Health
Bethesda, Maryland

STEVEN D. PASSIK, PH.D.
Director of Symptom Management and
Palliative Care
Markey Cancer Center
University of Kentucky
Lexington, Kentucky

AMY H. PETERMAN, PH.D.
Director of Research, Center on
Outcomes, Research and Education
Evanston Northwestern Healthcare
Research Assistant Professor, Institute
for Health Services Research and
Policy Studies
Northwestern University Medical School
Evanston, Illinois

RUSSELL K. PORTENOY, M.D.
Chairman, Department of Pain Medicine
and Palliative Care
Beth Israel Medical Center
Professor of Neurology
Albert Einstein College of Medicine
Bronx, New York

BARRY ROSENFELD, PH.D.
Associate Professor, Department of
Psychology
Fordham University
Bronx, New York

KENDRITH M. ROWLAND, JR., M.D.
Mayo Clinic and North Central Cancer
Treatment Group
Rochester, Minnesota

JEFF A. SLOAN, PH.D.
Mayo Clinic and North Central Cancer
Treatment Group
Rochester, Minnesota

THOMAS J. SMITH, M.D.
Chairman, Division of Hematology/
Oncology
Professor of Medicine and Health
Administration
VCU Health System
Richmond, Virginia

MILDRED Z. SOLOMON, ED.D.
Associate Clinical Professor of Social
Medicine and Anaesthesia
Harvard Medical School
Cambridge, Massachusetts
Vice-President, Education Development
Center, Inc.
Director, E.D.C.'s Center for Applied
Ethics and Professional Practice
Newton, Massachusetts

KELLI I. STAJDUHAR, R.N., PH.D.
CIHR/MSFHR Postdoctoral Fellow,
Center on Aging
Adjunct Assistant Professor, University of
Victoria
Research Associate, Vancouver Island
Health Authority
Adjunct Professor, University of British
Columbia, School of Nursing
Vancouver, British Columbia
Canada

ROSE STEELE, R.N., PH.D.
Assistant Professor, School of Nursing
Atkinson Faculty of Liberal &
Professional Studies
York University
Toronto, Ontario
Canada

NIGEL SYKES, M.D.
Consultant in Palliative Medicine
St. Christopher's Hospice
Honorary Senior Lecturer in Palliative
Medicine
King's College
University of London
London
United Kingdom

LYNNE I. WAGNER, PH.D.
Assistant Professor, Department of
  Psychiatry and Behavioral Sciences
Northwestern University Medical School
Faculty Fellow, Institute for Health
  Services Research and Policy Studies
Northwestern University
Clinical Research Scientist, Center on
  Outcomes, Research and Education
Evanston Northwestern Healthcare
Evanston, Illinois

DAVID E. WEISSMAN, M.D.
Professor of Medicine
Director, Palliative Care Program
Medical College of Wisconsin
Milwaukee, Wisconsin

MICHAEL A. WEITZNER, M.D.
Associate Professor of Interdisciplinary
  Oncology
University of South Florida
Chief, Palliative Care Service
Moffitt Cancer Center
Tampa, Florida

SIMON C. WESSELY, M.D.
Professor of Epidemiological and Liaison
  Psychiatry
Academic Department of Psychological
  Medicine
Guy's, King's and St. Thomas' School of
  Medicine and Institute of Psychiatry
London
United Kingdom

I

PAIN RESEARCH

1

Methodological Issues in the Design of Analgesic Clinical Trials

MITCHELL MAX

The treatment of pain was a major interest of Beecher, Lasagna, and Houde, three of the early proponents of randomized clinical trial methodology after its development in the late 1940s. These researchers called attention to challenges in analgesic studies that differed from those encountered in studying structural diseases, including the large magnitude of placebo effects, difficulty of symptom measurement, and frequent findings of negative results even with drugs known to be effective analgesics. In a classic textbook that discusses clinical trials to treat pain, insomnia, nausea, and other symptoms, Beecher[1] pointed out that the same challenges beset studies of diverse symptoms:

> The measurement of pain has never seemed to this writer to be only an end in itself, valuable as this end might be, but rather an area where he could learn how to attack other subjective responses.

Surprisingly, this insight has been neglected. There has been rather little interaction among investigators or regulators interested in clinical trials on different symptoms, who generally associate with others interested in the same group of diseases. I suggest that the accumulated literature of over 15,000 analgesic clinical trials as well as writings on study design[2–4] and pain measurement[5–7] may offer useful lessons for the design of studies of other symptoms. In this chapter, I discuss some of the firm conclusions from the experience of analgesic research and highlight areas of analgesic trial methodology that have had relatively little exploration, particularly repeated-dose studies in chronic pain, where an ongoing dialogue among symptom researchers might move all of these fields ahead. (An interactive, research case-based presentation of this material and research on other symptoms is available at http://symptomresearch.nih.gov[8]).

Explanatory versus Pragmatic Clinical Trials

One of the most useful distinctions for the design of clinical trials of all types was articulated by Schwartz and Lellouch,[9] who characterized two different purposes of clinical trials, which they called "explanatory" and "pragmatic." An *explanatory* approach seeks to elucidate a biological principle. The study population is considered to be a model from which one may learn principles of pharmacology or physiology that are likely to shed light on a variety of clinical problems. For example, the analgesic equivalency tables that guide opioid prescribing in a variety of conditions are largely based on studies of patients with pain from malignant tumors or from cancer surgery.[2,3] The investigators made the assumptions that the analgesics' relative potency in most pain conditions would be similar and that these patients provide a good predictive model for any pain condition. Their articles tend to refer to the drugs' "analgesic efficacy in humans" rather than in "cancer pain" or "postoperative pain." A *pragmatic* approach, in contrast, focuses on the question "What is the better treatment in the *particular clinical circumstances* of the patients in the study?"

As an illustration of how these approaches to design differ, consider a hypothetical analgesic that animal studies had shown to be effective in models of visceral pain. Looking first at patient selection, a palliative care researcher oriented toward the explanatory approach might select only a small subset of cancer patients in whom there was unequivocal radiological proof of hollow viscera involvement, while a pragmatic clinical researcher might open the study to patients with ill-defined abdominal pain. The explanatory approach would try to maximize the therapeutic response by selecting a high dose and monitoring patients frequently, while the pragmatically oriented investigator might choose an intermediate dose and provide the looser supervision common in clinical practice. The explanatory approach will usually mandate a placebo because even small amounts of pain relief over the placebo response may provide information about the mechanisms of visceral pain transmission and relief. The pragmatic approach, in contrast, generally compares the new treatment to the best treatment in clinical use.

Data analysis may also differ. In an explanatory trial, a few patients who discontinue the study medication after the first dose because of unpleasant side effects would provide no data about the biological effects of repeated dosing and are therefore excluded from the main analysis. (All patients should be analyzed in a secondary analysis, however, as some reviewers might be interested in this result.) In a pragmatically oriented trial, however, the primary analysis should be an "intent-to-treat" analysis, including either all patients who were randomized or all patients who received at least one dose because treatment failures due to side effects will weigh into the clinician's choice of treatment.

The dichotomous explanatory/pragmatic schema is an oversimplification, of course. The investigator usually wishes to address both theoretical and practical concerns. This distinction may, however, offer a useful perspective for making design choices in complex cases.

Choice of Treatments and Controls

Compared to trials of treatments for structural disease, symptom treatment trials are susceptible to both false-positive and false-negative results. A major source of false-positives is the placebo effect, which in analgesic trials is often substantial and may have a duration of weeks or months.[10] Essential steps to avoid false-positives are to maximize the effectiveness of blinding procedures and to check whether patients can guess their study assignment by the appearance, taste, or side effects of the treatments.[11] In studies of drugs that have unmistakable side effects, some investigators use "active" placebos, which mimic the side effects of the analgesic.[12–14] Potential drawbacks of active placebos include the possibility that the active drug may worsen the underlying symptom, thereby contributing to a false-positive result; improve the symptom, making it more difficult for the experimental drug to show an effect; or cause adverse reactions. If there is evidence that the active placebo does not affect the target symptom and the lowest dose that will produce some symptoms similar to the experimental drug is chosen, the resulting protection against accepting a truly ineffective drug should outweigh the risks.

The effectiveness of double-blinding may be checked by administering a brief questionnaire to the patient and study nurse (or another member of the research staff who has frequent contact with the patient and may have enough knowledge of the study to guess the treatment assignment). One should ask the subject to guess the treatment from the list of possibilities and to give the reason for the guess (important reasons are side effects and therapeutic effects). The results of such a questionnaire are clearest in the case where a drug produces immediate side effects and a delayed therapeutic effect. In that case, the questionnaire should be administered at an early time point, and identification of the treatments more frequently than chance suggests incomplete blinding of the study. Correct identification of the study drug based on therapeutic effect, however, can occur in a perfectly blinded study of an effective drug. Whatever the treatment, more patients with pain relief than without will suggest that an active treatment was given. One can factor out most of this bias if one stratifies the analysis to compare the frequency of correct responses within each level of pain relief reported by the patient.[15]

False-negative results may be due to a so-called lack of assay sensitivity, that is, inability of that particular study to distinguish drug from placebo even with an analgesic known to be effective in the study population.

To minimize these risks of false-positives and -negatives, analgesic researchers have developed a distinct logic regarding the choice of controls and the

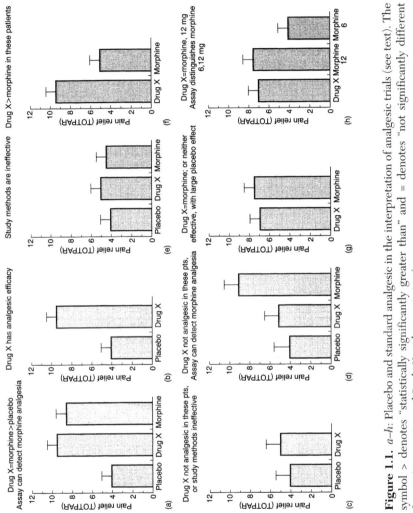

Figure 1.1. *a–h*: Placebo and standard analgesic in the interpretation of analgesic trials (see text). The symbol > denotes "statistically significantly greater than" and = denotes "not significantly different from." (From Max and Laska[16] with permission.)

interpretation of clinical trials. This framework, illustrated in Figure 1.1, is now widely applied to determine the validity of single-dose analgesic trials[8,16,17] and appears to be plausible for use in the study of other symptoms.

Interpreting analgesic studies: test drug, placebo, and positive control

Although the simplest of the classic designs consists of two treatments, the test medication and a placebo, most single-dose analgesic trials also include a standard analgesic "positive control." In single-dose trials, common positive controls include an opioid, a non-steroidal anti-inflammatory drug, or acetaminophen.

To demonstrate the value of these controls, consider a hypothetical study comparing the putative analgesic drug X to a morphine positive control and a placebo (Fig. 1.1a). Using summed pain relief scores as the measure of analgesia, drug X tended to be slightly, but not statistically significantly, more effective than morphine and both drug X and morphine were statistically superior to placebo. The conclusions are straightforward: drug X is an effective analgesic, and the study methods were sufficiently sensitive to distinguish morphine from placebo.

Omission of a positive control does not fatally flaw the study if drug X is superior to placebo (Fig. 1.1b), although one cannot be certain about the strength of the effect. The positive control serves as a yardstick against which to compare the magnitude of the analgesia produced by drug X. In pain syndromes for which there is no accepted effective treatment, the comparison of test drug to placebo must suffice. Should drug X fail to produce more analgesia than the placebo, however, omission of the positive control will render the study uninterpretable (Fig. 1.1c). One cannot reliably conclude that drug X is ineffective in this condition. Perhaps the drug is truly analgesic in patients with this condition, but the study methods were too insensitive to observe this effect. This could happen because patients were too stressed by the clinical setting to respond to medication, the pain questionnaires were insensitive, the procedures of the nurse observer were variable or confusing, or merely random variation. If a morphine positive control were included and shown to be superior to both placebo and drug X (Fig. 1.1d), this would validate the study methodology and indicate that drug X was not analgesic in this population. Alternatively, if morphine produced no more analgesia than drug X and the placebo (Fig. 1.1e), one could conclude that the study methods were inadequate to show the effects of even a strong analgesic.

What are the consequences of omitting the placebo and comparing drug X only to a standard analgesic? As in the previous case, this omission is less damaging when the assay shows a difference between the two treatments. The data in Figure 1.1f suggest that drug X is an effective analgesic in this population, although the proportion of analgesia attributable to the placebo effect cannot be determined for either drug X or morphine. If the responses to drug X and standard analgesic were similar, however (Fig. 1.1g), interpretation would be troublesome. The data might reflect either that drug X and morphine were both effective analgesics or that neither was effective and there was a large placebo effect.

If the use of a placebo group is difficult, an alternative approach is to use a second dose level of the standard analgesic. Figure 1.1h shows that morphine 12 mg surpassed morphine 6 mg, demonstrating the sensitivity of the study methods and implying that the effects of both drug X and morphine 12 mg were not merely placebo effects.

In addition to doses of a test drug, a standard analgesic, and a placebo, most analgesic studies include treatment groups or controls that are chosen to further elucidate the major research question. For example, when evaluating a range of doses of test analgesic, one might add additional doses of standard analgesic spanning that analgesic range, both to serve as a comparative yardstick and to verify that the study methods can separate high from moderate analgesic doses. (For further discussion of this point, see Max and Laska,[16] pp. 77–78.) To test the soundness of proposed designs, the investigator may wish to graph the possible outcomes as in Figure 1.1$a–h$. If the conclusion given a particular outcome is ambiguous, it may be wise to consider additional treatment groups that would distinguish among the alternative explanations. The addition of treatment or control groups is costly, however. One must either recruit more patients or reduce the size of each treatment group, lessening the statistical power of the comparisons. In many cases, particularly where negative results will not be of great interest, researchers may choose to omit controls whose main value is to clarify the interpretation of the negative result.

Placebo and positive controls in extended studies

In single-dose analgesic studies of cancer pain, there are rarely ethical objections to the use of placebos because patients understand that they can terminate the study and take additional analgesic at any time. In actual practice, many patients experience some placebo analgesia, and most tolerate the study for the 1–2 hours needed to evaluate the response to the placebo.

Chronic studies are a different matter, however. Although a placebo control has been considered to be appropriate in studies of pain syndromes in patients who have already failed all standard treatments, chronic administration of a placebo cannot be justified in pain syndromes that generally respond to therapy, such as most cancer pain syndromes. Moreover, attrition rates under such circumstances are likely to be high; for example, in a placebo-controlled drug trial among cancer patients,[18] 90% of the placebo group withdrew in the first day. The same problem exists for studies of discrete interventions, such as celiac block, that require a prolonged observation period after the treatment.

In these situations, therefore, the only feasible way to conduct placebo-controlled studies may be to give both placebo and active treatment groups access to a standard analgesic "rescue" dose. An example of a chronic placebo-controlled study of ibuprofen for metastatic bone pain is shown in Figure 1.2. Stambaugh and Drew[19] enrolled a group of inpatients whose bone pain required at least four daily doses of an oxycodone/acetaminophen (oxy/APAP) combination. Strong parenteral opioids were also given for severe breakthrough pain, but patients requiring more than one injection daily were dropped from the study. For the first 7 days of the study, no intervention took place; the daily dose of oxy/APAP was monitored, and patients assessed pain intensity and relief once a day. On days 8–14, half the patients received ibuprofen 600 mg po four times daily and the other half received placebo. Figure 1.2 shows that pain relief was better with ibuprofen than placebo and that the ibuprofen-treated group reduced their oxy/APAP consumption relative to the placebo group. This example illustrates how use of the background or rescue analgesic becomes another important outcome measure. Similar strategies have been used to study the analgesic effects of sustained-release morphine in cancer patients[20] and many types of intervention in postoperative pain.[21,22]

In these designs, the rescue analgesic may be given by any of a variety of routes, including oral, intramuscular, or intravenous (commonly by patient-controlled analgesia devices). Both pain report and rescue analgesic consumption should be examined as primary outcome measures. Although some investigators have used the amount of rescue drug consumed as the only outcome measure, many patients may not change their analgesic demands enough to completely offset any change in pain (as in Fig. 1.2 and Lehmann[22]). In addition, reduction of analgesic consumption alone is not a compelling clinical advantage unless pain or analgesic side effects can also be shown to be reduced. The power of a study to detect an effect of the experimental drug may be diluted if the therapeutic benefit shows up partly in reduced pain scores and partly in reduced use of rescue medication. For this reason, when doing an explanatory study to establish analgesic efficacy, many experts prefer a single-dose comparison in which patients agree to postpone taking rescue analgesic until pain becomes severe, after which time pain scores are imputed to be at the level at the time of rescue. In this type of study, there is generally a larger separation between pain scores among the treatment groups than when rescue medication is allowed. To recover the "lost power" of rescue dose paradigms, an analytic method has been proposed that integrates pain score and rescue analgesic consumption into a single summary variable,[23] but methodological study of this proposed method has not gone beyond the small number of patients in the original report.

In repeated-dose studies, just as in single-dose studies, positive controls or multiple levels of the test drug may also be used.[24,25] Provisions must generally be made for a rescue analgesic. In addition, the protocol should allow for lowering doses of the test drug or standard analgesic should drug toxicity occur.

Designing the appropriate control interventions may also be a challenge for nonpharmacological treatments. Control or sham interventions are possible with diverse treatments such as cognitive pain control techniques or acupuncture, but they are often open to criticism.[26] With more invasive methods, such as

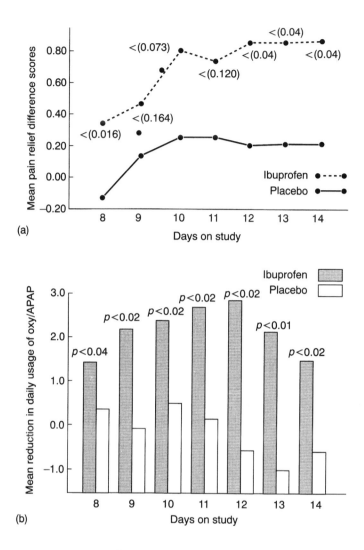

Figure 1.2. *a:* Comparison of mean pain relief differences of ibuprofen, 600 mg four times/day, versus placebo, both in combination with oxycodone/acetaminophen (oxy/APAP) as needed. Values in parentheses represent *p* values of ibuprofen versus placebo. Day 8 was the first day ibuprofen or placebo was added, after 7 days of baseline observations of pain and oxy/APAP consumption. *b:* Alterations of oxy/APAP use after addition of ibuprofen or placebo. Mean reduction scores were determined by comparing oxy/APAP use on days 6 and 7 with means for each of days 8–14. For each day, oxy/APAP use was reduced by addition of ibuprofen. (From Stambaugh and Drew[19] with permission.)

neuroablative procedures, placebo or sham procedures are generally considered inappropriate.

Parallel Group versus Crossover Designs

In a *parallel group* (also termed *completely randomized*) design, each patient receives a single treatment. In a *crossover* design, each patient receives some (incomplete block) or all (complete block) of the treatments being studied.

There are several obvious advantages to crossover designs. Analgesic studies often require large sample sizes because detection of a drug effect must compete with so many other causes of variation in pain report: the subject's painful lesion, tolerance to opioid medications, psychological makeup, previous pain experience, age, race, weight, interaction with the study personnel, etc. Much of this between-patient variation can be eliminated by using a crossover design, in which treatment comparisons are largely or entirely within the same patient.[27-31] Because of this reduction in variance and because each patient is used several times, crossover studies usually have greater statistical power for a given sample size than parallel group designs.[27] This is an important practical advantage, particularly when studies are performed in a single center. Crossover designs have been used frequently in studies of cancer pain.[2,3,32]

Such advantages notwithstanding, there may be problems with the use of crossover designs in palliative care settings. First, change in the painful lesions over time may introduce great variability into patient responses, thereby undermining the major potential advantage of the crossover design. This necessitates that the total duration of the crossover study be short enough to ensure that such within-patient variation will be less than the variation already existing between the patients enrolled. Changes in the underlying disease, as well as logistical factors and voluntary withdrawals, usually cause a higher dropout rate in crossover than in parallel group studies. Although the greater power of the crossover approach may compensate for a higher dropout rate, reviewers may doubt the general applicability of the results of a study completed by a minority of the patients entered.

Another major concern with crossover studies is the possibility of bias produced by unequal *carryover effects*, which are changes in the efficacy of treatments resulting from treatments given in earlier periods; they may be mediated by persistence of drug or metabolites, changes in brain or peripheral tissues caused by the treatment, or behavioral or psychological factors. The major problem with carryover effects occurs with the two-treatment, two-period design (2×2; Fig. 1.3, *left*). Results may be difficult to interpret whenever the treatment effect differs for the two periods. In this event, one cannot distinguish with any certainty whether this is due to a carryover effect (persistence of a pharmacological or psychological effect of the first treatment into the second period), a treatment $\times$ period interaction (the passage of time affects the relative efficacy of the treatments; for example, by the second period, patients who initially received placebo might be too discouraged to respond to any subsequent treatment), or a difference between the groups of patients assigned the two different orders of treatment. For this reason, regulatory agencies have been particularly reluctant to rely on data from such designs.

Fortunately, these statistical difficulties are largely limited to the 2 × 2 case (and Senn[31] argues that these difficulties have been exaggerated). If the investigator adds several other treatment sequences (Fig. 1.3, alternative 1) or a third treatment period (alternatives 2, 3), unbiased estimates of treatment effects are possible even in the presence of various types of carryover effect.[29,30] For studies involving three or more treatments, there are a variety of designs that allow these effects to be distinguished. Thus, although the relative brevity and simplicity of the 2 × 2 design may make it attractive for single-center pilot studies and for situations in which previous experience suggests that there is no significant carryover effect, the need to estimate treatment effects with greater certainty may recommend the use of alternative designs.

A variant of the crossover design, the enriched enrollment design, may be useful in studying treatments to which only a minority of patients respond.[33] If the results are not statistically significant in a conventional clinical trial, one cannot retrospectively point at the responders and claim that the treatment accounted for their relief. One can, however, enter them into a second prospective trial or a series of comparisons between treatment and placebo. If the results of the second trial considered alone are statistically significant, this suggests that the patients' initial response was not just due to chance. While statistically defensible, the enriched enrollment design is open to the criticism that prior exposure to the treatment may defeat the double-blind procedure (particularly with treatments that have distinctive side effects) and sometimes result in spurious positive results.

Parallel study designs are preferable when there are strong concerns about carryover effects or when the natural history of the pain syndrome makes

Standard 2 x 2	Alternative 1	Alternative 2	Alternative 3
A–B	A–B	A–B–B	A–B–B
B–A	B–A	B–A–A	B–A–A
	A–A		A–B–A
	B–B		B–A–B

Figure 1.3. Examples of crossover designs used to compare two treatments, A and B. Many statisticians have criticized the two-period, two-treatment design (*left*) for insensitivity in detecting carryover effects. The three designs at the *right* are examples of alternative designs that are better able to distinguish treatment from carryover effects.

disease-related changes in pain likely during the period required for a crossover study. Between-patient variability is the major problem posed by parallel group designs, and several approaches have been suggested to mitigate its impact.[34] For example, baseline pain scores may be subtracted from the treatment scores to yield pain intensity difference scores, or they may be treated as a covariate. This often eliminates a large part of the variance, thereby increasing the power of treatment comparisons. In single-dose analgesic drug trials, the baseline has generally been determined under "no treatment conditions," but as discussed above, a standard pain treatment regimen will generally be needed in palliative care contexts.

The investigator should also balance the treatment groups for variables that predict response, whenever these predictors are known or suspected.[35–37] If one wishes to examine response in specific subgroups, assignments must also be balanced appropriately. Groups can be balanced using stratification or various techniques of adaptive randomization.[38] In studies with sample sizes typical of single-center trials, 20–40 patients per group, these methods can significantly increase the study power if the prognostic variables are well chosen and the statistical methods take the balancing method into account.[34] If stratification is not feasible, post hoc covariate analyses or other statistical techniques may be an acceptable substitute if the variables in question are distributed fairly evenly among the treatment groups.

Other Issues in Analgesic Clinical Trials

Relative potency studies

One of the most useful tools in guiding the dosing of opioid analgesics has been the relative potency bioassays,[39] which compares two or more doses of a test drug with two or more doses of a standard (Fig. 1.4). A placebo may not be necessary in such trials because the demonstration of a statistically significant positive slope for the dose–response curves establishes assay sensitivity. A placebo is necessary, however, if one wishes to estimate the lowest dose at which analgesic efficacy might be detected.

There are several advantages to expressing the outcome of a study or group of studies in terms of relative potency.[40,41] First, such estimates allow clinicians to tailor the dosing of a new drug to the individual patient, based on the specific dose of the standard usually used by that patient. Second, this method eliminates the problem of expressing a drug's effect in units on an arbitrary analgesic scale, measurements whose absolute size may vary with the patient population, study methods, and placebo effect. Third, relative potency studies allow one to test whether a new analgesic or drug combination is superior to the standard in terms of toxicity as well as efficacy; the relative intensity of adverse effects can be estimated for the two treatments at doses providing the same analgesia.

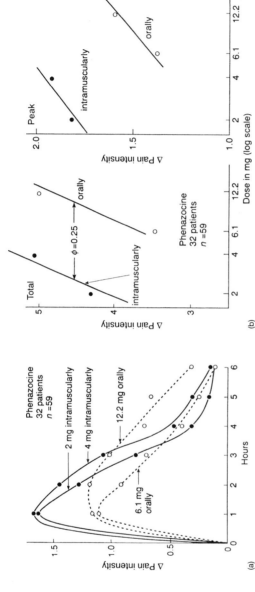

Figure 1.4. Four-point relative potency study comparing intramuscular (*filled circles*) and oral (*open circles*) phenazocine. *a*: Pain intensity difference (category scale) is plotted against time. Note the difference between the time course of analgesia for the two routes. *b*: Total (*left*) and peak (*right*) changes in pain intensity are plotted against dose. For total scores, oral phenazocine is one-fourth as potent as intramuscular drug. For peak scores, no relative potency can be calculated because there was no overlap between the level of response seen with the two routes. Because the time course of response differs between the routes, the relative potency calculated for total scores will change according to the length of the study; for example, if only the first 3 hours were considered, the disparity between the intramuscular and oral routes would have been even greater. (From Beaver et al.[40] with permission.)

There are also pitfalls in interpreting single-dose relative potency assays. If the dose–response curves of the test and standard drugs are not linear and parallel or the doses chosen are not in the same analgesic range, the calculated relative potency may be incorrect or meaningless. In addition, if the drugs to be compared have different kinetics, the relative potency may vary greatly depending on whether the peak pain relief or the summed scores over time are used. For example, using summed scores over time will favor a drug with longer duration (Fig. 1.4, *left*).

In addition, relative potency estimates derived from single-dose studies may not be sufficient to predict chronic dosing requirements, particularly when the pharmacokinetics of the treatments and their active metabolites differ. For example, the slowly metabolized analgesic methadone is equipotent to morphine as a single parenteral dose, but observations in cancer patients being converted from chronic treatment with one drug to the other suggest that methadone is more than 10 times more potent.[42] Additional repeated-dose relative potency studies of the common opioid analgesics are needed to provide a better basis for clinical treatment. One must be wary of several potential biases. If relative potency estimates are based on unidirectional shifts from opioid A to opioid B, the relative effectiveness of opioid B might be underestimated if opioid tolerance develops or if the underlying disease progresses in a way that tends to increase pain. One can avoid this bias by running the conversion in both directions.[8,43]

Another design feature that will enhance the validity of dose estimates in chronic dosing paradigms is multiple dose levels. If only one dose level of each drug is used, one may falsely conclude that these two doses are equivalent if there is minimal difference between pain levels and rescue dose medication for the two treatments. In contrast, if one randomly converts a patient from an adequate dose of one opioid to multiple dose levels of the other and then adjusts the dose up or down based on symptoms and need for rescue medication, one will approach the exact equivalent dose of the second opioid from either direction and facilitate an unbiased estimate.

Studies to assess whether two treatments are equivalent

A common error in study design is to assume that the demonstration of no significant difference between two analgesics proves that they are equivalent.[44] The error in this reasoning is illustrated by the following example. In a controlled trial, cancer patients received either intramuscular morphine 10 mg or intramuscular morphine 5 mg plus a peptide shown to potentiate opioid analgesia in animals. In the clinical trial, similar pain relief scores were observed for the two treatments, and the investigator concluded that the peptide doubled the analgesic effects of morphine. The data do not support this; without controls such as morphine 5 mg alone or placebo, there was no demonstration that the study methods would have been sensitive enough to detect a true difference between analgesics (Fig. 1.1g). Even if both morphine 10 mg and morphine 5 mg plus peptide had surpassed a control group, a convincing demonstration of equivalence would require demonstrating that the 95% confidence interval for the difference between the two treatments was also small.[45-47] This generally requires a much larger sample size than is needed to distinguish an active treatment from placebo.

Drug combinations

A number of types of drug, including opioids, α-adrenergic agonists, tricyclic antidepressants, sodium channel blockers, and gabapentin, have some effect in chronic pain; but pain levels are rarely reduced by more than 20%–25% below the persisting pain level in the placebo group. Many scientists speculate that unless a "magic bullet" finally arrives, improvement in pain treatment is likely to require drug combinations; but few analgesic combinations have been studied, particularly in chronic dosing trials. Controlled clinical trials of such combinations present particular challenges.[48-53] If a test drug is simply added to a standard regimen whose optimal dose is well known, the need for dose ranging is limited to the test drug.[54] Should uncertainty exist about the dose of each component, however, a rather complex study may be needed. For example, one might determine dose–response curves for each component alone and for several dose ratios of the combination.[55] Debate on the methodology for analgesic drug combination studies in animals has focused on whether the combination produces synergy, additivity, or subadditivity for analgesia. However, from the clinician's point of view, this emphasis is misplaced. The key issues are whether the combination has a better therapeutic ratio (ratio of analgesia to side effects) than either component or produces a higher maximal analgesic efficacy at tolerable doses. Treatment groups must be chosen to ensure that a comparison of side effects at equianalgesic doses will be possible.[50]

Several unsolved issues in pain measurement for clinical trials

Pain measurement is discussed at length in other sources,[5-7,20] but I would like to point out a few unsolved problems related to pain measurement in clinical trials. The relative sensitivity of several common pain scales has been well studied in single-dose analgesic trials. Littman et al.[56] compared a standard four-category pain intensity scale, a five-category relief scale, and a pain intensity visual analogue scale in 20 clinical trials in almost 1500 patients treated with the opioid agonist–antagonist dezocine, standard opioid analgesics, or placebo. The relief category scale was consistently the most sensitive to treatment differences, followed by the visual analogue scale, and finally the pain category scale. The relief category scale is more sensitive because it allows patients to make finer distinctions at low levels of pain relief; for example, patients often will report "slight" pain relief when pain has not changed enough to alter their report from "severe" to "moderate" pain intensity.

The sensitivity of pain intensity and relief scales in detecting treatment effects has not been directly compared in repeated-dose studies. A potential problem with relief scales is that as time passes patients may not be able to remember the baseline level of pain, so such ratings may be suspect. The first large studies to directly compare the sensitivity of the commonly used pain intensity scales in detecting treatment effects were carried out by Bellamy et al.,[57] who examined anti-inflammatory treatment in patients with osteoarthritis and rheumatoid arthritis. They found that a 0–10 numerical scale and a 100 mm visual analogue scale were equally sensitive, but considerably larger sample sizes would have been required to reach significance with the standard four-point pain intensity category scale or the McGill Pain Questionnaire. Because of the occasional confusion provoked by the more abstract visual analogue scale, we consider the 0–10 numerical scale best for chronic studies. Additional analyses of this scale have been done by Farrar et al.,[58] who suggested that a reduction of about 30% in the average intensity of this scale over a 2-month trial is the best "cut-off point" to suggest that the response is clinically meaningful to the patient.

In many repeated-dose analgesic trials, the primary outcome is pain measured at a single time point. Jensen and McFarland[59] suggested that because pain varies so much over the course of a week, this may risk introducing a large amount of unnecessary experimental variability. Based on data from patients with chronic nonmalignant pain, they showed that this error can be decreased by averaging one or two daily pain measurements over a period of 1 week.

One should also keep in mind that pain may have a number of components with different mechanisms. Clinical practice or scientific understanding may be enhanced if the relevant features of pain for the clinical trial are measured in isolation, in addition to an overall measure of pain relief. Recent work has focused on the various components of neuropathic pain[60] and incident or breakthrough pain in cancer patients.[61]

Conclusion

Several generations of analgesic researchers have come to a consensus on approaches to single-dose analgesic studies. Because the studies of other symptoms may share some of the same challenges, palliative care researchers may benefit from a familiarity with the analgesic study design literature. However, many clinical research problems with pain and other symptoms have received rather little study, including optimizing the sensitivity of symptom-based measures, combination studies, and the choice of control groups in repeated-dose studies. The solution to many of these problems may be facilitated by frequent discussions among clinical researchers working in different symptom areas.

Acknowledgments

Portions of this chapter are adapted with permission from Max MB, Laska EM. Single-dose analgesic comparisons. In: Max MB, Portenoy RK, Laska EM, eds. The Design of Analgesic Clinical Trials. New York: Raven Press, 1991; and Max MB, Portenoy RK: Pain research: designing clinical trials in palliative care. In: Doyle D, Hanks GW, MacDonald RN, eds. Oxford Textbook of Palliative Medicine, 2d ed. Oxford: Oxford University Press, 1998.

References

1. Beecher HK. Measurement of Subjective Responses: Quantitative Effects of Drugs. New York: Oxford University Press, 1959.
2. Houde RW, Wallenstein SL, Beaver WT. Evaluation of analgesics in patients with cancer pain. In: Lasagna L, ed. Clinical Pharmacology. International Encyclopedia of Pharmacology and Therapeutics, sect 6. New York: Pergamon Press, 1966: 59–97.
3. Houde RW, Wallenstein SL, Beaver WT. Clinical measurement of pain. In: de Stevens G, ed. Analgetics. New York: Academic Press, 1965:75–122.
4. Max MB, Portenoy RK, Laska EM, eds. The Design of Analgesic Clinical Trials. New York: Raven Press, 1991.
5. Price DD. Psychological Mechanisms of Pain and Analgesia. Seattle: IASP Press, 1999.
6. Chapman CR, Loeser JD, eds. Issues in Pain Measurement. New York: Raven Press, 1989.
7. Turk DC, Melzack R, eds. Handbook of Pain Assessment. New York: Guilford Press, 1992.
8. Max MB, Lynn J, eds. Interactive Textbook of Symptom Research. Bethesda, MD: National Institute of Dental and Craniofacial Research, http://symptomre-search.nih.gov, 2002.
9. Schwartz D, Lellouch J. Explanatory and pragmatic attitudes in therapeutic trials. J Chronic Dis 1967; 20:637–648.
10. Turner JA, Deyo RA, Loeser JD, et al. The importance of placebo effects in pain treatment and research. JAMA 1994; 271:1609–1614.
11. Moscucci M, Byrne L, Weintraub M, et al. Blinding, unblinding, and the placebo effect: an analysis of patients' guesses of treatment assignment in a double-blind trial. Clin Pharmacol Ther 1987; 41:259–265.
12. Max MB. Neuropathic pain. In: Max MB, Portenoy RK, Laska EM, eds. The Design of Analgesic Clinical Trials. Advances in Pain Research and Therapy, vol 18. New York: Raven Press, 1991:193–220.
13. Greenberg RP, Fisher S. Seeing through the double-masked design: a commentary. Control Clin Trials 1994; 15:244–246.
14. Max MB. Small clinical trials. In: Gallin JI, ed. Principles and Practice of Clinical Research. New York: Academic Press, 2002:207–224.
15. Shlay JC, Chaloner K, Max MB, et al. A randomized placebo-controlled trial of a standardized acupuncture regimen and amitriptyline for pain caused by HIV-related peripheral neuropathy. JAMA 1998; 280:1590–1595.

16. Max MB, Laska EM. Single-dose analgesic comparisons. In: Max MB, Portenoy RK, Laska EM, eds. The Design of Analgesic Clinical Trials. Advances in Cancer Research and Therapy, vol 18. New York: Raven Press, 1991:55–95.

17. Food and Drug Administration. Guideline for the Clinical Evaluation of Analgesic Drugs. Rockville, MD: US Department of Health and Human Services, 1992.

18. Stambaugh JE, McAdams J. Comparison of intramuscular dezocine with butorphanol and placebo in chronic cancer pain: a method to evaluate analgesia after both single and repeated doses. Clin Pharmacol Ther 1987; 42:210–219.

19. Stambaugh JE, Drew J. The combination of ibuprofen and oxycodone/acetaminophen in the management of chronic cancer pain. Clin Pharmacol Ther 1988; 44:665–669.

20. Portenoy RK. Cancer pain. In: Max MB, Portenoy RK, Laska EM, eds. The Design of Analgesic Clinical Trials. Advances in Cancer Research and Therapy, vol 18. New York: Raven Press, 1991:233–266.

21. VadeBoncouer TR, Riegler FX, Gautt RS, et al. A randomized double-blind comparison of the efficacy of interpleural bupivicaine and saline on morphine requirements and pulmonary function after cholecystectomy. Anesthesiology 1989; 71:339–343.

22. Lehmann KA. Patient-controlled intravenous analgesia for postoperative pain relief. In: Max MB, Portenoy RK, Laska EM, eds. The Design of Analgesic Clinical Trials. New York: Raven Press, 1991:481–506.

23. Silverman DG, O'Connor TZ, Brull SJ. Integrated assessment of pain scores and rescue morphine use during studies of analgesic efficacy. Anesth Analg 1993; 77:168–170.

24. Jadad AR, Carroll D, Glynn CJ, et al. Morphine responsiveness of chronic pain: double-blind randomized crossover study with patient-controlled analgesia. Lancet 1992; 339:1367–1371.

25. Max MB. Challenges in the design of clinical trials of drug combinations. In: Gebhart GF, Hammond DL, Jensen TS, eds. Proceedings of the VII World Congress on Pain. Seattle: IASP Publications, 1994:569–586.

26. Chapman CR, Donaldson GW. Issues in designing trials of nonpharmacological treatments for pain. In: Max MB, Portenoy RK, Laska EM, eds. The Design of Analgesic Clinical Trials. New York: Raven Press, 1991:699–711.

27. Louis TA, Lavori PW, Bailar JC, et al. Crossover and self-controlled designs in clinical research. N Engl J Med 1984; 310:24–31.

28. James KE, Forrest WH, Rose RL. Crossover and noncrossover designs in four-point parallel line analgesic assays. Clin Pharmacol Ther 1985; 37:242–252.

29. Jones B, Kenward MG. Design and Analysis of Cross-Over Trials. London: Chapman and Hall, 1989.

30. Ratkowsky DA, Evans MA, Alldredge JR. Cross-Over Experiments: Design, Analysis, and Application. New York: Marcel Dekker, 1993.

31. Senn S. Cross-Over Trials in Clinical Research. Chichester: John Wiley and Sons, 1993.

32. Bruera E. Cancer pain: chronic studies of adjuvants to opioid analgesics. In: Max MB, Portenoy RK, Laska EM, eds. The Design of Analgesic Clinical Trials. New York: Raven Press, 1991:267–281.

33. Byas-Smith MG, Max MB, Muir J, et al. Transdermal clonidine compared to placebo in painful diabetic neuropathy using a two-stage "enriched enrollment" design. Pain 1995; 60:267–274.

34. Lavori PW, Louis TA, Bailar JC, et al. Designs for experiments—parallel comparisons of treatment. N Engl J Med 1983; 309:1291–1298.

35. Kaiko RF, Wallenstein SL, Rogers AG, et al. Sources of variation in analgesic responses in cancer patients with chronic pain receiving morphine. Pain 1983; 15:191–200.

36. Thaler HT. Outcome measures and the effect of covariates. In: Max MB, Portenoy RK, Laska EM, eds. The Design of Analgesic Clinical Trials. New York: Raven Press, 1991:106–111.

37. Bruera E, MacMillan K, Hanson J, et al. The Edmonton staging system for cancer pain: preliminary report. Pain 1989; 37:203–210.

38. Friedman LM, Furberg CD, DeMets DL. Fundamentals of Clinical Trials, 3rd ed. Littleton, MA: PSG Publishing, 1996.

39. Laska EM, Meisner MJ. Statistical methods and applications of bioassay. Annu Rev Pharmacol Toxicol 1987; 27:385–397.

40. Beaver WT, Wallenstein SL, Houde RW, et al. A clinical comparison of the effects of oral and intramuscular administration of analgesics: pentazocine and phenazocine. Clin Pharmacol Ther 1968; 9:582–597.

41. Laska EM, Sunshine A, Mueller F, et al. Caffeine as an analgesic adjuvant. JAMA 1984; 251:1711–1718.

42. Lawlor PG, Turner KS, Hanson J, et al. Dose ratio between morphine and methadone in patients with cancer pain: a retrospective study. Cancer 1998; 82: 1167–1173.

43. Heiskanen T, Kalso E. Controlled-release oxycodone and morphine in cancer related pain. Pain 1997; 73:37–45.

44. Temple R. Government viewpoint of clinical trials. Drug Info J 1982; 16:10–17.

45. Detsky AS, Sackett DL. When was a "negative" clinical trial big enough? How many patients you needed depends on what you found. Arch Intern Med 1985; 145:709–712.

46. Makuch R, Johnson M. Issues in planning and interpreting active control equivalence studies. J Clin Epidemiol 1989; 42:503–511.

47. Makuch RW, Johnson MF. Some issues in the design and interpretation of "negative" clinical studies. Arch Intern Med 1986; 146:986–989.

48. Carter WH Jr, Carchman RA. Mathematical and biostatistical methods for designing and analyzing complex chemical interactions. Fundam Appl Toxicol 1988; 10: 590–595.

49. Plummer JL, Short TG. Statistical modelling of the effects of drug combinations. J Pharmacol Methods 1990; 23:297–309.

50. Max MB. Divergent traditions in analgesic clinical trials. Clin Pharmacol Ther 1994; 56:237–241.

51. Berenbaum MC. What is synergy? Pharmacol Rev 1989; 41:93–141.

52. Sethna NF, Liu M, Gracely RH, et al. Analgesic and cognitive effects of intravenous ketamine–alfentanil combinations vs. either drug alone after intradermal capsaicin in normal subjects. Anesth Analg 1998; 86:1250–1256.

53. Lavigne GJ, Hargreaves KM, Schmidt EA, et al. Proglumide potentiates morphine analgesia for acute surgical pain. Clin Pharmacol Ther 1989; 45:666–673.

54. Beaver WT. Combination analgesics. Am J Med 1984; 77(3A):38–53.

55. Levine JD, Gordon NC. Synergism between the analgesic actions of morphine and pentazocine. Pain 1988; 33:369–372.

56. Littman GS, Walker BR, Schneider BE. Reassessment of verbal and visual analog ratings in analgesic studies. Clin Pharmacol Ther 1985; 38:16–23.

57. Bellamy N, Campbell J, Syrotuik J. Comparative study of self-rating pain scales in rheumatoid arthritis patients. Curr Med Res Opin 1999; 15:121–127.

58. Farrar JT, Young JP Jr, LaMoreaux L, et al. Clinical importance of changes in chronic pain intensity measured on an 11-point numerical pain rating scale. Pain 2001; 94:149–158.

59. Jensen MP, McFarland CA. Increasing the reliability and validity of pain intensity measurement in chronic pain patients. Pain 1993; 55:195–203.

60. Galer BS, Jensen MP. Development and preliminary validation of a pain measure specific to neuropathic pain: the Neuropathic Pain Scale. Neurology 1997; 48: 332–338.

61. Portenoy RK, Payne D, Jacobsen P. Breakthrough pain: characteristics and impact in patients with cancer pain. Pain 1999; 81:129–134.

II

RESEARCH IN ANOREXIA AND GASTROINTESTINAL DISORDERS

2

Methodological Issues Regarding Cancer Anorexia/Cachexia Trials

CHARLES L. LOPRINZI, JEFF A. SLOAN, AND KENDRITH M. ROWLAND, JR.

This chapter reviews information regarding developing, conducting, and analyzing trials designed to test potential agents for alleviating cancer-related anorexia/cachexia. The information is derived from experience generated by the North Central Cancer Treatment Group (NCCTG) in conducting a series of 10 trials which, to date, have entered over 2000 patients. A summary of these trials is provided in Table 2.1.

Patient Selection

Patients selected for most of our clinical trials have lost at least 5 pounds in weight over the preceding 2 months or less excluding perioperative weight loss; alternatively, patients could have had an estimated daily intake of less than 20 calories per kilogram (physician-judged, not necessarily requiring dietary measurements). In addition, each patient must have perceived weight loss as a problem, and both the patient and the attending physician must have determined that weight gain would be beneficial for the patient. Our trials require that patients have histological or cytological evidence of cancer and be considered incurable with available therapies. Patients must have an intact gastrointestinal tract without evidence of obstruction, malabsorption, or intractable vomiting (>5 episodes per week). They must not be receiving tube feedings or parenteral nutrition.

In an effort to include patients who would be living for an appreciable enough period to provide study end points, a few criteria must be met. These include an Eastern Cooperative Oncology Group performance status of 0–2, a physician-judged life expectancy of at least 3 months, and no history of brain

Table 2.1. North Central Cancer Treatment Group experience with cancer anorexia/cachexia trials

Trial description	Enrolled patients
Cyproheptadine vs. placebo	295
Megestrol acetate vs. placebo	133
Megestrol acetate/dose–response trial	342
Megestrol acetate/body composition trial	12
Pentoxifylline vs. placebo	70
Megestrol acetate vs. dexamethasone vs. fluoxymesterone	180
Megestrol acetate vs. dronabinol vs. both	265+
Hydrazine sulfate vs. placebo/colorectal cancer	127
Hydrazine sulfate vs. placebo/lung cancer	243
Megestrol acetate vs. placebo in newly diagnosed small cell lung cancer	243
Total patients	2100+

metastases. Patients are required to be alert, mentally competent, and able to take oral medication. We have excluded patients with evidence of ascites, given the effect of ascites on the gastrointestinal tract. In early studies, we excluded patients with edema but allowed this in later studies, to analyze the effect of particular drugs on appetite, as opposed to relying on nonfluid weight gain (discussed below under Study End Points).

Our studies of certain steroid medications have excluded patients with breast, ovarian, endometrial, and/or prostate cancer because of the effects of these medications on the primary tumor process.

Stratification Factors

Stratification factors in our trials have generally included the following:

- Primary malignant disease: lung cancer versus gastrointestinal cancer versus other
- Severity of weight loss (excluding perioperative weight loss) in the preceding 2 months: <10 pounds versus >10 pounds
- Planned chemotherapy at the time of study entry: none versus cisplatin versus noncisplatin chemotherapy
- Sex: male versus female
- ECOG performance status: 0–1 versus 2
- Patient age <50 versus ≥50 years
- Planned concurrent radiation therapy: yes versus no
- Physician estimate of survival: 3–4 months versus 4–6 months versus >6 months

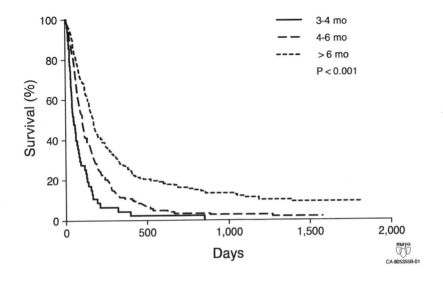

Figure 2.1. Kaplan-Meier survival curves for patients entered on a cancer anorexia/ cachexia clinical trial[33] segregated by physician estimate of survival at the time of study entry.

This relatively large number of stratification factors can be accommodated via procedures developed by Therneau et al.[1] Of particular interest is the information we have generated from a series of trials requiring physicians to estimate survival (without specific instructions on how to do this). Figure 2.1 illustrates how well physicians differentiate patient survival of 3–4 months versus 4–6 months versus >6 months.

Required Testing

In our cooperative oncology group trials evaluating cancer anorexia/cachexia, we believe that simplicity is desirable; thus, we have worked at having our protocols be as user-friendly as is feasible. We have moved away from requiring blood work as measures of nutritional parameters. We rely primarily on patient-completed questionnaires to measure appetite and quality of life (QOL). In the past, these were required at baseline and at monthly intervals, but more recently we have requested them at weekly intervals for the first month of study participation. This is based on information demonstrating that appetite stimulants, such as megestrol acetate, can alleviate symptoms in a matter of days as opposed to weeks.[28] Patient history, physical examination, weight, edema presence, and performance status are requested at baseline and at monthly intervals.

Study End Points

When we began studying cancer anorexia/cachexia, we felt that body composition was probably the most important study end point. There are a number of means for accomplishing this, including plethysmography and skinfold thickness. However, these measurements are not easily obtained in cooperative oncology group settings. In our initial trials, patient weight gain (excluding patients who had evidence of ascites or edema in these measurements) was our primary measure of efficacy. With experience, we have recognized that there is a relatively tight correlation between patient nonfluid weight and appetite as measured by patient questionnaires.[3] At present, we feel that patient appetite is the most important and most easily obtained parameter. The patient appetite instrument used in our initial trial, which has basically been kept intact through 10 studies, has provided substantial information to support its validity and reliablility. These data include the following:

- Six different questions addressing appetite/food intake variations provide reproducible information.[3–5]
- Appetite changes as measured by these questionnaires correlate with non-fluid weight gain.[3]
- Several different trials evaluating megestrol acetate and using different instruments have reported positive results.[2–7]

In addition, along with the ease of measuring appetite compared to body composition changes, reversal of anorexia is probably more important in terms of patient QOL than is reversal of cachexia.

It is difficult to measure directly the entities that represent clinical anorexia/cachexia. Many intangible constructs, such as pain, are easily recognizable subjectively but difficult to quantify objectively. We all know what pain is, but we are unable to directly observe and measure pain in the same consistent and reliable fashion that we measure tumor response. We are left, as a result, with having to use surrogate measures of the construct under study. For example, although the research on pain measurement is large and impressive in its scope and science,[8] at the end of the day we are left with measuring pain by asking patients to give us a number between 1 and 10, supplemented possibly by descriptive adjectives.

Much has been written about the difficulties of defining and measuring the primary end points for anorexia/cachexia.[9] Loss of weight and appetite would at first seem to be simple enough end points, but the issue is complicated.[10,11] It is difficult to obtain detailed and reliable food intake data from seriously ill patients,[12] and in many clinical settings this would represent an undue, unethical burden. Furthermore, the dietary intake of advanced cancer patients is highly variable, both within and among patients.[13]

Loss of appetite is not interpreted the same way by all people.[12] It is also difficult to discern whether the loss of interest in food is due to the cancer or a concomitant problem, such as depression.[14] Several other symptoms can be considered a trigger for anorexia/cachexia.[15] The mechanism of anorexia/cachexia is clearly more complex than simple weight and appetite loss itself.[16] Unfortunately, attempts at compartmental modeling of the complex structure of anorexia/cachexia by describing body composition have produced confusing and conflicting results.[17–21]

Recent publications have begun to focus on the development of specific tools to measure anorexia/cachexia and the related impact it has on a patient's QOL. Most of these tools have been simple questionnaires or single-item instruments using visual analogue scales.[22,23] At the heart of this research is the assumption that improvements in the more objective measures of weight gain and increased food intake will coincide with a sense of overall well-being, which can be captured by the use of simple QOL measurement tools.[24] Unfortunately, while substantial work has been done in recent years to produce standardized and usable measures of patient QOL, there remains uncertainty regarding the accuracy, utility, and clinical significance of measuring patient QOL.[25]

It is important to keep the points of the directly preceding paragraphs in mind as one considers the various ways we have chosen to measure anorexia/cachexia and the related analytical procedures we have used. Despite the aforementioned provisos, it is necessary to "do something" so that potential treatments for anorexia/cachexia can be evaluated.

We believe that in the presence of substantial barriers, such as those delineated above, it is important to observe the KISS (keep it simple and straightforward) principle in designing and analyzing anorexia/cachexia trials. As such, we incorporate measures that are simple, brief, and targeted at the global constructs of appetite improvement, weight gain, and overall QOL. Our objective is to obtain global measures of each of these three constructs in every trial in an efficient manner without causing undue burden to the patients.

One primary objective efficacy end point is a patient's weight. Like others, we have used a comparison between baseline and post-treatment weights (either an absolute difference, percentage change, or percentage of ideal weight) to serve as the basis for analysis. Weight data are excluded if a patient has concurrent evidence of edema or ascites.

Appetite improvement is typically the primary subjective end point involved in anorexia/cachexia trials. It is difficult for a physician or patient to subjectively or objectively assess changes in appetite by the absolute amount of nourishment consumed. We have focused primarily on the patient's perception of whether or not the appetite has improved. Simple Likert scaling provides, in our opinion, the best degree of precision that can be elicited from most patients to assess whether the appetite has improved or worsened a small, moderate, or large amount.

A series of short questionnaire items facilitates this approach. A sample of such a tool used in a recent anorexia/cachexia trial is given in the Appendix. Each item can be summed up on a "was it worth it" (WIWI) or a "did it work" (DIW) scale. We have used the Spitzer Uniscale single-item visual analogue tool to obtain a measure of global QOL over a number of treatment trials.[26] The single item has proven to be more sensitive to changes in QOL than larger, more complex instruments.[27] Use of a simple visual analogue scale for obtaining global measures of generic constructs has long been established in the psychosocial literature.[27,28]

The end points for an anorexia/cachexia trial need to be multivariate in nature by encompassing the triad of patient weight gain, appetite improvement, and QOL. Although each of these end points may be complex in nature, we have stressed the importance of keeping the instrumentation as simple as possible. In essence, each construct within the triad of the complex end point can be measured by a single value. Once these mechanisms are in place, it becomes important to decide a priori what shift in each of these three constructs will be considered a clinically significant improvement.

Power Considerations

Once the end points have been defined, the next critical step is to define how much of an effect is important. This simple question can be answered in many complicated ways. We will take each construct within the triad primary end point defined in the previous section in turn and discuss power considerations for each.

Weight gain may seem at first to be the easiest construct for which to determine a clinically significant effect. It is arguable, however, given the confounding factors of co-morbidities and concomitant cancer treatment, as to what degree weight realistically can be expected to be augmented in patients with advanced cancer. We have operationally defined relative success classifications for the weight end point as a percentage of baseline weight. If a patient achieves, by the end of the treatment period, an increase of 5% or 10% over the baseline weight, then it is reasonable to declare such a situation a success.

Using the above definitions of success and failure in terms of the weight gain end point, power calculations are a simple matter, analogous to standard phase II treatment trial binomial end points. All that is needed for sample size specification is a decision as to what proportion of patients are declared a "success" for a particular treatment. Megestrol acetate, for example, produced success rates in our trials of between 9% and 15%.[3,4] Any new treatment would have to produce at least similar success percentages with a more limited toxicity profile to be considered a reasonable alternative. Our recently completed comparison of megestrol acetate versus fluoxymesterone versus dexamethasone had 158 patients per treatment arm, which provided 80% power to detect a difference of 10% in the percentage of successful patients between megestrol acetate and either of the two alternative treatments using a two-sided test for equality of proportions with a 5% type I error rate. Any smaller study would not be able to detect small enough effect sizes.

A similar approach is suggested for the other two subjective constructs within the triad primary end point for anorexia/cachexia. Appetite and QOL improvement that will be considered clinically significant need to be specified in advance so that the trial is appropriately sized and powered. While this may seem daunting at first, there are data in the literature that can provide starting point estimates for effect sizes. For example, in a megestrol acetate trial,[3] we observed a change in appetite effect size for megestrol acetate of 33%, defined as a one-category improvement in the Likert item used for appetite improvement. The power calculation is a straightforward application of inference for the standard Wilcoxon rank sum test. For example, in our megestrol acetate, fluoxymesterone, and dexamethasone trial,[33] we had 80% power to detect a one-category shift for 29% of the population in the appetite gain item using a two-sided testing procedure with a 5% type I error rate.

An average shift in the responses to Spitzer's QOL item of 10% seems a reasonable benchmark that a treatment has had a moderately large impact on overall patient QOL.[21] Other authors are comfortable with an average 1.5-point difference on a 10-point scale or a half-point difference in a 5-point Likert tool.[29] As will be seen below, these suggested effect sizes are comparable to what we have suggested.

We have developed an approach that marries the theoretical range of the QOL instrument used with a framework put forward by Cohen[30] for measuring intangible constructs in the behavioral sciences.[31] In brief, we assume that all "soft" end points measured by a Likert or similar subjective format have an underlying theoretical continuum running from the best to worst possible scenarios. We then are able to transform any such measurement onto a 0–100 scale that represents a patient's position along this theoretical continuum relative to the best (100) and worst (0) situations. We subsequently use, as an estimate for the standard deviation of the end point, a fraction of the theoretical range of 100 units based on the empirical rule from statistical theory. The empirical rule states that the range of a distribution is roughly equivalent to six standard deviations. Hence, any QOL measure that has been transformed onto a 0–100 scale will have a standard deviation of around 16.7% (100/6). The power calculations are then based on the Cohen[30] framework of small, moderate, and large effect sizes for soft end points, such as one encounters routinely in the social sciences.

For our anorexia/cachexia trials, producing power calculations for comparing the average scores on the appetite and QOL constructs (transformed onto the 0–100 scale) between two treatments now is simply a function of Wilcoxon procedures, as previously described, or simple two-sample *t*-tests. Cohen[30] described small, moderate, and large effect sizes for this procedure as being 0.2, 0.5, and 0.8 standard deviations. Multiplying these by our estimate for the standard deviation of 16.7%, we find that for the appetite and QOL constructs small, moderate, and large shifts on average between, for example, megestrol acetate and dexamethasone, would represent differences of 3, 8, and 13 units, respectively. Our megestrol acetate trial,[4] for example, had 80% power to detect a difference of 8 units between two treatments, which would be a moderate effect size.

The primary advantage of this approach is its simplicity. Certainly, if better estimates of the standard deviation for these soft end points are available in the literature, they would produce more accurate power calculations. At present, however, this is not the case. Further, if one were to use the previously mentioned effect sizes of a 1.5-point shift on a scale of 10 units or a half-point shift on a 5-point scale, these correspond to roughly 0.9 standard deviations by our classification system, which would represent a large effect size. Hence, one would produce required sample sizes likely to be too small to detect any but very profound shifts in QOL.

Once the power and sample size requirements have been calculated for all three constructs within the triad primary end point, we recommend taking the maximum of the three sample sizes to ensure that the trial is powered sufficiently for each primary measure (weight, appetite, QOL). Typically, shifts in QOL will require fewer observations than the other two constructs. Some authors have recommended the collection of QOL data on a subset of patients to alleviate patient burden and conserve system resources.[28,29] We do not recommend this for anorexia/cachexia trials, however, because the burden is a single question per patient and the resources saved by sampling a subset of patients are most likely spent in the random allocation of QOL tools to patients, especially given the missing data, which will be discussed in subsequent sections.*

Clinical Realities

The most important clinical reality for anorexia/cachexia trials is that the patient population is seriously ill. Hence, one cannot expect the patients to be willing or able to consistently produce a large amount of data. As discussed previously, we have tried to minimize the clinical data points to enhance both the proportion of patients who will provide data and the length of time that patients will be able to produce data. Despite such precautions, a substantial proportion of patients will not produce valuable data. As this is a reality of measuring anorexia/cachexia, it is important to keep it in mind for the design and analysis of the trial.

First, in terms of eligibility criteria, a number of patients will not have documented evidence of weight loss. We have adopted the policy that as long as the patient's physician is satisfied that the definition of the anorexia/cachexia syndrome is appropriate for the patient, the patient is eligible for the trial.

Second, and perhaps more importantly, one must design the trial to accommodate situations that will arise in patients who are terminally ill. For example, we have made it possible for patients to take home copies of the appetite, QOL,

---

*The computer code via the SAS system for the missing data and power calculations of this chapter are available via e-mail (jsloan@mayo.edu).

and supportive questionnaire items once they leave the clinical setting. This is done so that if they are unable to return to the clinic for some reason, they can complete these simple items via a phone call. This adds between 10% and 20% to the amount of completed data on a trial. Use of surrogate scores (such as asking the spouse of the patient to fill out the questionnaire) is a further alternative, but we do not recommend using this approach until it has been demonstrated via pilot testing that the scores one obtains from the surrogates are indeed comparable to those one would have obtained from the patients themselves.[28]

Missing Data

The reality of working with seriously ill patients is that some will die during the course of the trial. There are several ways to handle this eventuality in the design and analysis phase of the trial.

In the design phase, one can choose among several methods to adjust for missing data.[32] Recent QOL research has focused on multiple imputation methods. The number of alternative approaches here is staggering. One can choose to impute missing data by carrying forward the last score obtained, the minimum score obtained, the maximum score obtained, the average value obtained, or a zero to reflect the fact that the patient is no longer living. Each of these approaches has application. Figure 2.2 displays the profile of QOL scores for 104

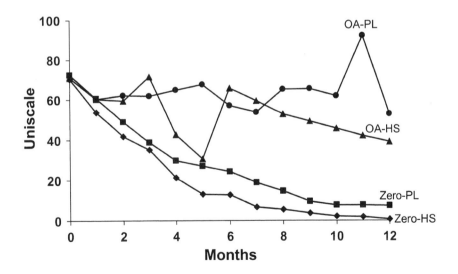

Figure 2.2. Mean quality-of-life scores for 104 patients in a trial[34] who were randomized to receive hydrazine sulfate (HS) or placebo (PL) (*1*) using observations available (OA) or (*2*) imputing zeros for patients who had died (Zero).

patients over 12 separate time points receiving a treatment (hydrazine sulfate) or a placebo using either the observations that are available (OA) at each time point or imputing zeroes for any patient who has died and therefore provided missing data (Zero). As one can see, there may be very different inferences drawn, depending on the method chosen. The two profiles using all available data only (the OA lines) overlap and seem to indicate that the QOL for both treatment groups is the same. In this particular trial, however, the attrition rate was considerable so that the number of patients available at time point 12 is less than 5% of the original number of patients that began the trial. Hence, the OA QOL scores are representative of the "good performers" in this trial. These data are not "wrong" but need to be interpreted within the context that the QOL for the subpopulation of patients who survive through all 12 time points is basically the same for both treatment groups. If one were to consider the average QOL for all patients who had originally begun the trial, then the Zero curves are of interest. The marked drop in average QOL for the group of 104 patients that began this study incorporates consideration for the attrition observed. Furthermore, the placebo group was consistently higher in terms of average QOL, due in part to a differential in survival between the two treatment groups. Either of these two sets of treatment comparison curves is relevant, depending on which context is more appropriate for a particular analysis.

Figure 2.3 shows how the average patient QOL profile is profoundly impacted by the manner in which the missing data are imputed. The lines plotted depict the QOL profiles obtained if missing data were inputed using only the available observations at each point (OA); carrying forward the average value (AVCF), the last value (LVCF), the minimum value (MVCF), or a zero (Zero); or using only the people who provided complete data (Complete). While it is encouraging to see that the profiles are relatively consistent across a number of imputation methods, the stark contrast between the Zero and OA lines indicates that any analysis of such end points needs to be done with great regard given to the imputation procedure used. We have taken the approach of using several imputation procedures on the same data to obtain an indication of the sensitivity of results to the imputation method.

Imputation of scores between observation points is handled most easily by assuming some form of trend from point A to point C and estimating where the patient would have been on average at point B. The amount of difference seen in results from such imputation is likely to be slight unless the amount of missing data is tremendous. We once again recommend using a number of alternative approaches to test the robustness of results relative to imputation methods and assumptions. It has been our experience that imputation of values between observed data points for particular patients is needed less frequently than filling out the profile after patients have ceased to provide data.

Another popular approach is to use multiple imputation methods.[32] Unfortunately, such methods are assumption-laden and perhaps contradictory to

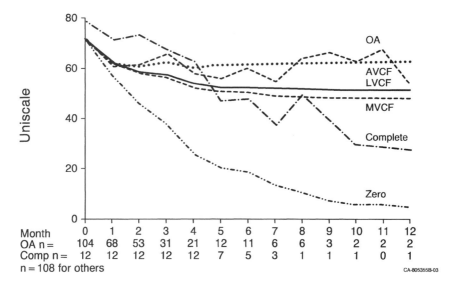

Figure 2.3. Mean quality-of-life scores on a clinical trial[34] based on the following imputation methods for missing data: (*1*) observations available (OA), (*2*) average value carried forward (AVCF), (*3*) last value carried forward (LVCF), (*4*) minimum value carried forward (MVCF), (*5*) imputing zeros for deaths (Zero) using LVCF for interval missing data or off study without death, or (*6*) using only patients who provided complete data (Complete).

the KISS principle. Unless more than 20% of the data are missing, the results one gets from any imputation approach will likely be the same.[32]

Statistical Methods

Statistical methodology for anorexia/cachexia trials is similar to that involved in other clinical trials. As seen previously under Power Considerations, typical group comparisons using standard *t*-test, Wilcoxon test, and equality of proportions test procedures can be applied to anorexia/cachexia trials with appropriate definition of end points and effect sizes.

Statistical methods used on anorexia/cachexia data have often included high-power statistical procedures, such as repeated-measures analysis of variance, polynomial effects models, and other multivariate analyses.[17] Our approach has been to use more simple, straightforward procedures and to hold the more complicated analyses in abeyance until the basic questions have been answered. The assumptions required for generalizability of results for the more involved procedures are both numerous and complex. Further, the assumptions are not tenable for measuring intangible constructs with inherent measurement error, a lack of normality, and a measurement level somewhere between ordinal and interval level data. More importantly, as mentioned above, the amount of missing data one can expect to see in an anorexia/cachexia trial is nontrivial, which severely restricts the applicability of several of the more complicated statistical routines.

A key issue for the handling of data from an anorexia/cachexia trial is the classification of whether each patient has experienced treatment success according to a priori specified definitions for the three constructs that make up the primary end point. We have taken the approach that if a patient fails to provide evidence of treatment success, regardless of the reason, we classify the case as a treatment failure. This intent-to-treat type of analysis produces efficacy estimates that are "worst-case scenario" in that the proportion of successes one can expect to see in the clinical environment will be at least the level reported from the anorexia/cachexia trial. It is true that some patients will have been classified as not having had a treatment success when in fact they did but were unable or unwilling to report it. Given the patient population, however, it is more reasonable to assume that the vast majority of patients who died or failed to complete the study did not receive sufficient benefit from the study regimen to be classified as a success.

Summary

As with any research endeavor, the study of anorexia/cachexia is difficult and fraught with potential pitfalls. Our experience may aid in the standardization of design and analytic approaches for anorexia/cachexia trials so that meta-analytic process, formal or otherwise, may be facilitated. Our overriding principle has been to keep the process as simple as possible due to the many potentially concomitant confounding influences. The rationale for this approach is that if the treatments applied to anorexia/cachexia do not produce profound results in the presence of substantial systemic noise, then they are not likely to be seen as efficacious in the community clinical environment beyond the pristine clinical trials setting. Since the community oncology setting is the final and true arbiter for the success or failure of a particular anorexia/cachexia treatment, we feel the justification for such a realistic approach to anorexia/cachexia research is self-evident.

References

1. Therneau TM. How many stratification factors are "too many" to use in a randomization plan? Control Clin Trials 1993; 14:98–108.
2. Bruera E, Macmillan K, Kuehn N, et al. A controlled trial of megestrol acetate on appetite, calorie intake, nutritional status, other symptoms in patients with advanced cancer. Cancer 1990; 66:1279–1282.

3. Loprinzi CL, Michalak JC, Schaid DJ, et al. Phase III evaluation of four doses of megestrol acetate as therapy for patients with cancer anorexia and/or cachexia. J Clin Oncol 1993; 11:762–767.

4. Loprinzi CL, Ellison NM, Schaid DJ, et al. A controlled trial of megestrol acetate in patients with cancer anorexia and/or cachexia. J Natl Cancer Inst 1990; 82:1127–1132.

5. Kardinal CG, Loprinzi CL, Schaid DJ, et al. A controlled trial of cyproheptadine in cancer patients with anorexia and/or cachexia. Cancer 1990; 65:2657–2662.

6. Cleeland CS, Nakamura Y, Mendoza TR, et al. Dimensions of the impact of cancer pain in a four country sample: new information from multidimensional scaling. Pain 1996; 67:267–273.

7. Tchekmedyian NS, Hickman M, Siau J, et al. Megestrol acetate in cancer anorexia and weight loss. Cancer 1992; 69:1268–1274.

8. Zamora PO, Garcia de Paredea ML, Montero JM. Usefulness of megestrol acetate in cancer cachexia and anorexia. Am J Clin Oncol 1992; 15:436–440.

9. Burman R Chamberlain J. The assessment of the nutritional status, caloric intake, and appetite of patients with advanced cancer. In: Bruera E, Higinson I, eds. Cachexia–Anorexia in Cancer Patients. London: Oxford University Press, 1996:83–93.

10. Donnelly S, Walsh D. The symptoms of advanced cancer. Semin Oncol 1995; 22:67–72.

11. Donnelly S, Walsh D, Rybicki L. The symptoms of advanced cancer: identification of clinical and research priorities by assessment of prevalence of severity. J Palliat Care 1995; 11:27–32.

12. Nelson K, Walsh D, Sheehan Fa. The cancer anorexia–cachexia syndrome. J Clin Oncol 1994; 12:213–225.

13. Walsh TD, Bowman KB, Jackson GP. Dietary intake of advanced cancer patients. Hum Nutr 1983; 37A:41–45.

14. Grosvenor M, Bulcavage L, Chlebowski RT. Symptoms potentially influencing weight loss in a cancer patient population. Cancer 1989; 63:330–334.

15. Costa G, Bewley P, Aragon M. Anorexia and weight loss in cancer patients. Cancer Treat Rep 1981; 65:3–7.

16. Von Meyenfeldt MF, Soeters PB. Mechanisms of anorexia in cancer and potential ways for intervention. Clin Oncol 1986; 5:293–306.

17. Shigal HM. Body composition of patients with malnutrition and cancer. Cancer 1985; 55:250–253.

18. Cohn SH, Gartenhaus W, Vartsky D, et al. Body composition and dietary intake in neoplastic disease. Am J Clin Nutr 1981; 34:1997–2004.

19. Watson WS, Sammon AM. Body composition in cachexia resulting from malignant and non-malignant diseases. Cancer 1980; 46:2041–2046.

20. MacFie J, Burkinshaw C. Body composition in malignant disease. Metabolism 1987; 36:290–294.

21. Heymsfield SD, McManus CB. Tissue components of weight loss in cancer patients: a new method of study and preliminary observations. Cancer 1985; 55:238–241.

22. Osoba D, Murray N, Gelmon K. Quality of life, appetite and weight change in patients receiving dose-intensive weekly chemotherapy. Oncology 1994; 8:61–65.

23. Cella DF, Von Roenn J, Lloyd S, et al. The Bristol-Myers Anorexia/Cachexia Recovery Instrument (BACRI): a brief assessment of patients' subjective response to treatment for anorexia/cachexia. Qual Life Res 1995; 4:221–231.

24. Cella DF, Bonomi AE, Leslie WT, et al. Quality of life and nutritional well-being: measurement and relationship. Oncology 1993; 7:105–111.
25. Leplege A, Hunt S. The problem of quality of life in medicine. JAMA 1997; 278: 47–50.
26. Spitzer WO, Dobson AJ, Hall J, et al. Measuring the quality of life of cancer patients: a concise QL-index for use by physicians. J Chronic Dis 1981; 34:585–597.
27. Sloan JA, Loprinzi CL, Kuross SA, Miser AW, O'Fallon JR, Mahoney MR, Heid IM, Bretscher ME, Vaught NL. Randomized comparison of four tools measuring overall quality of life in patients with advanced cancer. J Clin Oncol 1998; 16: 3662–3673.
28. Spilker B. Quality of Life and Pharmacoeconomics in Clinical Trials. New York: Lippincott-Raven Press, 1996.
29. Cella DF, Bonomi AE. Measuring quality of life: 1995 update. Oncology 1995; 9: 47–60.
30. Cohen J. Statistical Power Analysis for the Behavioral Sciences. Hillsdale, NJ: Lawrence Erlbaum Associates, 1988.
31. Sloan JA, O'Fallon JR, Suman VJ, Sargent DJ. Incorporating quality of life measurement in oncology clinical trials. Proc Am Stat Assoc, 1998; Biometrics Section: 282–287.
32. Fairclough D. Summary measures and statistics for comparison of quality of life in trials of cancer therapy. Stat Med 1997; 16:1197–1209.
33. Loprinzi CL, Kugler J, Sloan J, et al. Phase III randomized comparison of megestrol acetate, dexamethasone, and fluoxymesterone for the treatment of cancer anorexia/cachexia. Proc Am Soc Clin Oncol 1997; 16:48a.
34. Loprinzi CL, Goldberg RM, Su JQ, et al. Placebo-controlled trial of hydrazine sulfate in patients with newly diagnosed non-small cell lung cancer. J Clin Oncol 1994; 6:1126–1129.

Appendix

PATIENT QUESTIONNAIRE
Pretreatment

1. Do you have presistent swelling of your legs or abdomen? (Check one)
   _____ Yes
   _____ No

2. How would you compare your appetite now to what it was before your present illness? (Check one)
   _____ The same
   _____ Increased
   _____ Slightly reduced (about 75% of normal)
   _____ Moderately reduced (about 50% of normal)
   _____ Markedly reduced (about 25% of normal or less)

3. What is your current food intake in comparison to before your present illness? (Check one)
   _____ The Same
   _____ Increased
   _____ Slightly reduced (about 75% of normal)
   _____ Moderately reduced (about 50% of normal)
   _____ Markedly reduced (about 25% of normal or less)

4. How would you rate/describe your appetite? (Check one)
   _____ Very good
   _____ Good
   _____ Fair
   _____ Poor
   _____ Very poor

5. How do you presently feel about your weight status? (Check one)
   _____ I would like to stabilize or increase my weight
   _____ My weight status is not a problem
   _____ I would like to lose weight
   _____ Other (please describe) _____

6. How much nausea have you had on an average over the previous week? (Check one)
   _____ None
   _____ Mild, able to eat reasonably well
   _____ Moderate, significantly decreased oral intake
   _____ Severe, no significant oral intake

PATIENT QUESTIONNAIRE
Pretreatment

7. How many times have you vomited over the past week? (Check one)

_____ 0 times

_____ 1–3 times

_____ 4–10 times

_____ >10 times

8. **Please mark with an "X" the appropriate place within the bar below to indicate how you would rate your own quality of life during the past week.**

   Lowest quality applies to someone completely dependent physically on others, seriously troubled mentally, unaware of surroundings, and in a hopeless position.

   Highest quality applies to someone physically and mentally independent, communicating well with others, able to do most of the things enjoyed, pulling own weight, with a hopeful yet realistic attitude.

LOWEST QUALITY   HIGHEST QUALITY

(Please mark one X within the bar)

3

Assessment of Novel Therapies for Constipation: Focus on Opioid Analgesics

JOSEPH F. FOSS

Pain control is a primary goal of palliative care. The World Health Organization (WHO) guidelines for pain control specify an escalating series of therapies, but the ultimate resource for the control of severe pain remains the opioids.

Forty to forty-five percent of patients presenting for hospice care complain of constipation on admission.[1–3] There are multiple factors that may account for this in the palliative care population, including the patient's primary disease process; decreased mobility, fluid intake, food intake, and fiber intake; and non-opioid drug use.[4] The prevalence of constipation in those receiving strong opioids is markedly higher, however, in the range 80%–90%. Constipation may result in undesired outcomes, ranging from an increase in abdominal pain with increased drug requirements to obstipation with the potential for bowel obstruction or perforation. It may be severe enough to limit use of analgesics even when medically indicated.[2,5]

Many caregivers now prophylactically initiate a bowel maintenance program, usually including recommendations for increased activity and fluid intake and regular use of stool bulking agents, stool softeners, and bowel stimulants, when opioid therapy is initiated.[6] Although many patients will have acceptable bowel habits with this program, others will continue to be troubled by the problem. Unfortunately, these seemingly simple measures may be difficult for the patient at the end of life, already faced with low energy levels, anorexia, and an occasionally dizzying array of medications to take during the day. Some patients will develop significant side effects due to the constipation or its treatment or will decrease their use of opioids and tolerate the pain in preference to the constipation. Neither of these outcomes is acceptable; hence, there is a need for ongoing research into the prevention and treatment of opioid-induced constipation.

Current research is focused on many areas. Work is needed to define the mechanisms by which opioids produce constipation. While the motility effects have been well documented, the antisecretory effects bear additional study with regard to their facilitating constipation. The secondary effects of opioid receptor activation also may be further defined and present new opportunities for pharmacological intervention. Those developing opioid alternatives, especially opioids with differing receptor affinities, have been unable to separate the analgesic properties from the side effects of opioids. Methods to optimize opioid use (for example, rotating opioid type, alternative routes of administration) and traditional bowel care methods are being examined, but it is difficult at times to compare the results of interventions as the model and definition of success vary widely between publications. New therapies, including the use of opioid antagonists in the gut, also are being studied. Translation of data from animal studies to humans is difficult, however, due to differences in the physiology of the opioid systems.

Research Goals

The short-term goals for research include the refinement of our definition and measurement of constipation in the target population and perhaps the development of a model in human volunteers to study new therapies prior to bringing them into the palliative care arena. Longer-term goals will focus on the further elucidation of the mechanisms of opioid-induced constipation and the development of specific therapies that will allow for the use of opioids to achieve adequate analgesia while minimally impacting gastrointestinal function. Specific areas include antagonism of the opioid receptors in the gut or alteration of the secondary mechanisms by which these receptors change gastrointestinal function.

Research Methodologies

Definition and measurement of constipation

Current approach
There are very few similarities across reports in the literature that examine the issue of opioid-induced constipation. Patient questionnaires are frequently used but are not standardized. They generally include a self-assessment of constipation and a series of questions that attempt to describe the nature of the stool (firmness, etc.) and the act of defecation (straining, pain, etc.). Stool frequency is usually assessed, but there is a wide variation of "normal" or acceptable values in the population (three times per day to three times per week), and it can be difficult to set a single frequency such as <1 stool/48 hours as a cut-off (even though this type of number is often seen in therapeutic schemes for advancing to more aggressive therapy). Stool characteristics such as mass, volume, water content, and firmness have been examined in the gastroenterology literature.[7]

Laxative use is frequently reported as an indicator of constipation, but the use of laxatives in hospice patients (63% of patients not receiving opioids) exceeds the number of patients reporting constipation (45%).[8] Thus, in study environments, one must examine whether there were specific indications for laxative use before and after the study intervention to assess the validity of any changes in laxative use patterns.

The history and physical exam can provide a good indication in both subjective (patient self-report) and objective (abdominal distention or masses, hard stool on rectal exam) terms of the presence of constipation. Unfortunately, the lack of standards for describing the signs and symptoms has limited the usefulness of this approach. Additionally, the examination for constipation is rarely performed and documented in clinical practice, where specific protocols do not exist.

The abdominal plain film has been proposed as an indicator of the presence and degree of constipation.[9] It can definitely demonstrate the presence of stool and its distribution in the colon. The technique needs to be further correlated with a standard description of constipation and its ability to document successful therapy.

Ingestion of radiopaque markers has been used to enhance the value of the abdominal radiograph in the study of gut transit and constipation. Markers must be taken and then followed with serial radiographs (with the attendant increase in radiation exposure), or a series of markers of different shapes may be taken over a period of days with a single film examining their location to demonstrate motility. The stool may even be radiographed to track the passage of the markers. Barium is used to demonstrate the anatomy of the gut and may be followed for motility studies. It may, however, contribute to the formation of hard stools, which may be difficult to pass. Radiolabeled meals or markers have the advantage of being able to demonstrate gut function without affecting gastrointestinal physiology.[10] Their use is limited by the need for specialized imaging equipment and the special handling of the radioisotopes both going into the subject and after their excretion.

The oral–cecal transit time assessed by the pulmonary hydrogen (H_2) measurement technique is based on the observation of an increase in H_2 that is produced when carbohydrate is fermented by colonic bacteria. This H_2 production is reflected by a concomitant increase the concentration of H_2 excreted in exhaled breath.

The time between ingestion of an unabsorbable sugar such as lactulose and the rise in breath H_2 represents the oral–cecal transit time.[11-13] The earliest detectable and sustained rise in pulmonary H_2 excretion, that is, a sudden rise to the peak (>25 ppm) or an increase of at least 2 ppm above the baseline maintained and increased in three consecutive samples, indicates that some of the lactulose has reached the cecum.[14,15] This then represents primarily the oral–cecal transit time and only indirectly correlates with motility in the colon. This technique is limited by a sensitivity to diet (requiring a low-residue diet for

12–24 hours pre-examination), the ability of repeated or larger doses of lactulose to act as a laxative, and differences in gut flora. Approximately 12% of the population does not produce H_2 after ingestion of the sugar.

Surface gut myoelectric tracing reflects the changes induced by opioids on gut activity. The technique is technically challenging in the separation of the gastrointestinal signals from those of overlying muscle. It also represents activity over gut regions and may not distinguish between the large and small bowel.

Proposed approach

We propose that the research community begin to move toward a more uniform set of measures for constipation and the efficacy of therapy. In many ways, the subjective response of patients should weigh most prominently in our assessment (see Table 3.1 for a suggested set of questions). Addition of one of the objective measures cited should be considered, to demonstrate that the changes in the patient assessment of constipation correlate with a physiological effect on gut motility.

Models of constipation

Animal models of constipation in lower mammals, whether in vitro or in vivo, are troubled by the well-documented differences between the species in receptors and the subsequent differences in response to opioids. This can be particularly challenging when extrapolating dose information to humans. Primates are much more representative but have the attendant difficulties of cost. In all animal models, many physiological processes may be measured both invasively and non-invasively. The ability to assess subjective effects (for example, dissatisfaction with stool frequency or consistency) is limited, however, with behavioral studies providing limited translation to human responses.

Acute or subacute dosing of opoids in normal volunteers has been used in the study of opioid effects and their treatment. This model has the advantage of

Table 3.1. Suggested assessment questions for constipation

Patient self-assessment
  Have you been constipated over the last *n* months? (Y/N)
    (where *n* is a period appropriate to the study)
  How often are your stools (or how many stools per week)?
  What would you consider an acceptable number per week?
    (Achieving the acceptable level could be used in a binary assessment of treatment success.)
  How often are your bowel movements (rated on a five-point scale: never, rarely, sometimes,
    mostly, always):
    Accompanied by straining?
    Hard?
    Painful?

---

studying subjects free of co-morbidities and other potential causes of gastrointestinal dysfunction. Furthermore, subjects may be studied with somewhat more invasive measures than those that would be tolerated by the terminally ill patient in a palliative care setting. They likely will be better able to report their subjective sense of treatment effects without confounding pain or other discomfort. These benefits are offset by the knowledge that chronic opioid use initiates physiological changes that result in tolerance to opioids and increased sensitivity to antagonists.

Patients treated chronically with opioids also take much larger doses than those that can be given safely to the opioid-naive volunteer. As most of the antagonists being studied are believed to be competitive, the dose ratio may be an important part of their use.

We have recently analyzed a population of volunteers on methadone maintenance programs to study antagonists in the treatment of constipation. These subjects must be monitored closely for illicit drug use, but a subgroup relatively free of significant co-morbidity can be identified and studied.

The target population presents many challenges to these studies. The primary disease process is rarely static, and studies which require more than a few days may be confounded by other physiological changes or even loss of participants due to death. These patients and their caregivers are also frequently interested in minimizing the invasiveness and intrusiveness of any study or therapeutic intervention. This pushes the investigator toward the use of subjective measures, but these may also be confounded by the "good days and bad days" effect, which can be seen in the terminally ill population.

Opioid agonists and antagonists in opioid-induced constipation

The delineation of opioid receptor subtypes has led researchers to explore their differential activity in an effort to produce a selected set of effects.[16] To date, there has been limited success with this approach, and there are no potent μ-opioid analgesics clinically available which do not affect the gut. Other receptor types, such as κ opioids, have been studied; and mixed agonists, such as butorphanol, are available.

Kappa-opioid agonists do not appear to slow gastrointestinal motility. Clinical experience with κ opioids to date has been frustrated by the appearance of dose-limiting central nervous system side effects.[17] ADL 10-0101 (Adolor Corporation, Exton, PA) is in clinical trials for the treatment of visceral pain. A recent trial in six patients with pain due to chronic pancreatitis refractory to treatment with traditional μ opioids demonstrated efficacy with no significant associated central nervous system side effects.[18]

Tertiary opioid antagonists (naloxone, naltrexone, and nalmefene) have been used intravenously, epidurally, and orally to control opioid-induced side effects. The hallmark of this approach is the use of careful titration to reverse the undesirable effects of the opioids, such as respiratory depression, pruritus, or constipation, without reversing the desired analgesic effect. Interindividual variation and the sensitivity of patients who may be tolerant to the opioids, and hence more sensitive to the antagonists, may yield a varying therapeutic threshold for the use of these drugs.

Selective antagonism of opioid gastrointestinal side effects by tertiary compounds, such as naloxone or naltrexone, has been attempted but has been limited by the propensity for these compounds to reverse analgesia or to induce opioid withdrawal.[19–21] In trials of oral naloxone to treat opioid-induced constipation, 2/10 subjects exhibited symptoms associated with withdrawal.[22] Naltrexone also crosses the blood–brain barrier and, thus, blocks both the beneficial pain-relieving effects and the adverse effects of morphine.

Methylnaltrexone is a quaternary derivative of naltrexone. It does not penetrate into the brain[23] and has the potential to block undesirable opioid effects predominantly mediated by peripheral receptors (for example, in the gastrointestinal tract), while sparing opioid effects, including analgesia, mediated at receptors in the central nervous system.[24] It appears to have limited effects in opioid-naive volunteers.[25]

The ability of methylnaltrexone to reverse the effects of acutely administered opioids on oral–cecal transit time without affecting analgesia has been demonstrated in human volunteers.[26] More recently, the ability to induce defecation in chronically constipated methadone users without inducing signs or symptoms of opioid withdrawal has demonstrated the potential of this approach for even patients tolerant to opioids.[27]

In animal models, even quaternary opioids may exhibit reversal of analgesia when given in large doses or over prolonged periods. The picture is clouded, however, by the ability of some animals to demethylate methylnaltrexone, yielding the much more active tertiary compound. This metabolic pathway does not appear to be present in humans with acute dosing. Studies of the pharmacokinetics and pharmacodynamics of long-term methylnaltrexone administration in humans are needed. The problem may be obviated by the use of intermittent dosing or unique dosage forms to limit the probability of producing active metabolites.

Alvimopan (ADL 8-2698, Adolor Corporation) is a novel peripherally restricted opioid antagonist. In development for oral administration, it has activity specific to the gastrointestinal tract, with very limited absorption. In healthy subjects, alvimopan antagonized loperimide-induced changes in gastrointestinal transit and prevented morphine-induced delays in oral–cecal transit time without antagonizing centrally mediated analgesia. In patients treated with opioids for chronic pain or opioid addiction, oral doses of 0.5–3.0 mg alvimopan reversed opioid bowel dysfunction. Common side effects, seen primarily at higher doses, included abdominal discomfort, flatulence, and diarrhea; supramaximal doses (≥ 3.0 mg) produced side effects indicative of a localized gastrointestinal withdrawal response. No signs of loss of analgesia or central withdrawal were observed. Alvimopan is currently in phase III trials for opioid bowel dysfunction.[28]

Additional study into the best mode of using these drugs is also needed. It is not clear at this time whether providing persistent antagonism of the gut receptors and thus attempting to maintain normal gastrointestinal activity is optimal or if providing acute antagonism once each day or every other day, much as with a laxative, is sufficient to control opioid-induced constipation. This pattern of use may also play a role if chronic blockade of gut receptors by an antagonist leads to loss of sensitivity, requiring potential alterations in dose or frequency of administration.

Non-opioid receptor–mediated therapy of opioid-induced constipation

Cisapride has been studied as a promotility agent to treat constipation.[29] The effects of stimulant laxatives on reversing opioid-induced decreases in gut motility have also been studied. These agents do not restore normal patterns of motility but increase motility with compensatory mechanisms.

Cisapride has multiple drug interactions (antibiotics, antidepressants, antifungals, and protease inhibitors) and potentially severe adverse side effects, which contraindicate the drug's use in patients with certain disorders, such as congestive heart failure, multiple organ failure, chronic obstructive pulmonary disease (which causes serious respiratory problems), and advanced cancer. Cisapride was withdrawn from the US market on July 14, 2000, due to the risk of serious cardiac arrhythmias in certain patients.

Given the existence of numerous drugs other than opioids that are implicated in producing constipation, such as anticholinergics, calcium channel blockers, and serotonin agonists, it would seem possible to use pharmacological approaches to these systems to enhance gut motility. Circulating hormones and peptides such as angiotensin, vasopressin, catecholamines, serotonin, histamine, acetylcholine, somatostatin, vasoactive intestinal polypeptide, neuropeptide Y, substance P, and others also have effects on the secretory and motility effects of the gut.

These nonopioid targets generally represent transmitter families with widespread distribution in the body. If new drugs are to be developed with efficacy and limited side effects, their activity would need to be limited to the gut. Identification of gut-specific receptor subtypes and synthesis of compounds targeted specifically at those is the most elegant, and perhaps the most difficult, approach. The unique anatomy of the gut suggests the search for compounds with an effect localized by physiochemical properties that might limit absorption or pharmacological properties such as high first-pass metabolism that would limit systemic effects.

Table 3.2. Site-specific concerns in palliative care

Hospital

Requires assessment tools that are quickly completed. Hospital setting may allow for higher degree of invasiveness.

Rapid institution and evaluation of therapy to minimize in-hospital time.

Hospice

Requires assessment tools that are easily and quickly completed.

Availability of several modes of administration as many patients do not have parenteral access and may have limited ability to tolerate oral medications.

Home

Requires assessment tools that are easily and quickly completed, preferably by noninvestigator caregivers or family members.

Availability of several modes of administration as many patients do not have parenteral access and may have limited ability to tolerate oral medications.

Dosing and time course of action that allow for providing appropriate assistance when the drug causes defecation.

Problems Unique to Palliative Care

The palliative care model is challenging in that it spans a variety of environments (Table 3.2) and a variety of patient types. Patients are in a dynamic situation as they near the end of life. While many would optimally spend time in the home setting, they may frequently have to move to more acute-care settings. If the goal is return to the home, they may not be available for prolonged studies in a facility. Their disease processes are also rarely static, with changing therapeutic needs that may confound the ability to control use of a given intervention or the measure of its efficacy if the study period is at all prolonged. Constipation is best measured over days to weeks, not minutes to hours.

No discussion in the current healthcare environment is complete without addressing cost issues. The cost of end-of-life care has come under increasing scrutiny as the population ages and palliative care becomes more sophisticated. New drug therapies are likely to be costly when compared to very inexpensive interventions, such as fiber and over-the-counter laxatives; but to the extent that they decrease facility admissions for more intensive care, either for constipation complications or for inadequate pain control, the overall cost–benefit analysis may favor their use. Very sophisticated models are required to assess their value in terms of reducing pain or suffering and improving quality of life.

Translational Research

Exploring and translating opioid research in animal models is challenging. The opioid receptors demonstrate differences both in specificity for agonists and antagonists and in the distribution of receptors. In spite of this, animal models have provided many insights into mechanisms by which opioids act, and there may be more commonality in the secondary actions that are produced, which have not been explored for their therapeutic potential.

Clinical Research

De Luca and Coupar[30] have reviewed recent research into the antidiarrheal effects of opioids. An important part of this recent work is the renewed interest in the antisecretory effects of opioids, as well as the changes in transit they induce. Normalizing the secretory/absorption balance in the gut may be valuable in the treatment of opioid-reduced constipation. The success of the use of nonabsorbable, orally administered osmotic agents may be in part related to this phenomenon. Stool water content can give insight into this aspect of constipation.

Nitric oxide and L-arginine have been implicated as a modulator of morphine-induced constipation.[31] L-Arginine has stereospecific peripheral action in reversing morphine effects in mice. This may warrant further investigation in humans.

Endogenous antagonists of opioids (corticotropin) have been demonstrated to block morphine-induced changes or gut motility in guinea pigs.[32] These agents also may antagonize analgesia and must be studied with regard to their ability to selectively affect the gut.

Preclinical studies indicate that non-mu opioid–mediated antinociception through the kappa-opioid receptor is possible in models of colorectal distention, uterine cervical nociception, and urinary bladder distention. Ongoing research on compounds with the ability to separate these effects from kappa opioid–induced central nervous system effects[33] may yield alternative therapies for these types of visceral and inflammatory pain.

Acknowledgments

The author is currently an employee of Adolor, the company developing alvimopan and ADL 10-0101. The author also holds a proprietary interest in methylnaltrexone.

References

1. Walsh TD. Oral morphine in chronic cancer pain. Pain 1984; 18:1–11.
2. Glare P, Lickiss JN. Unrecognized constipation in patients with advanced cancer: a recipe for therapeutic disaster. J Pain Symptom Manage 1992; 7:369–371.
3. Sykes NP. Current approaches to the management of constipation. Cancer Surv 1994; 21:137–146.
4. Portenoy RK. Constipation in the cancer patients: causes and management. Med Clin North Am 1987; 71:303–311.

5. McCaffrey M, Beebe A. Managing your patients' adverse reactions to narcotics. Nursing 1989; 19:166–168.

6. Cameron JC. Constipation related to narcotic therapy. A protocol for nurses and patients. Cancer Nurs 1992; 15:372–377.

7. Harari D, Gurwitz JH, Avorn J, et al. How do older persons define constipation? J Gen Intern Med 1997; 12:63–66.

8. Sykes NP. A volunteer model of comparison of laxatives in opioid-related constipation. J Pain Symptom Manage 1996; 11:363–369.

9. Bruera E, Suarez-Almazor M, Velasco A, et al. The assessment of constipation in terminal cancer patients admitted to a palliative care unit: retrospective review. J Pain Symptom Manage 1994; 9:515–521.

10. Kaufman PN, Krevsky B, Malmud LS, et al. Role of opiate receptors in the regulation of colonic transit. Gastroenterology 1988; 94:1351–1356.

11. Bond JH, Levitt MD. Investigation of small bowel transit time in man utilize pulmonary hydrogen (H_2) measurements. J Lab Clin Med 1975; 85:546–555.

12. Yuan CS, Foss JF, O'Connor M, et al. Methylnaltrexone prevents morphine-induced delay in oral–cecal transit time without affecting analgesia: a double-blind randomized placebo-controlled trial. Clin Pharmacol Ther 1996; 59:469–475.

13. Yuan CS, Foss JF, Moss J, et al. Gut motility and transit changes in patients receiving long-term methadone maintenance. J Clin Pharmacol 1998; 38:931–935.

14. Read NW, Al-Janabi MN, Bates TE, et al. Interpretation of the breath hydrogen profile obtained after ingesting a solid meal containing unabsorbable carbohydrate. Gut 1985; 26:834–842.

15. Basilisco G, Camboni G, Bozzani A, et al. Oral naloxone antagonizes loperamide-induced delay of orocecal transit. Dig Dis Sci 1987; 32:829–832.

16. Shook JE, Lemcke PK, Gehrig CA, et al. Antidiarrheal properties of supraspinal mu and delta and peripheral mu, delta and kappa opioid receptors: inhibition of diarrhea without constipation. J Pharmacol Exp Ther 1989; 249:83–90.

17. Pande AC, Pyke RE, Greiner M, et al. Analgesic efficacy of enadoline versus placebo or morphine in postsurgical pain. Clin Neuropharmacol 1996; 19:451–456.

18. Eisenach JC, Carpenter R, Curry R. Analgesia from a peripherally active kappa-opioid receptor agonist in patients with chronic pancreatitis. Pain 2002 (accepted for publication).

19. Gowan JD, Hurtig JB, Fraser RA, et al. Naloxone infusion after prophylactic epidural morphine: effects on incidence of postoperative side-effects and quality of analgesia. Can J Anaesth 1988; 35:143–148.

20. Jaffe JH, Martin WR. Opioid analgesics and antagonists. In: Gilman AF, Rall TW, Nies AS, et al., eds. The Pharmacological Basis of Therapeutics. New York: Pergamon Press, 1990:485–521.

21. Culpepper-Morgan JA, Inturrisi CE, Portenoy RK, et al. Treatment of opioid-induced constipation with oral naloxone: a pilot study. Clin Pharmacol Ther 1992; 52:90–95.

22. Sykes NP. An investigation of the ability of oral naloxone to correct opioid-related constipation of patients with advanced cancer. Palliat Med 1996; 10:135–144.

23. Russel J, Bass P, Goldberg LI, et al. Antagonism of gut, but not central effects of morphine with quaternary narcotic antagonists. Eur J Pharmacol 1982; 78:255–261.

24. Brown DR, Goldberg LI. The use of quaternary narcotic antagonists in opiate research. Neuropharmacology 1985; 24:181–191.
25. Foss JF, O'Connor M, Yuan CS, et al. Safety and tolerance of methylnaltrexone in healthy humans: a randomized placebo-controlled intravenous ascending-dose and pharmacokinetic study. J Clin Pharmacol 1997; 37:25–30.
26. Foss JF. A review of the potential role of methylnaltrexone in opioid bowel dysfunction. Am J Surg 2001; 182:19S–26S.
27. Yuan CS, Foss JF, O'Connor M, et al. Methylnaltrexone for reversal of constipation due to chronic methadone use. JAMA 2000; 283:367–372.
28. Schmidt WK. Alvimopan (ADL 8-2698) is a novel peripheral opioid antagonist. Am J Surg 2001; 182:27S–38S.
29. Gardner VY, Beckwith JV, Heyneman CA. Cisapride for the treatment of chronic idiopathic constipation. Ann Pharmacother 1995; 29:1161–1163.
30. De Luca A, Coupar IM. Insights into opioid action in the intestinal tract. Pharmacol Ther 1996; 69:103–115.
31. Calignano A, Moncada S, Di Rosa M. Endogenous nitric oxide modulates morphine-induced constipation. Biochem Biophys Res Commun 1991; 181:889–893.
32. Poggioli R, Arletti R, Vergoni AV, et al. ACTH-(1-24) antagonizes the cholestatic and constipating effects of morphine. Arch Int Pharmacodyn 1988; 293:265–272.
33. DeHaven-Hudkins DL, Gaunter EK, Gottshall SL, et al. Peripheral restrictions of kappa opioid receptor agonists as defined by pharmacokinetic parameters correlates with behavioral indices of sedation in the rat. Soc Neurosci 2000; 26:915.

4

Measurement of Constipation

NIGEL SYKES

In gastroenterology, chronic idiopathic constipation has been the subject of considerable investigation. The results form a large body of fundamental research into the physiological control of intestinal function, a range of techniques by which to investigate and describe the patterns of motility disorder associated with constipation, and a somewhat less extensive literature assessing the clinical effectiveness of existing or innovative treatments. Pediatric and geriatric specialties have generated their own literature on therapeutic interventions and on the clinical investigation of the underlying gut dysfunction.

In palliative care, research on constipation has attracted much less enthusiasm than investigations of symptoms such as pain and breathlessness. The greatest part of the work describes the extent of the problem and audits the treatments currently used for it. A small number of studies assess the effectiveness of these or alternative treatments. Research into the causation of constipation in the terminally ill is negligible. As in other areas of therapeutics in palliative care, much knowledge is extrapolated, not necessarily inappropriately, from the results of studies performed on other patient groups. However, there is a need for more research that is truly relevant to palliative care patients.

It has been clearly demonstrated that constipation is widespread in the palliative care population and inadequately relieved by current treatment regimes. Case note reviews in several hospices show consistently that about 50% of patients admitted complain of constipation. Twycross and Lack[1] used the same approach, applied to 460 patients, to find that about 75% of hospice inpatients receive at least one oral laxative drug and that, despite this, 40% require ongoing rectal laxative interventions in addition. Similar results have been reported from Holland.[2] Therefore, it may not be surprising that interview/questionnaire studies have found that constipation causes a level of distress rivaling that of pain,[3,4] especially as most patients dislike the rectal procedures to which so many of them are subjected (N.P. Sykes, unpublished observation).

How constipation should be identified is a question to which little attention has been paid in palliative care. In gastroenterology, constipation is widely defined for research purposes according to what are sometimes called the "Rome criteria,"[5] which state that constipation is present if two or more of the following symptoms have existed for over 3 months:

- Straining at least 25% of the time
- Hard stools at least 25% of the time
- Incomplete evacuation at least 25% of the time
- Three or fewer bowel movements per week

These criteria are informed by epidemiological studies showing that 95%[6] to 99%[7] of a healthy population defecate at least three times per week.

From within palliative care, it has been suggested that the use of abdominal radiographs can improve the diagnosis of constipation over physician and nursing assessment alone.[8] This study has not yet been followed up to define the extent of radiology use that is therapeutically beneficial. The diagnosis of constipation in the palliative care studies mentioned so far is based on patients' self-report or inference from the need to use laxatives. Given the ethos of the specialty and its context of incurable, fatal disease, it is indeed appropriate that constipation should, as a non-life-threatening condition, be identified as a symptom rather than a disease.

There has been some work on how hospice patients identify themselves as constipated (N.P. Sykes, unpublished observation); the results are generally consistent with gastroenterological studies and indicate that difficulty in defecation and reduced stool frequency, in that order, are the most important determinants in the symptom complex. However, it is clear that significant numbers of patients would consider themselves constipated without satisfying the quantitative dimensions of the Rome criteria.

No physiological investigations of constipation appear to have been performed on this population apart from a single report of the investigation of transit time in hospice patients.[9] Considerably prolonged transit was shown in about half of the patients, all of whom were receiving a supposedly therapeutic dose of laxatives.

The etiology of constipation in palliative care has been little examined. Opioid analgesics are often blamed, but a prospective study of laxative and analgesic use found that, although opioids were the most readily identifiable causative factor, a considerable residual level of constipation remained in those who did not take this class of drug.[10] The origins of the remainder of the constipation can be deduced from gut physiology, that is, reduced food and fluid intake and reduced activity; but the relative contribution of each factor has not been defined. One study found an inverse correlation between performance status and constipation;[11] another, using a different activity scale and in a perhaps sicker population, did not (N.P. Sykes, unpublished observation).

The pattern of laxative use in a hospice has been described,[12] but a survey of nurses in different hospices revealed a wide variety of drugs used singly and in various combinations (N.P. Sykes, unpublished observation). There remains a lack of clarity regarding the relative efficacy of the available agents, which is not addressed by the trials performed in other areas of medicine.[13] This is partly because of the different populations included in the trials but also the varying conditions under which they were performed. In addition, many trials use dietary fiber or a bulking laxative as a comparator; a study of the use of dietary fiber supplementation in radiotherapy patients (a relevant population) showed that it was poorly tolerated in the amounts required to influence stool frequency,[14] while clinical experience indicates that the volume of water required for the safe administration of bulking agents is hard for many terminally ill patients to handle. The combinations of senna/lactulose and danthron/poloxamer have been compared in an open-label crossover trial,[15] and senna has been compared with lactulose[16] or an Ayurvedic formulation[17] in open, parallel group trials, all in palliative care units. Outcome measures differed between the trials, two of which claimed to find a difference in therapeutic efficacy and the other not.

Even if opioids do not account for the total of constipation in palliative care, they are its most distinctive component. An alternative approach to patient-based trials has been to mimic opioid-induced constipation in healthy volunteers, using loperamide. In this model, senna, lactulose, and a danthron/docusate combination were reported to have the same laxative effectiveness but to differ in the frequency of adverse effects and the medication burden required, the softener/stimulant combination being superior.[18]

An innovative line of treatment for the opioid component of constipation is the use of opioid antagonists given orally, by which route they have low systemic availability but retain the potential to act locally at gut opioid receptors without significantly affecting the central nervous system (CNS) receptors that mediate analgesia. Effectiveness has been shown in several clinical trials using naloxone.[19-22] However, a substantial minority of patients in several of these trials experienced symptoms of opioid withdrawal, and a large multicenter study of naloxone in constipation has recently been abandoned.

There is interest in quaternary and glucuronide derivatives of native opioid antagonists, which should have a reduced likelihood of crossing the blood–brain barrier and, hence, of causing systemic withdrawal. Methylnaltrexone has been shown to reverse opioid-induced constipation in volunteers and methadone addicts when given by mouth[23] and appears to pose a very low risk of reversing opioid analgesia.[24] The peripherally selective mu antagonist ADL8-2698 has shown minimal systemic absorption or CNS penetration when given orally. In volunteers who had been given morphine, ADL8-2698 enhanced gastrointestinal motility and increased stool weight, while in patients receiving postoperative opioid analgesia, it has reduced the duration of constipation.[25]

Goals of Clinical Research in Constipation

Short-term goals

There is evidence that patients (British ones, anyway) dislike enemas and suppositories but often end up receiving them in addition to subtherapeutic doses of oral laxatives. There is also evidence that laxatives are the most common cause of diarrhea in palliative care.[26] Other than by extrapolation from data obtained from different groups of patients, there is currently little basis on which to design a laxative regime in palliative care or evidence regarding strategies that might minimize or avoid laxative use. Rather than conduct multiple comparisons of individual drugs, it might be more time- and cost-effective to examine how to use different classes of drug, as identified by their mechanism of action.

In Britain, there is some clinical consensus that there are advantages of efficacy and reduced adverse effects in combining stimulating (gut muscle irritant) and softening (osmotic, surfactant, or lubricating) agents, and proprietary preparations exist that do this. However, the evidence for this is small, and the practice is clearly not accepted everywhere. Patients do not find all laxatives equally acceptable, and poor compliance will limit the clinical effectiveness of a preparation regardless of its intrinsic potency. Laxatives differ also significantly in cost. Hence, there remains the need to conduct comparisons of individual laxatives and to include measures of patient acceptability and expense among the outcomes.

How often should laxatives be given and how should the doses be titrated to relieve constipation without causing diarrhea? One study found that a dose-titration schedule significantly reduced the use of rectal agents;[15] can this be replicated? Rectal laxatives will remain necessary for some patients, yet little is known about their effectiveness save that microenemas and phosphate enemas are said to be of equal effectiveness,[27,28] while glycerine suppositories are less effective than bisacodyl suppositories.[29] This evidence, although of indifferent quality, might be enough; but patients receive enemas and suppositories in multiple combinations, with either a full rectum or an empty one (N.P. Sykes, unpublished observation). It is easy to ignore this chaotic state of affairs, but it gives rise to costs, both financial and in patient discomfort, and needs examination.

Stratagems for minimizing laxative use require attention. Are there acceptable ways of increasing the fiber content of terminally ill patients' diets to an extent that will aid bowel function? Do alternative approaches, such as abdominal massage or heat application, have any validity? Can the opioid-induced component of constipation be reduced by the use of opioids other than morphine? Opioids may vary in their constipating potency. There is now reasonable evidence that transdermal fentanyl is somewhat less constipating than morphine,[30] possibly because of the smaller doses that have to be given to achieve CNS penetration. Reduction in laxative use has also been reported after changing from morphine to methadone but, to date, only on a case history basis.[31]

Indeed, it is still unclear to what extent tolerance to the constipating effects of opioids occurs over time. Conventional clinical teaching is that significant tolerance does not develop and, experimentally, mu$_2$ receptor–mediated opioid actions, such as delaying intestinal transit, show less development of tolerance than mu$_1$-mediated analgesia does.[32] However, there are patients who have taken substantial doses of morphine over a period of months and maintain a normal bowel habit on little or no laxative. Have they become tolerant, or do they lie at one extreme of the dose–response relationship for morphine constipation?

There are drugs with laxative potential outside the usual armamentarium. The current trials of opioid antagonists must be brought to a conclusion as these drugs may relieve not only opioid analgesic–induced constipation but also, because of the involvement of endogenous opioids in the control of gut motility,[33] other elements of constipation.[34]

There are also drugs that show properties that make them potential alternatives to existing laxatives used in palliative care. Examples include the prostaglandin analogue misoprostol,[35] the motilin agonist macrolide antibiotic erythromycin (and potentially other non-antibacterial macrolides),[36] and colchicine, which inhibits microtubule formation but whose mode of stimulating intestinal transit is unclear.[37] In addition, polyethylene glycol solution is relatively well established in other areas of medicine[38] but has not been tested in a palliative care population. Of these, misoprostol might have inadequate potency and polyethylene glycol may impose an unacceptable volume burden; but all of these drugs are eligible for investigation of their laxative efficacy in palliative care patients (Table 4.1).

Long-term goals

Although constipation is such a prominent symptom in palliative care, we know little of its etiology. Opioid analgesics are often blamed, but 63% of patients not

Table 4.1. Goals of Clinical Research in Constipation

- Which laxative agents offer the best combination of efficacy, low incidence of adverse effects (colic, diarrhea, bloating), acceptability, and cost?
- Are there advantages in using laxative combinations? If so, what combinations?
- How should dose titration be performed to relieve constipation without causing diarrhea and to minimize the use of rectal laxatives?
- How should suppositories and enemas be used? Which preparations and in what combinations?
- Are there viable alternatives to laxatives, such as abdominal massage or heat application?
- Do alternative opioids to morphine really have a significantly lower constipating effect?
- Does opioid-induced constipation disappear with time?
- What is the therapeutic place of opioid antagonists?
- What is the therapeutic place of current drugs with potential laxative power, for example, macrolides, colchicine, and polyethylene glycol?

---

taking such drugs nevertheless need laxatives.[10] Therefore, a long-term aim would be to develop a greater understanding of the pattern of gastrointestinal dysfunction in patients with advanced disease and the mediating factors that underlie it. In one sample, 84% of palliative care patients reported that they had been rarely or never constipated prior to their illness although 53% of them now experienced constipation at least half the time (N.P. Sykes, unpublished observation). Thus, the vast majority who are constipated have had normal bowel function in their preillness lives, but the behavior of their intestinal tract has now changed.

In 17 hospice patients with cancer who were receiving laxatives, the mean whole-gut transit time was 124 hours (range 34–289),[9] in eight of whom it was longer than 96 hours, the outer limit of normality for a Western population.[39] However, the distribution of any transit delay between different bowel segments is not known nor is the source of constipation in those who have a normal transit time. It is understood that distension and gastric emptying stimulate colonic peristalsis, and hence, impaired appetite will tend to constipate. Reduced fluid intake will result in less fluid secretion into the gut lumen and a harder, smaller fecal mass that is difficult to expel. Generalized muscular weakness will impair the ability to strain at stool effectively. Autonomic neuropathy impairing gastrointestinal transit is associated with some cancers, particularly of the lung or pancreas,[40] and certain chemotherapies (particularly vincristine[41]). In population studies, depression is associated with constipation,[6] and low mood has been associated physiologically with colonic relaxation:[42] these findings may be relevant in the 25% or so of palliative care patients who show evidence of clinical depression.

The physiological role of tachykinins in modulating intestinal motility is now well established, in particular the contractile role of substance P (through acetylcholine release) and the relaxant activity of vasoactive intestinal peptide (via nitric oxide release). Individuals with idiopathic slow-transit constipation have reduced rectal mucosal levels of substance P,[43] while another neuropeptide, peptide YY, has shown raised levels in colonic samples from constipated patients;[44] in dogs it has been found to mediate the gut slowing observed in response to a fatty meal.[45] Scope exists here for comparative studies in palliative care patients in collaboration with other disciplines.

There is increasing interest in the possible role of cytokines in mediating not only cancer cachexia and anorexia but also other symptoms of advanced disease. A wide variety of cytokines are produced by intestinal endothelium[46] and have been implicated in several pathological processes affecting the gut, such as necrotizing enterocolitis, celiac disease, and inflammatory bowel disease. Interleukin-1β and tumor necrosis factorα are secretory mediators in the human colon,[47] and the former has been found to inhibit small intestinal acetylcholine release in rats via production of another cytokine, leukemia-inhibitory factor.[48] Therefore, there is potential for cytokines to be influential in mediating the underlying level of constipation observed in patients with advancing cancer or other debilitating, nonmalignant conditions. As cytokines begin to be investigated in a palliative care setting, their possible gastrointestinal actions must not be overlooked.

Methodologies

All research in palliative care is hampered by the frailty of the patient population. Their condition is unstable and deteriorating, rendering invasive or lengthy investigations intolerable and producing a high dropout rate from prospective studies. Multiple confounding variables are usually present, and the prevalence of mental impairment is high, reducing the reliability of outcome measures. In consequence, case note reviews are a tempting research method but limited in scope. There may be more to be learned in this way about laxative requirements in relation to opioid doses and about the pattern of use of rectal laxatives, but in practice the quality of outcome in terms of constipation relief is usually hard to judge and the patient perspective is frequently almost entirely absent. Urgently required are more prospective studies, with all of the difficulties these entail. An additional handicap is the relative isolation of some palliative care services from investigational facilities, such as radiology, and this factor will influence the type of studies that individual centers can perform (Table 4.2).

A prime methodological consideration is how to measure constipation and, hence, what end point is taken to indicate its relief.[49] Viewing constipation as a symptom, the most important assessment is that of the patient, who will define when he or she is constipated and when not. A discrete response modification of a visual analogue scale and an adjectival scale both showed concurrent validity in

Table 4.2. Constipation Research Methodologies in Palliative Care

- Questionnaires
- Patient diaries
- Constipation scales
- Case note reviews
- Transit time assessment
- Stool frequency, defecation-free interval
- Stool form
- Abdominal radiology
- Randomized controlled trials (not necessarily blinded)
- Functional assessments
- Depression/anxiety assessment scales

measuring constipation in hospice patients (N.P. Sykes, unpublished observation) and can be extended to assess the adverse effect of diarrhea.

Alternatively, the questionnaire-based Constipation Assessment Scale was validated through administration to patients receiving opioids and, thus, is directly relevant to palliative care.[50] This scale defines the components of the constipation experience that are prominent for the individual and can be completed within 2 minutes in cancer patients. Subsequently a five-item version of the original eight-item scale was validated but in a different population.[51] Neither version can show the impact of diarrhea nor can other questionnaire-based constipation assessments that have been validated more rigorously elsewhere but are longer.[52,53] These assessments can be administered either face to face or in diary format. Although simple to conduct and indicative of the impact of constipation on the patient, they do not provide objective indices of bowel function and are inadequate for drug-regulatory purposes.

Attempts to relate the severity of constipation to functional or emotional factors have used the Eastern Cooperative Oncology Group Performance Scale,[11] the Barthel Activities of Daily Living Scale, and the Hospital Anxiety and Depression Scale (N.P. Sykes, unpublished observation). All of these are open to objections of being insufficiently discriminatory for this purpose or of not having been validated in this population. These are areas of assessment that have wider relevance within palliative care and require the development of useful and properly validated measurement tools.

In addition to assessing the patient's view of constipation, laxative studies should gather information about adverse effects (in particular, nausea and vomiting, diarrhea, bloating, and colic), the acceptability of the preparations (taste and texture of liquids or size and shape of pills or capsules), compliance in home-based studies, the costs both of the doses found to be required and of any additional professional interventions needed (such as home nurse visits to administer suppositories or visits to hospital emergency rooms because of constipation). To date, such data have been collected variably.

An objective indicator of the presence of constipation is a plain abdominal radiograph. A scoring system to describe the amount of stool present was described and tested by Bruera et al.[8] in a palliative care study. Similar systems of more[54] or less[55] complexity have been described elsewhere and are claimed to show high interobserver reliability and good correlation with stool frequency. Radiographs are, of course, a static measure of current fecal loading and give no information about the speed of transit or about performance of different colonic segments. In a large pediatric study, Barr scores[54] showed poor correlation with transit time and too great a variability to be reliable in diagnosing chronically constipated subjects.[56] However, scoring of pre- and postintervention radiographs could aid the objectivity of assessment in badly needed trials of the efficacy of suppositories and enemas in palliative care.

A commonly used index of bowel function is stool frequency, which, for the sake of reliability, should be assessed prospectively either by ward observation or by patient diary and not by recall at clinic appointments.[57] Consistent stool frequencies of three or less per week are accepted to indicate constipation.[5] A variant that has been used in a palliative care setting is the number of defecation-free 72-hour intervals. This is based on a clinical perception of the longest time reasonable for a patient to be allowed to remain without a bowel action and constitutes a measure of the "failure rate" of the laxative.[16]

However, a constipated person may still have a normal stool frequency by virtue of passing relatively frequent small stools. Frequency tells nothing about intestinal activity, which is revealed by measures of stool consistency and bowel transit time. Stool consistency can be measured directly,[58] which is clinically impractical, or by formal grading of the stool appearance,[59] which correlates well with transit time in terminally ill patients[9] and in those with irritable bowel syndrome, who are able to judge the form score reliably themselves.[60] Stool consistency may thus be useful as a proxy measure of colonic peristaltic function for studies performed in situations where there is no access to the radiographic facilities required for direct estimation of transit.

In our population, transit time has been measured directly using radiopaque markers.[9] For logistical reasons, this study collected and radiographed the stools, but it is more pleasant and reliable to take an abdominal radiograph if facilities permit. This could also allow the estimation of segmental transit time, to reveal whether there is any differential slowing of peristalsis in the four colonic regions, an investigation that has never been performed in opioid-induced constipation. Because of the time taken to reach steady state in very constipated patients, repeated X-rays may be needed, posing ethical or practical problems.[61] Segmental and overall transit times can also be measured by scintigraphy,[62] which minimizes the oral marker burden for the patient but involves equipment and facilities that are unlikely to be readily available for most palliative care services.

The desirable characteristics of the randomized controlled trial, which must be the basic design of laxative comparisons, are well known; but the widely differing physical characteristics of available preparations often make blinding or the provision of a placebo impossible. In the minds of many in palliative care, an emphasis on patient comfort also poses ethical difficulties over the use of placebo or treatment-withholding arms. There is also the related question over the point at which "rescue" laxation should be allowed and what form this should take. Because of the latency of action of oral laxatives, a trial must last at least a week and preferably longer; but as trials progress, the dropout rate can be considerable (56% in one 2-week trial[15] and 58% in a 5-week trial[16]). Both parallel group and crossover designs have been used; the latter limits the sample size required and avoids accidental differences between trial groups but requires statistical allowance for order effects.[63]

An approach to overcoming the confounding variables of deteriorating patient condition (resulting in fluid and dietary changes as well as loss of numbers to the study) and medication alterations for evolving symptoms has been the use of loperamide to mimic opioid-induced constipation in healthy volunteers.[18]

Although it is tempting to suppose that in the presence of similar dietary and bowel histories among the participants such studies should produce standardized levels of constipation against which laxative potency and efficacy could be judged, the highly variable individual responses to either the analgesic or constipating effects of opioids make this unlikely in practice. However, the effects of any one dose of loperamide should be constant in an individual, so trials involving random sequencing of laxatives, with appropriate washout periods, against a set loperamide dose should yield one of the best indications of relative potency we are likely to get. Thus far, the model has not been used in this way.

Improvement in knowledge of the physiology of constipation in palliative care requires collaborative work with other disciplines but involves increasing degrees of invasiveness. Analysis of segmental contributions to colonic transit delay has been mentioned. The technique of rectal manometry[61] could clarify the extent to which morphine reduces rectal sensation, making fecal impaction more likely to occur, in a patient group whose sensation may often already be reduced by advanced age. Colonic biopsies might be assayed for tachykinin and cytokine levels for comparison with normal subjects and those with other forms of constipation.

Conclusion

Research into constipation is rarely easy and never glamorous, but it is important to tackle a persistent symptom that causes very many of our patients considerable distress.

References

1. Twycross RG, Lack SA. Constipation. In: Twycross RG, Lack SA, eds. Control of Alimentary Symptoms in Far Advanced Cancer. Edinburgh: Churchill Livingstone, 1986:166–207.
2. Schoorl J, Zylicz Z. Laxantiabeleid bij terminale patienten ondelmatig. Ned Tijdschr Geneeskd 1997; 141:823–826.
3. Holmes S. Use of a modified symptom distress scale in assessment of the cancer patient. Int J Nurs Stud 1989; 26:69–79.
4. Dunlop GM. A study of the relative frequency and importance of gastrointestinal symptoms and weakness in patients with far advanced cancer: student paper. Palliat Med 1989; 4:37–44.
5. Thompson WG, Longstreth GF, Drossman DA, et al. Functional bowel disorders and functional abdominal pain. Gut 1999; 45:1143–1147.
6. Drossman DA, Sandler RS, McKee DC, et al. Bowel patterns among subjects not seeking health care. Gastroenterology 1982; 83:529–534.
7. Connell AM, Hilton C, Irvine G, et al. Variation in bowel habit in two population samples. BMJ 1965; ii:1095–1099.

8. Bruera E, Suarez-Almazor M, Velasco A, et al. The assessment of constipation in terminal cancer patients admitted to a palliative care unit. J Pain Symptom Manage 1994; 9:515–519.

9. Sykes NP. Methods of assessment of bowel function in patients with advanced cancer. Palliat Med 1990; 4:287–292.

10. Sykes NP. The relationship between opioid use and laxative use in terminally ill cancer patients. Palliat Med 1998; 12:375–382.

11. Fallon M, Hanks G. Morphine, constipation and performance status in advanced cancer patients. Palliat Med 1999; 13:159–160.

12. Twycross RG, Harcourt JM. The use of laxatives at a palliative care centre. Palliat Med 1991; 5:27–33.

13. NHS Centre for Reviews and Dissemination. Effectiveness of laxatives in adults. Eff Health Care 2001; 7:1–12.

14. Mumford SP. Can high fiber diets improve the bowel function in patients on a radiotherapy ward? In: Twycross RG, Lack SA, eds. Control of Alimentary Symptoms in Far Advanced Cancer. Edinburgh: Churchill Livingstone, 1986:183–184.

15. Sykes NP. Clinical comparison of laxatives in a hospice. Palliat Med 1991; 5:307–314.

16. Agra Y, Sacristan A, Gonzalez M, et al. Efficacy of senna versus lactulose in terminal cancer patients treated with opioids. J Pain Symptom Manage 1998; 15:1–7.

17. Ramesh PR, Suresh Kumar K, Rajagopal MR, et al. Managing morphine-induced constipation: a controlled comparison of an Ayurvedic formulation and senna. J Pain Symptom Manage 1998; 16:240–244.

18. Sykes NP. A volunteer model for the comparison of laxatives in opioid-induced constipation. J Pain Symptom Manage 1997; 11:363–369.

19. Sykes NP. Oral naloxone in opioid associated constipation. Lancet 1991; 337:1475.

20. Culpepper-Morgan JA, Inturrisi CE, Portenoy RK, et al. Treatment of opioid-induced constipation with oral naloxone: a pilot study. Clin Pharmacol Ther 1992; 52:90–95.

21. Sykes NP. An investigation of the ability of oral naloxone to correct opioid-related constipation in patients with advanced cancer. Palliat Med 1996; 10:135–144.

22. Latasch L, Zimmermann M, Eberhardt B, et al. Aufhebung einer Morphin-induzierten Obstipation durch orales Naloxon. Anaesthesist 1997; 46:191–194.

23. Yuan CS, Foss JF. Oral methylnaltrexone for opioid-induced constipation. JAMA 2000; 284:1383–1384.

24. Yuan CS, Foss JF, O'Connor M, et al. Methylnaltrexone prevents morphine-induced delay in oral-cecal transit time without affecting analgesia: a double-blind randomized placebo-controlled trial. Clin Pharmacol Ther 1996; 59:469–475.

25. Taguchi A, Sharma N, Saleem RM, et al. Selective postoperative inhibition of gastrointestinal opioid receptors. N Engl J Med 2001; 345:935–940.

26. Twycross RG, Lack SA. Diarrhea. In: Twycross RG, Lack SA, eds. Control of Alimentary Symptoms in Far Advanced Cancer. Edinburgh: Churchill Livingstone, 1986:208–229.

27. Gass OC. Clinical evaluation of Index single use enema and phosphate enema. In: Proceedings of a Symposium on the Clinical Evaluation of a New Disposable Microenema, New Brunswick, NJ. Atlantic City: Chalfonte-Haddon Hall, 1963:6.

28. Postlethwait RW. Microenema as evacuant before proctoscopy. Curr Ther Res 1965; 7:7–9.

29. Sweeney WJ. The use of disposable microenema in obstetrical patients. In: Proceedings of a Symposium on the Clinical Evaluation of a New Disposable Microenema, New Brunswick, NJ. Atlantic City: Chalfonte-Haddon Hall, 1963:7–8.

30. Radbruch L, Sabatowski R, Loick G, et al. Constipation and the use of laxatives: a comparison between transdermal fentanyl and oral morphine. Palliat Med 2000; 14:111–119.

31. Daeninck PJ, Bruera E. Reduction in constipation and laxative requirements following opioid rotation to methadone. J Pain Symptom Manage 1999; 18:303–309.

32. Ling GS, Paul D, Simontov R, et al. Differential development of acute tolerance. Life Sci 1989; 45:1627–1636.

33. Puig MA, Gascon P, Craviso GL, et al. Endogenous opiate receptor ligand: electrically induced release in the guinea pig ileum. Science 1977; 195:419–420.

34. Kreek MJ, Paris P, Bartol MA, et al. Effects of short term oral administration of the specific opioid antagonist naloxone on fecal evacuation in geriatric patients. Gastroenterology 1984; 86:1184.

35. Roarty TP, Weber F, Soykan I, et al. Misoprostol in the treatment of chronic refractory constipation: results of a long-term open label trial. Aliment Pharmacol Ther 1997; 11:1059–1066.

36. Hasler W, Heldsinger A, Soudah H, et al. Erythromycin promotes colonic transit in humans; mediation via motilin receptor. Gastroenterology 1990;98:A358.

37. Verne GN, Eaker EY, Davis RH, et al. Colchicine is an effective treatment for patients with chronic constipation. Dig Dis Sci 1997; 42:1959–1963.

38. Freedman MD, Schwartz HJ, Roby R, et al. Tolerance and efficacy of polyethylene glycol 3350/electrolyte solution versus lactulose in relieving opiate induced constipation: a double-blinded placebo-controlled trial. J Clin Pharmacol 1997; 37: 904–907.

39. Read NW, Timms JM. Defaecation and the pathophysiology of constipation. Clin Gastroenterol 1986; 15:937–965.

40. Sodhi N, Camilleri M, Camoriano JK, et al. Autonomic function and motility in intestinal pseudoobstruction caused by paraneoplastic syndrome. Dig Dis Sci 1989; 34:1937–1942.

41. Chabner BA, Allegra CJ, Curt GA, et al. Antineoplastic agents. In: Hardman JG, Limbird LE, eds. The Pharmacological Basis of Therapeutics, 9th ed. New York: McGraw-Hill, 1996:1233–1288.

42. Snape WJ. Physiology of colonic motility: methods of evaluation. In: Fisher RS, Krevsky B, eds. Motor Disorders of the Gastrointestinal Tract. New York: Academic Press, 1993:103–107.

43. Tzavella K, Riepl RL, Klauser AG, et al. Decreased substance P levels in rectal biopsies from patients with slow transit constipation. Eur J Gastroenterol Hepatol 1996; 8:1207–1211.

44. Sjolund K, Fasth S, Ekman R, et al. Neuropeptides in idiopathic chronic constipation (slow transit constipation). Neurogastroenterol Motil 1997; 9:143–150.

45. Lin HC, Zhao X-T, Wang L, et al. Fat-induced ileal brake in the dog depends on peptide YY. Gastroenterology 1996; 110:1491–1495.

46. Nilsen EM, Johansen FE, Jahnsen FL, et al. Cytokine profiles of cultured microvascular endothelial cells from the human intestine. Gut 1998; 42:635–642.

47. Bode H, Schmitz H, Fromm M, et al. IL-1beta and TNF-alpha, but not IFN-alpha, IFN-gamma, IL-6 or IL-8, are secretory mediators in human distal colon. Cytokine 1998; 10:457–465.

48. Van Assche G, Collins SM. Leukemia inhibitory factor mediates cytokine-induced suppression of myenteric neurotransmitter release from rat intestine. Gastroenterology 1996; 111:674–681.

49. Sykes NP. Methods for clinical research in constipation. In: Max M, Lynn J, eds. Symptom Research: Methods and Opportunities. An Interactive Textbook. Bethesda, MD: National Institutes of Dental and Craniofacial Research. www.symptomresearch.com/chapter_3/index.htm, 2001.

50. McMillan SC, Williams FA. Validity and reliability of the Constipation Assessment Scale. Cancer Nurs 1989; 12:183–188.

51. Broussard BS. The Constipation Assessment Scale for pregnancy. J Gynecol Neonat Nurs 1998; 27:297–301.

52. Osterburg A, Graf W, Karlbom U, et al. Evaluation of a questionnaire in the assessment of patients with faecal incontinence and constipation. Scand J Gastroenterol 1996; 31:575–580.

53. Agachan F, Chen T, Pfeifer J, et al. A constipation scoring system to simplify evaluation and management of constipated patients. Dis Colon Rectum, 1996; 39: 681–685.

54. Barr RG, Levine MD, Wilkinson RH, et al. Occult stool retention: a clinical tool for its evaluation in school aged children. Clin Pediatr (Phila) 1979; 18:674–679.

55. Blethyn AJ, Verrier Jones K, Newcombe R, et al. Radiological assessment of constipation. Arch Dis Child 1995; 73:532–533.

56. Benninga MA, Buller HA, Staalman CR, et al. Defecation disorders in children, colonic transit time versus the Barr score. Eur J Pediatr 1995; 154:277–284.

57. Manning AP, Wyman JB, Heaton KW. How trustworthy are bowel histories? Comparison of recalled and recorded information. BMJ 1976; 2:213–214.

58. Exton-Smith AN, Bendall MJ, Kent F. A new technique for measuring the consistency of faeces. Age Ageing 1975; 4:58–62.

59. Davies GJ, Crowder M, Reid B, et al. Bowel function measurements of individuals with different eating patterns. Gut 1986; 27:164–169.

60. O'Donnell LJ, Virjee J, Heaton KW. Detection of pseudodiarrhoea by simple clinical assessment of intestinal transit rate. BMJ 1990; 300:439–440.

61. Mollen RM, Claassen AT, Kuijpers JH. The evaluation and treatment of functional constipation. Scand J Gastroenterol 1997; 32(Suppl223):8–17.

62. Notghi A, Hutchinson R, Kumar D, et al. Simplified method for the measurement of segmental colonic transit time. Gut 1994; 35:976–981.

63. Hills M, Armitage P. The two-period cross-over clinical trial. Br J Clin Pharmacol 1979; 8:7–20.

5

Clinical Trials of Antiemetics in the Palliative Care Setting: Research Issues

ALICE INMAN AND STEVEN D. PASSIK

Considering the effect nausea and vomiting have on the quality of life of terminally ill patients, it is surprising that little research attention has been given these symptoms outside of that related to chemotherapy. Nausea and vomiting are reported to occur in up to 62% of terminally ill patients, with 40% experiencing these symptoms in the last 6 weeks of life.[1] Most of these studies suggest a higher incidence in the female population. Since the pathophysiology and mechanism involved in chemotherapy-induced nausea and vomiting differ from those in advanced disease, research dealing with the former may not be applicable to the latter. The majority of studies looking at nausea and vomiting in advanced disease have been case studies.

Etiology of Emesis

There are four general physiological mechanisms involved in nausea and vomiting: visceral or gastrointestinal tract disorders, chemical triggers, central nervous system (CNS) disturbances, and vestibular disturbances.[2] Treatment should be directed at the cause of the emesis; therefore, successful treatment of the nausea and/or vomiting depends on identifying the underlying mechanism. Once the mechanism is identified, drug therapy may be selected based on the pharmacological properties of the drug. Nausea in advanced illness, such as cancer, is likely to involve multiple mechanisms, generally requiring a combination of multiple drugs and other interventions.[3]

Nausea may be caused by disorders that directly affect the gastrointestinal tract, such as distension, stasis, or obstruction of gastric, bowel, biliary, or genitourinary tracts; constipation; cancer of the stomach, pancreas, and liver; peritoneal metastases; gastric irritation from drugs or blood; and external pressure.[2,4,5] Dopamine (D_2) and serotonin (or 5-hydroxytryptamine$_3$, 5-HT$_3$) receptors in the gut signal the vomiting center via vagal and sympathetic afferents. Therefore, drugs of choice in nausea mediated by this mechanism include dopamine antagonists (prokinetic agents) and serotonergic antagonists.[1,5]

Chemical causes of nausea and vomiting include medications (opioids, digitalis, estrogens, aspirin, and alcohol), metabolic abnormalities (hypercalcemia, uremia, hyponatremia), and toxins (abnormal cancer metabolites, infection, radiation, peptides from cancer).[1] These chemicals stimulate the chemoreceptor trigger zone (CTZ) via D_2 and 5-HT_3 receptors.[6] Treatment would target the source of the problem, which might be as simple as discontinuing or changing a medication or more complex, as in targeting the receptors involved using D_2 (neuroleptic and prokinetic agents) and 5-HT_3 antagonists.[1]

Factors within the CNS that may cause nausea and vomiting include primary or metastatic brain tumors, meningitis (carcinomatous, infectious, or chemical), and elevated intracranial pressure. These factors directly stimulate the vomiting center (VC) by inflammation with increased prostaglandin synthesis or increased intracranial pressure.[6] Receptors involved include histamine (H_1), muscarinic cholinergic, and 5-HT_3. Depending on the factor involved, anti-inflammatory agents, anxiolytics, corticosteriods, or antihistamines may be indicated.[5,6] Psychological and emotional factors (such as pain, fear, and anxiety) also play an important role.

Vestibular disturbances due to medications (aspirin, opioids), local tumors (acoustic neuroma, primary or secondary brain tumors), labyrinthitis, motion sickness, or Meniere's disease may also cause nausea and vomiting. These problems may activate the VC through the vestibular apparatus.[5] Some medications, such as aspirin and opioids, directly stimulate the vestibular area that provides input to the VC. Receptors involved in this process include those in the vestibular nuclei, such as 5-HT_3, H_1, and muscarinic cholinergic.[1] This has led to the use of antihistamines and belladonna alkaloids to alleviate nausea and vomiting arising from this source.[5]

Management of nausea and vomiting should be based on an assessment of probable cause, with drugs selected based on their pharmacological properties. The classes of drugs frequently used to treat nausea and vomiting include the D_2 antagonists and prokinetic agents, H_1/muscarinic (cholinergic, parasympathetic) receptor blockers, 5-HT_3 antagonists, corticosteroids, cannabinoids, antianxiety agents, and somatostatin analogues. Most of the research available on these drugs pertains to treatment of nausea and vomiting associated with chemotherapy, with little attention paid to controlled trials in the palliative care setting.

Antiemetics

Dopamine antagonists

Dopamine antagonists include neuroleptic agents and prokinetic drugs. The neuroleptic agents include the butyrophenones, which block dopamine receptors at the CTZ, and phenothiazines, which block both dopamine and serotonin receptors at the CTZ and act at the VC and the vestibular center.[7] These medications can cause extrapyramidal symptoms; the phenothiazines can also cause hypotension.[4]

Prokinetic agents, such as metoclopramide and domperidone, block dopamine receptors in the CTZ at regular dosages and, in high doses, increase peristalsis in the upper gut by blocking 5-HT_4 receptors.[1,6] Their action on the 5-HT_4 receptors stimulates the myenteric plexus to release acetylcholine. The cholinergic effects that result from this release increase the tone of the lower esophageal sphincter, promote gastric emptying, and increase motility of the gastrointestinal tract.[4,6,8] Adverse effects include mild sedation, dystonic reactions (particularly in patients under 30 years of age), akathisia, tardive dyskinesias, and diarrhea.[4]

Histamine₁/muscarinic receptor blockers

The antihistamines that provide the most control of nausea and vomiting (diphenhydramine, hydroxyzine) possess significant antimuscarinic and sedative effects.[9] The H_1 (cyclizine and meclizine) and muscarinic (belladonna alkaloids, such as hyoscine and scopolamine) antagonists act on their corresponding receptors in the VC and the vestibular center.[6] Common side effects of the antihistamines include dry mouth, drowsiness, and constipation.[10] Anticholinergic crisis can occur and is more common in elderly patients or patients receiving other medications with anticholinergic properties.[4]

Serotonin receptor antagonists

The serotonin receptor antagonists (ondansetron, granisetron, and dolasetron) block 5-HT_3 receptors in the gastrointestinal tract, the CTZ, and the nucleus tractus solitarius.[6] These drugs have proven to be highly effective in acute chemotherapy-induced nausea and vomiting but are not effective at preventing delayed emesis induced by anticancer drugs, such as doxorubicin (Adriamycin), cyclophosphamide (Cytoxan), cisplatin, and CPT-11 (irinotecan); by motion sickness; or by dopamine receptor agonists.[6] Their use for intractable vomiting associated with terminal illness is based only on clinical experience, not empirical research.[1] Their efficacy is estimated in the 15% range, which is problematic given their expense.

Corticosteroids

The mechanism of the antiemetic activity of corticosteroids is unclear but may involve inhibition of the synthesis of prostaglandins, cellular permeability changes, and/or reduction of edema associated with gastrointestinal or cerebral tumors.[10] Reduction of cerebral edema may decrease the intracranial pressure responsible for nausea and vomiting in some patients. Reduction of edema associated with gastrointestinal tract tumors may relieve obstruction. These agents are seldom used alone to control nausea and vomiting and are more commonly administered in conjunction with other antiemetics. Although few adverse effects are associated with short courses of corticosteroids, insomnia, mood changes, agitation, psychotic behavior, edema, peptic ulceration, and hyperglycemia may occur.[10]

Cannabinoids

The exact mechanism by which cannabinoids control nausea and vomiting is unknown but appears to involve receptors in the CTZ.[4,9] Dronabinol is the only legally available cannabinoid in the United States; nabilone is available and used in other countries.[1] Adverse effects are common but generally manageable and include sedation, dry mouth, orthostatic hypotension, ataxia, mood changes, anxiety, and cognitive and memory impairment.

Antianxiety agents

Benzodiazepines may have some antiemetic properties but are used predominantly as adjuncts to other antiemetics because of their anxiolytic, amnestic, and sedative properties.[10] They have received considerable attention in relation to their use in patients receiving chemotherapy, especially if anticipatory nausea and vomiting are problems. Side effects include drowsiness and lethargy.

Somatostatin analogues

Octreotide is a long-acting peptide that inhibits the release and activity of gastrointestinal hormones.[11,12] Secretion of growth hormone, gastrin, secretin, vasoactive intestinal peptides, pancreatic polypeptides, insulin, and glucagon is inhibited; and secretion of gastric acid, pepsin, pancreatic enzyme, bicarbonate, intestinal epithelial electrolytes, and water is blocked.[13,14] The result of these actions is modulation of gastrointestinal function, with reduced secretions, slowed motility, diminished bile flow, increased production of mucus, and reduced splanchnic blood flow.[11,13,15] Although it has a more powerful effect than somatostatin, it has less influence on insulin secretion. When surgery is not an option for bowel obstruction, octreotide has been highly effective at controlling vomiting by decreasing intestinal secretions.[1]

Atypical antipsychotics

Clinical experience and results of recent studies and a case report[16] suggest that there may be a role for atypical antipsychotics, such as olanzapine in the treatment of a wide variety of cancer-related nausea and vomiting cases. Passik et al.[17]

reported benefits of olanzapine for advanced cancer patients with opioid-induced nausea. These agents act at multiple dopaminergic, serotonergic, muscarinic, and histaminic sites and may be particularly efficacious against nausea arising from multiple etiologies. Olanzapine has shown tolerability and efficacy in the treatment of delayed emesis induced by chemotherapy.[18] This agent offers the additional advantages of appetite stimulation and low rates of extrapyramidal symptoms.

Review of Antiemetic Research in Terminally Ill Patients

Research on antiemetics in patients with advanced disease has followed the pattern of treatment for emesis at other stages but predominantly comprises retrospective case studies. The scant research available on antiemetics in advanced illness has targeted visceral/gastrointestinal and chemical origins of nausea and vomiting, with less attention to vestibular or CNS origins. Medications that have received research attention as antiemetics in terminal illness include the dopamine antagonists, serotonin receptor antagonists, and somatostatin analogues.

Dopamine antagonists

Baines et al.[19] found that phenothiazines and butyrophenones are most effective at treating vomiting due to intestinal obstruction in a study of 40 patients with far-advanced abdominal and/or pelvic malignant disease. However, only five of the 40 treated patients ceased vomiting. Twenty-nine patients reported no more than one episode of vomiting per day and little or no nausea. Four patients reported moderate to severe vomiting, even with treatment.

Bruera et al.[20] reviewed the incidence and intensity of nausea and vomiting in 100 advanced-cancer patients being treated according to a metoclopramide-based therapeutic ladder. Patients were assessed using a visual analogue scale twice a day for various symptoms, including nausea and vomiting. If nausea or vomiting was present, the patient was started on metoclopramide 10 mg every 4 hours orally or subcutaneously (sc). If symptoms were not controlled, the metoclopramide was augmented with dexamethasone 10 mg twice daily. If symptoms continued, continuous sc infusion of metoclopramide 60–120 mg daily was given along with the dexamethasone. Finally, if response was still poor, other antiemetics were administered. Twenty-five percent required other antiemetics due to bowel obstruction ($n = 18$), extrapyramidal symptoms ($n = 3$), allergy ($n = 1$), renal failure ($n = 1$), or unknown causes ($n = 2$). In the absence of bowel obstruction, good control of nausea and vomiting was provided by metoclopramide and/or metoclopramide plus dexamethasone. Four percent developed adverse reactions consisting of akathisia ($n = 3$) and rash ($n = 1$).

Serotonin receptor antagonists

Marsden[21] presented three cases in which dramatic results were seen in patients started on ondansetron. The first patient (renal cell carcinoma metastatic to bone and liver) ceased vomiting within 4–5 days and the other two (carcinoma of rectum metastatic to bone and liver and pancreatic carcinoma), within 24 hours. Vomiting recurred in patient 2 when she developed a bowel obstruction. The obstruction was treated with conservative measures (increased steroids and enemas). After resolution, the vomiting was again controlled with ondansetron. Previous treatment with domperidone, cyclizine, stemetil, and dexamethasone failed to control the vomiting in patient 3; vomiting ceased within 24 hours of starting ondansetron 8 mg three times a day. Nausea and vomiting remained well controlled in patients 1 and 2 until death and in patient 3 until within 48 hours of death. All three patients had been unsuccessfully treated previously with a wide range of antiemetics. Patient 2 remained on steroids during her treatment with ondansetron. Since the report did not indicate the dose of ondansetron for patients 1 and 2, it is not possible to ascertain whether the difference in timing of cessation of vomiting in patient 1 was due to the quantity of medication given or the disease process. Use of ondansetron allowed two of the patients to remain comfortably at home.

Cole and colleagues[22] presented a case in which therapeutic doses of haloperidol (1.5 mg at bedtime) and ondansetron (8 mg three times a day) provided relief of intractable nausea and vomiting in a woman with advanced cancer and decreased liver function receiving morphine. Neither agent alone controlled the vomiting, but in combination complete control was maintained until the last 2 weeks of life, when she experienced occasional vomiting.

Andrews et al.[23] presented two cases in which ondansetron, a 5-HT$_3$ antagonist, provided relief of vomiting within 24 hours in renal failure. In the first case, a 76-year-old woman with polycystic kidney disease developed uncontrolled nausea and vomiting. Within 24 hours of starting on oral ondansetron 8 mg twice daily, the vomiting ceased. The vomiting recommenced within 24 hours of stopping the ondansetron, and reinstatement of the medication again led to improvement. The second case was a 76-year-old man with symptomatic uremia. He was unresponsive to intravenous metoclopramide but obtained complete relief of vomiting within 24 hours of starting on oral ondansetron 8 mg twice daily. No adverse effects were observed in either case. Since both unchanged drug and liver metabolites of ondansetron are excreted in the urine, caution should be exercised in using it in patients with renal dysfunction.

Currow and colleagues[24] reported a retrospective study of 16 patients treated for nausea and vomiting associated with either advanced human immunodeficiency virus/acquired immunodeficiency syndrome (HIV/AIDS) or malignancy. These patients were nonresponsive to standard antiemetics. Two investigators independently reviewed the response of patients to ondansetron 48 hours after starting treatment. Eighty-one percent (13/16) of patients benefited from treatment with ondansetron. Response was rapid, sustained, and well tolerated. The authors suggested that ondansetron should not be reserved for third- or fourth-line therapy but started at earlier stages. Cost was justified by increased quality of life and the opportunity to be treated at home.

Porcel and Schoenenberger[25] studied 10 terminal cancer patients with persistent nausea and vomiting not associated with chemotherapy or radiotherapy. All 10 patients had been unsuccessfully treated with a combination of metoclopramide 20 mg every 6 hours sc and haloperidol 25 mg every 8 hours sc. Four patients also received dexamethazone (8 mg daily sc in three patients and 4 mg every 6 hours sc in one patient). Each patient had a different type of advanced cancer, six had liver metastases, and one had brain metastasis. After stopping all other antiemetics, patients were started on a 5-HT_3 receptor antagonist (either ondansetron 4 mg every 8 hours sc or granisetron 3 mg per day sc). Within a few hours of starting the medication, vomiting ceased in seven patients, was partially controlled in two patients (unresectable esophageal carcinoma and metastatic renal carcinoma diagnoses), and remained unchanged in one patient (bowel obstruction). The authors concluded that 5-HT_3 receptor antagonists are effective at controlling nausea and vomiting in terminal cancer patients unless bowel obstruction is present.

Somatostatin analogues

Khoo et al.[26] first reported using octreotide in terminally ill patients with intestinal obstruction who were nonsurgical candidates. All five patients experienced vomiting that was unresponsive to conventional therapy, including prochlorperazine, metoclopramide, cyclizine, and dexamethasone. Vomiting ceased within 1 hour of starting octreotide, and symptom relief continued until death in three patients. Various regimens were used, generally starting with sc injection and proceeding to continuous infusion. Medication was stopped in two patients due to lack of supplies. In those two patients with interrupted treatment, vomiting recurred within 12 hours after stopping the octreotide. Vomiting ceased again once treatment was reinstated. There were no important adverse reactions.

Mercadante et al.[15] obtained good control of vomiting in 12 of 14 advanced-cancer patients with intestinal obstruction with sc bolus or continuous infusion of octreotide. Octreotide was generally initiated after conventional drugs, such as haloperidol, chlorpromazine, and ranitidine, failed to control the vomiting. Dosage ranged from 0.3 mg to 0.6 mg per day. Half of the patients reported painful injection. No other adverse reactions were noted.

Khoo et al.[27] found that continuous sc infusion of octreotide controlled or markedly reduced the amount of vomiting or nasogastric aspirate in 18 of 24 patients with malignant intestinal obstruction. Fourteen patients achieved complete control of vomiting, two still experienced some nausea, and two others had transient vomiting. Vomiting was generally controlled within 2–4 hours of achieving the correct dose and maintained until death in 16 patients. Dosage varied from 150 μg to 700 μg per day in responders. Six patients did not respond. No adverse effects were noted.

Mangili et al.[14] studied 13 patients with terminal ovarian cancer and found that octreotide controlled vomiting in all cases. Symptom relief was achieved within 3 days, with no reported adverse effects. Although this medication is expensive, treatment allowed the patients to be followed at home, thereby eliminating hospital costs.

Cannabinoids

Green et al.[28] presented a 52-year-old with AIDS and intractable nausea and vomiting who was treated with nabilone. Despite treatment with prochloperazine, cyclizine, domperidone, and high-dose intravenous infusions of metoclopramide, he continued to vomit until started on oral nabilone 1 mg twice daily. Complete control of the vomiting was maintained until death 4 days later.

Flynn and Hanif[29] presented a 38-year-old man with AIDS and refractory nausea and vomiting treated with nabilone. Treatment with scopolamine disk and dimehydrinate proved ineffective, and he was started on nabilone 2 mg orally twice per day. Nausea and vomiting were rapidly controlled, and after 7 days, the dose was reduced to 1 mg orally twice daily. He maintained good control of the nausea and vomiting until death 12 days later.

Methodological Issues

Self-report

Most of the studies of antiemetics in terminally ill patients to date have involved retrospective narratives. There is substantial individual variation in the presentation of emesis in terminally ill patients. There are usually a number of factors that may influence one or more of the mechanisms known to cause nausea and vomiting. These factors result from different and sometimes multiple disease processes, progression of disease, polypharmacy, and personality factors. The interaction of all of these variables makes researching specific etiologies difficult and generalization of results tenuous.

A few of the studies used self-report, which is appropriate for the measurement of a subjective symptom; nevertheless, self-report in advanced illness may be compromised by methodological limitations. Measures may not be completed in a timely manner, and the delay between the event and the time of the report may color the patient's perception of the event. The tendency of a patient to exaggerate or minimize symptoms may affect the reporting of an event. The cognitive status of the patient may be impaired, from either advanced disease or medication, and he or she may not accurately remember events. The patient may enlist the help of family members in completing the measure, thereby compounding the problem with the perceptions of the "helper(s)."

Eliciting self-report in patients with advanced disease may also be subject to bias. Differences in interviewing styles, rapport, gender of patient and/or interviewer, type of questions asked, and timing of questions may also affect results. With small case studies, there is apt to be little or no training of the interviewers, creating the potential for discrepancy in responses. If adequate training and/or written protocol is not provided, even responses to structured interviews may vary considerably. The amount of time allotted to each question and the encouragement, verbal or nonverbal, given patients to completely respond to questions may differ. Rapport often determines the amount of information a patient will give to an interviewer. There is also the possibility of the patient wanting to present a certain image to a particular interviewer and coloring responses accordingly, that is, trying to please the researcher who is also the treating physician. The wording of questions may affect the quality and quantity of information elicited. Asking a patient if he or she was bothered by nausea may elicit a very different response from asking how many times he or she felt the need to vomit. If inquiries are made immediately after eating, exposure to nauseous odors, or the wearing off of medication, the responses may be biased.

Gender-based differences related to language or prior symptom-related experience may play a role in both reporting and interpreting the severity of symptoms. In a prospective study of 100 patients (55 male and 45 female) with advanced cancer, Curtis et al.[30] found that women reported more frequent and severe gastrointestinal problems than men.

Co-morbidities

Nausea and vomiting are particularly difficult to study in isolation as they are often accompanied by multiple related symptoms. Of the six most common symptoms reported by patients admitted to St. Christopher's Hospice, five (weakness, anorexia, pain, constipation, and cough) were related to nausea/vomiting, either contributing to or resulting from it.[31] Weakness leads to decreased activity, which may increase the incidence of constipation. Constipation contributes to nausea and vomiting through receptors in the gut, which signal the vomiting center via vagal and sympathetic afferents.

Medications used to relieve pain symptoms are a frequent cause of nausea and vomiting. Opioids activate the CTZ to produce nausea and vomiting. Since movement often increases the nausea and vomiting, a vestibular component may also be involved.[32] Opioids compound the lowered gastric motility experienced by many terminally ill patients and can contribute to the anorexia/cachexia syndrome. This syndrome involves decreased gastrointestinal motility, early satiation, and nausea.

Nausea and vomiting also may exacerbate an already poor appetite in the terminally ill patient. The resultant decrease in food and fluid intake along with the loss of electrolytes due to the vomiting further compromise the body's electrolyte balance, resulting in metabolic abnormalities. Uncontrolled coughing, with its forceful contraction of abdominal muscles, also can instigate vomiting.

Polypharmacy

Polypharmacy complicates the study of antiemetics in advanced disease. The average number of medications being taken by residents of long-term care facilities varies between 6.6 and 7.7.[33] The percentage of patients with adverse drug reactions increases from 10% when taking a single drug to 100% when 10 medications are taken.[33] Most terminally ill patients require multiple medications, and many experience adverse drug reactions. The decline in function of the various organs involved in drug metabolism, storage, and excretion, due to both aging and disease processes, and the number of medications taken make optimal dosing and the prevention of adverse effects complicated. Adverse effects of the many drugs along with interactions among drugs increase the problems associated with advanced disease.

Limitations/Considerations in Designing Nausea and Vomiting Studies in Palliative Care

The very nature of terminal illness mandates that research methods be selected on both methodological and practical grounds. Although the double-blind, placebo-controlled, randomized study is considered standard in research, one encounters many difficulties when considering such methods in studying terminally ill patients. This is especially true with nausea and vomiting, in which case practitioners are reluctant to assign a control due to the physiological and psychological impact of the symptoms.

The World Medical Association Declaration of Helsinki[34] established principles for conducting medical research. It stated that the physician must always be free to use whatever methods he or she feels necessary to save a life, restore health, or alleviate suffering. Since alleviating suffering is of primary importance in palliative care, it becomes difficult to justify the use of a placebo in such research. Without standards for the treatment of nausea and vomiting in this population, deciding on a comparator arm for randomized trials is difficult.

Other problems associated with empirical studies in terminally ill patients include under-representation of patients with the most advanced disease and the number of participants accrued. Patients may be too ill to participate in interviews or complete questionnaires, the course of the illness may advance rapidly and lead to a high attrition rate, and the numbers of patients willing to participate in research at the end of life may be too few to provide sufficient power to demonstrate efficacy. Family members (and/or health-care providers) may be unwilling or ambivalent about "bothering" the patient with study requirements when time and energy are limited. This is especially true if there is no immediate benefit to the dying person. The family may have to be called upon to provide proxy consent, which may, therefore, not be readily forthcoming.

Controlled trials are difficult to plan in the last days of life because of the uncertainty of the course of the disease, the myriad symptoms, limited time remaining, and/or unwillingness of the patient or family to enter a study at that time. As the disease progresses, more of the pathways leading to nausea and vomiting may be triggered. Treatment of the nausea and vomiting becomes more complicated, with increasing interactions between the various treatments and the progressing illness. In such situations, it is difficult to control variables or isolate effects. The episodic nature of nausea and vomiting and the declining overall condition of the patient make it difficult to evaluate symptoms prior to and during treatment. It would be unethical to withhold antiemetics at such a time. Many terminally ill patents are cared for at home, and it is difficult to control a drug regimen in such cases.

Future Research

There is a need for empirically supported interventions to treat nausea and vomiting in patients with advanced illness. To date, most of the research evaluating antiemetics in this population has comprised retrospective narratives often based on only case notes. Treatment has been based on anecdote or physician preference and the narrative written after the fact. The field needs to focus on prospective, or "live," studies, in which events are recorded as they occur. In prospective studies, more attention is focused on understanding the problem in depth and carefully observing changes as they occur in response to specific clinical interventions.

There are specific challenges to incorporating and adapting study designs considered standard in mainstream healthcare to the palliative care setting. These challenges have been previously discussed and relate to the condition of the terminally ill patient, concerns of family and healthcare providers, and accruing a sufficient number of participants. However, these are only challenges, not impossibilities.

There is a need for research focusing on evaluating current treatments and developing new approaches, pharmaceutical and otherwise, to treating nausea and vomiting in terminally ill patients. New and more efficient methods of drug delivery specifically designed to circumvent the problems associated with the usual routes of administration in patients with nausea and vomiting are needed. Well-designed studies with randomized control groups designed to evaluate new pharmaceutical agents or new uses for existing agents that control nausea and vomiting based on the specific mechanisms triggering the symptoms are needed. Studies need to be designed to accrue sufficient numbers of patients to provide adequate statistical power. Such a design may involve multisite participation, a short study period to compensate for the inevitable attrition in such a population, and observations/documentation predominantly done by healthcare profession-als to avoid burdening the patient or family. With the growth and changes in home hospice, there is a wealth of opportunity to involve the hospice team in such research.

There is ongoing research into integrative therapies for resolving nausea and vomiting associated with chemotherapy. These can be investigated for use in nausea and vomiting associated with advanced disease. Among the integrative therapies currently being studied and used by chemotherapy patients are behav-ioral interventions, such as hypnosis, relaxation, guided imagery, and distraction. The benefits of complementary therapy are fewer side effects, increased self-care by patients, ease of administration, and less expense. Published studies exist that support the effectiveness of all of these methods at reducing nausea and vomiting.[35,36]

Summary

Nausea and vomiting occur at some point in approximately 62% of patients with advanced disease, and 40% experience such symptoms during the last 6 weeks of life.[37] In spite of these percentages, little empirical research is available to assist in managing these symptoms. Most of the existing research on antiemetics involves chemotherapy-induced or radiation-induced nausea and vomiting and may not be relevant to the treatment of symptoms resulting from advanced disease.

Most of the studies in the literature are retrospective. Various medications are tried, and then one retraces the history of the symptoms to determine which medications were effective. Prospective studies with symptomatology docu-mented at entrance to a palliative care program or hospice care and careful re-porting of symptoms and treatment thereafter are needed.

There are numerous problems inherent in the study of people with advanced disease. Such patients have a myriad symptoms interacting with each other and each requiring treatment. Treating one symptom may exacerbate or improve an-other or cause entirely new problems. Determining whether improvement or ex-acerbation is part of the disease process, the treatment, or another emerging problem is often very difficult.

References

1. Tyler LS. Nausea and vomiting in palliative care. J Pharm Care Pain Symptom Control 2000; 8:263–281.
2. Lichter I. Results of antiemetic management in terminal illness. J Palliat Care 1993; 9:19–21.
3. Bruera E, Chadwick S, Brenneis C, et al. Methylphenidate associated with narcotics for the treatment of cancer pain. Cancer Treat Rep 1987; 71:67–70.

4. Waller A, Caroline NI. Handbook of Palliative Care in Cancer, 2nd ed. Boston: Butterworth Heinemann, 2000.

5. Fallon BG. Nausea and vomiting unrelated to cancer treatment. In: Berger A, Portenoy RK, Weissman DE, eds. Principles and Practice of Supportive Oncology. Philadelphia: Lippincott-Raven, 1998:179–189.

6. Lichter I. Which antiemetic? J Palliat Care 1993; 9:42–50.

7. Baines MJ. ABC of palliative care: nausea, vomiting, and intestinal obstruction. BMJ 1997; 315:1148–1150.

8. Pappano AJ. Cholinoceptor-activating and cholinesterase-inhibiting drugs. In: Katzung BG, ed. Basic and Clinical Pharmacology. Stamford, CT: Appleton and Lange, 1998:90–104.

9. Altman DF. Drugs used in gastrointestinal diseases. In: Katzung BG, ed. Basic and Clinical Pharmacology. Stamford, CT: Appleton and Lange, 1998:1017–1029.

10. Rousseau P. Antiemetic therapy in adults with terminal disease: a brief review. Am J Hospice Palliat Care 1995; 5:13–18.

11. Reichlin S. Medical progress: somatostatin. N Engl J Med 1983; 309:1495–1501.

12. Kutz K, Nuesh E, Rosenthaler J. Pharmacokinetics of SMS 201-995 in healthy subjects. Scand J Gastroenterol 1986; 21(Suppl 119):65–72.

13. Mercadante S, Maddaloni S. Octreotide in the management of inoperable gastrointestinal obstruction in terminal cancer patients. J Pain Symptom Manage 1992; 7:496–498.

14. Mangili G, Franchi M, Mariana A, et al. Octreotide in the management of bowel obstruction in terminal ovarian cancer. Gynecol Oncol 1996; 61:345–348.

15. Mercadante S, Spoldi E, Caraceni A, et al. Octreotide in relieving gastrointestinal symptoms due to bowel obstruction. Palliat Med 1993; 7:295–299.

16. Pirl WF, Roth AJ. Remission of chemotherapy-induced emesis with concurrent olanzapine treatment: case report. Psychooncology 2000; 9:84–87.

17. Passik S, Lundberg J, Kirsh K, et al. A pilot exploration of the anti-emetic activity of olanzapine for the relief of nausea in patients with advanced cancer and pain. J Pain Symptom Manage 2002; 23:526–532.

18. Passik S, Loehrer P, Navari R, et al. A phase I trial of olanzapine (Zyprexa) for the prevention of delayed emesis in cancer patients: a Hoosier Oncology Group study. In: Program, Proceedings of American Society of Clinical Oncology, 38th Annual Meeting, May 18–21, 2000, Orlando, FL.

19. Baines M, Oliver DJ, Carter RL. Medical management of intestinal obstruction in patients with advanced malignant disease. Lancet 1985; ii:990–993.

20. Bruera E, Seifert L, Watanabe S, et al. Chronic nausea in advanced cancer patients: a retrospective assessment of a metoclopramide-based antiemetic regimen. J Pain Symptom Manage 1996; 11:147–153.

21. Marsden SC. Use of ondansetron (Zofran). N Z Med J 1993; 106:1666.

22. Cole RM, Robinson F, Harvey L, et al. Successful control of intractable nausea and vomiting requiring combined ondansetron and haloperidol in a patient with advanced cancer. J Pain Symptom Manage 1994; 9:48–50.

23. Andrews PA, Quan V, Ogg CS. Ondansetron for symptomatic relief in terminal uraemia [letter]. Nephrol Dial Transplant 1995; 10:140.

24. Currow DC, Coughlan M, Fardell B, et al. Use of ondansetron in palliative medicine. J Pain Symptom Manage 1997; 13:302–307.

25. Porcel JM, Schoenenberger JA. Antiemetic efficacy of subcutaneous 5-HT$_3$ receptor antagonists in terminal cancer patients [letter]. J Pain Symptom Manage 1998; 15:265–266.

26. Khoo D, Riley J, Waxman J. Control of emesis in bowel obstruction in terminally ill patients. Lancet 1992; 339:375–376.

27. Khoo D, Hall E, Motson R, et al. Palliation of malignant intestinal obstruction using octreotide. Eur J Cancer 1994; 30A:28–30.

28. Green ST, Nathwani D, Goldberg DJ, et al. Nabilone as effective therapy for intractable nausea and vomiting in AIDS. Br J Clin Pharmacol 1989; 28:494–495.

29. Flynn J, Hanif N. Nabilone for the management of intractable nausea and vomiting in terminally staged AIDS. J Palliat Care 1992; 8:46–47.

30. Curtis EB, Krench R, Walsh D. Common symptoms in patients with advanced cancer. J Palliat Care 1991; 7:25–29.

31. Baines M. Nausea and vomiting in the patient with advanced cancer. J Pain Symptom Manage 1988; 3:81–85.

32. Way WL, Fields HL, Way EL. Opioid analgesics and antagonists. In: Katzung BG, ed. Basic Clinical Pharmacology. Stamford, CT: Appleton and Lange, 1998:496–515.

33. Katzung BG. Special aspects of geriatric pharmacology. In: Katzung BG, ed. Basic Clinical Pharmacology. Stamford, CT: Appleton and Lange, 1998:989–998.

34. World Medical Association. Declaration of Helsinki. In: Handbook of Declarations. London: World Medical Association, 1989.

35. King CR. Nonpharmacologic management of chemotherapy-induced nausea and vomiting. Oncol Nurs Forum 1997; 24(Suppl):41–48.

36. Burish TG, Tope DM. Psychological techniques for controlling the adverse side effects of cancer chemotherapy. J Pain Symptom Manage 1992; 7:287–301.

37. Reuben DB, Mor V. Nausea and vomiting in terminal cancer patients. Arch Intern Med 1986; 146:2021–2023.

III

RESEARCH IN
RESPIRATORY SYMPTOMS

6

Multidimensional Assessment of Dyspnea

DEBORAH DUDGEON

Dyspnea, an awareness of breathing discomfort, is a very common symptom that accompanies many illnesses and pathological conditions. In a longitudinal study[1] of women and men aged 65 years and older, the prevalence of dyspnea was 19.4%–29.2% and associated with a significant risk for loss of mobility within 4 years. In people with mild to moderate cardiovascular disease, breathlessness limits physical activity, and people with advanced cardiovascular disease are dyspneic even at rest.[2] Approximately 50% of a general outpatient cancer population describe some breathlessness,[3] with this number rising to 45%–70% in the terminal phases of cancer.[4-9] Muers and Round[10] noted that breathlessness was a complaint at presentation in 60% of 289 patients with non-small cell lung cancer and that this number increased to almost 90% just prior to death.

In a study of late-stage cancer patients, Roberts et al.[11] found that almost 62% of the patients with dyspnea had been short of breath for a duration exceeding 3 months. This study showed that the patients universally responded by decreasing their activity to whatever degree would relieve their shortness of breath. Various activities intensified dyspnea for these patients: climbing stairs, 95.6%; walking slowly, 47.8%; getting dressed, 52.2%; talking or eating, 56.5%; and resting, 26.1%. Brown et al.[12] found that 97% of lung cancer patients studied had decreased their activities and 80% believed they had socially isolated themselves from friends and outside contacts to cope with their dyspnea. Others have found that the quality of life of patients with cardiovascular disease is equally affected by the presence of breathlessness. Breathlessness has also been associated with increased mortality in patients with chronic obstructive pulmonary disease (COPD), vascular disease, and terminal cancer.[8,13,14]

Effectiveness of Treatment

Unfortunately, despite the prevalence, severity, and impact on people's lives, the treatments available for the management of dyspnea when reversible causes are not present are relatively ineffective. Higginson and McCarthy[15] found that dyspnea was the main symptom in 21% of 86 terminal cancer patients cared for at home and that there was no change in dyspnea scores over time; they suggested that existing methods for control of the symptom were ineffective and that new interventions were needed. Dudgeon et al.[16] also found that the dyspnea of patients admitted to an acute-care palliative care unit was not effectively controlled, with a median score on a 100 mm visual analogue scale for breathlessness remaining at 50 mm after 7 days of intervention.

Difficulties in Assessing Dyspnea

Management of dyspnea requires an understanding of the multidimensional nature and the pathophysiological mechanisms that cause this distressing symptom. Dyspnea, like pain, is a subjective experience that involves many factors that modulate both the quality and the intensity of its perception. Distinct sensations of breathing are produced by stimulation of various neurophysiological pathways, the conscious perception of the stimuli, and the interpretation in the context of lifelong previous experience and learning. Unfortunately, the neuropathways underlying the sensation of dyspnea are not well understood.[17] There is difficulty defining the precise physical stimulus that causes the discomfort, and the understanding of the pathophysiology has largely been derived from induced respiratory sensation in healthy subjects or people with COPD. Stimuli to induce dyspnea have included hypoxia or hypercapnia, added respiratory load (such as breathing through a straw or strapping a chest), breath holding, and exercise. The relationship between these experimental models and spontaneous breathlessness is unclear.[17,18]

When discussing the multidimensional assessment of dyspnea, we need to ask the question "assessment for what?" Clinical assessments are usually directed at determining the underlying pathophysiology, to determine the appropriate treatment and to evaluate the response to therapy. Research questions may be epidemiological, to determine the prevalence of the symptom and associated factors, the natural history of breathlessness, and the pathophysiology, or related to clinical trials to evaluate treatment modalities. The assessment tools and methods depend on the setting and the questions that are being asked.

Clinical Assessment

Clinical assessment of dyspnea should include a complete history of the symptom, including its temporal onset (acute or chronic), whether it is affected by positions, qualities, associated symptoms, precipitating and relieving events or activities, and response to medications. A past history of smoking, underlying lung or cardiac disease, concurrent medical conditions, allergy history, and details of previous medications or treatments should be elicited.[19,20]

A careful physical examination focused on possible underlying causes of dyspnea should be performed. Particular attention should be directed at signs associated with certain clinical syndromes that are associated with common causes of dyspnea. An example of this would be the dullness to percussion, decreased tactile fremitus, and absent breath sounds associated with a pleural effusion in a person with lung cancer. Another example would be the findings of congestive heart failure with an elevated jugular venous pressure, an S_3 heart sound, and bilateral crackles audible on chest exam.[19,20]

Dyspnea, like pain, is a subjective experience that may not be evident to an observer. *Tachypnea*, rapid respiratory rate, is not dyspnea. Medical personnel must learn to ask for and accept the patient's assessments, often without measurable physical correlates. When patients say that they are having discomfort with breathing, we must believe they are dyspneic. Gift et al.[21] studied the physiological factors related to dyspnea in subjects with COPD with high, medium, and low levels of breathlessness. There were no significant differences in respiratory rate, depth of respiration, or peak expiratory flow rates at the three levels of dyspnea. There was, however, a significant difference in the use of accessory muscles between patients with high and low levels of dyspnea. This suggests that this is a physical finding which reflects the intensity of dyspnea.

Diagnostic tests helpful in determining the etiology of dyspnea include chest radiograph; electrocardiogram; pulmonary function tests; arterial blood gases; complete blood counts; serum potassium, magnesium, and phosphate levels; cardiopulmonary exercise testing; and tests specific for the suspected underlying pathologies (echocardiogram for suspected pericardial effusion).[19] The choice of appropriate diagnostic tests should be guided by the stage of disease, the prognosis, the risk/benefit ratios of any proposed tests or interventions, and the desires of the patient.

Dyspnea and Psychological Factors

Dyspnea incorporates not only physical neuroanatomical elements but also affective components, which are shaped by previous experience.[22,23] Individuals with comparable degrees of functional lung impairment may experience considerable differences in the intensity of dyspnea they perceive.[22] This lack of correlation and predictability may be due to any one or a combination of factors, including adaptation, differing physical characteristics, and psychological conditions.[22] Anxious, obsessive, depressed, and dependent persons appear to experience dyspnea that is disproportionately severe relative to the extent of pulmonary disease.[22] Burns and Howell[24] found that patients with airway disease who had disproportionately severe breathlessness were more likely to manifest symptoms of a psychiatric disorder (most commonly depression) and that their breathlessness resolved with resolution of the psychiatric disorder. Gift et al.[21] found that anxiety was higher during episodes of high or medium dyspnea levels compared with low dyspnea. Others have found that anxiety and depression seem to perpetuate episodes of disproportionate breathlessness.[25] Kellner et al.[26] found that in multiple regression analyses depression was predictive of breathlessness. Studies in cancer patients by Dudgeon and Lertzman[27] and others[3,9,28] have also shown that, although the correlation coefficients are low, anxiety is significantly correlated with the intensity of dyspnea.

Qualitative Dimensions of Dyspnea

In discussing the assessment of dyspnea, it is important to understand that it is not a single sensation. As clinicians, we have not been taught to determine the qualitative components of the symptom as with pain, where descriptions such as "burning," "stabbing," and "shooting" suggest neuropathic pain. Simon et al.[29] developed a list of phrases describing the discomfort of breathlessness solicited from patients with cardiopulmonary disease. The list was subsequently given to 53 patients with breathlessness due to pregnancy and a variety of cardiopulmonary disorders.[30] Cluster analysis identified that discreet groupings of words were associated with different pathophysiological conditions ("chest tightness," "exhalation," and "deep" with asthma). Each condition was characterized by more than one cluster, suggesting that more than one physiological mechanism might be responsible for the breathlessness of that condition. Some clusters were associated with more than one condition, suggesting that some of the mechanisms were common to more than one condition. This work suggests that dyspnea mediated by similar receptors evokes common word descriptors.[31] From the research to date, it is, however, not known whether the dyspnea questionnaire is useful in establishing the diagnosis of a specific cardiopulmonary disease.[31] O'Donnell et al.[32–34] found that while descriptor choices were clearly different between health and disease states, they provided no discrimination, for example, between COPD, restrictive lung disease, and congestive heart failure.

Measurement of Dyspnea

As dyspnea is a complex, subjective experience, it is difficult to quantify. Standardized pulmonary function tests are usually poorly correlated with measures of the intensity of dyspnea.[35] There is no known organic correlate of dyspnea, and it is difficult to document exactly what is being measured (for example, fatigue).[36,37] The intensity of dyspnea varies with the magnitude of the task and associated effort (walking on flat or climbing stairs and speed of walking).[31] There are measures that tap into the qualitative components of dyspnea (both subjective and objective quantitative measures, functional or quality-of-life measures) and others that address the multifaceted nature of dyspnea and its expression. Most of the measurement instruments for breathlessness were developed for use in patients with a chronic pulmonary disease. Only a few have been validated in patients with cancer.

Visual analogue scale

The visual analogue scale (VAS) is one of the most popular techniques for measuring the perceived intensity of the symptom. This scale is usually a 100 mm vertical or horizontal line, anchored at each end by descriptions such as "not at all breathless" and "not very breathless." Unfortunately, there are no standards for anchoring the ends of the scale or for administration. At times, it is used with a specific dyspnea-producing task;[38] at others, people are asked to quantify their "usual" breathlessness.[12] Subjects are asked to mark the line at the point which best describes the intensity of their breathlessness; therefore, it is a global rating scale. The VAS is not appropriate for comparing dyspnea in different patients as there are no standard principles that allow the scales to be used consistently by different subjects. The scales can be used as an initial assessment, to monitor progress, and to evaluate the effectiveness of treatment in an individual patient.[37]

Test–retest reliability was established for the VAS in people with stable asthma[39] and in a cancer population.[12] Aitken[40] and Gift and colleagues[21] established the validity of the scale with external resistive loading of respiration and in asthmatics and COPD patients, respectively. Dhand et al.[39] found the VAS correlated highly with peak expiratory flow rate percentage ($r = -0.72$) in people with stable asthma but less well in acutely ill asthmatics ($r = -0.32$). In two studies, the vertical VAS had greater sensitivity to change than the horizontal scale.[37,41,42]

Likert scales

Guyatt et al.[43] found that a seven-point Likert scale (with responses 1, all the time; 2, most of the time; 3, a good bit of the time; 4, some of the time; 5, a little of the time; 6, hardly any of the time; and 7, none of the time) was more quickly understood than a VAS for dyspnea anchored by "none of the time" and "all of the time." The responsiveness to change following a pulmonary rehabilitation program was similar with both methods. Reuben and Mor[4] used a 0–4 Likert scale with "none," "mild," "moderate," "severe," and "horrible" in the National Hospice Study to grade the intensity of breathlessness. Dudgeon et al.[3] compared this scale with a VAS ($r = 0.82$, $p = 0.0001$) in an outpatient cancer population. The category "horrible" was chosen infrequently; therefore, it was suggested that the "horrible" and "severe" categories be collapsed.

Magnitude estimation scales

Some scales use a ratio scaling technique that measures the relationship between the intensity of a physical stimulus and its perceived magnitude.[44,45] These scales attempt to estimate absolute sensory intensity and to allow comparison of intensity across individuals.[46]

The Borg scale

The Borg scale was developed in 1962[47] to rate perceived exertion and effort during exercise. The modified Borg scale is a category scale with ratio properties that was adapted by Burdon et al.[48] to measure the intensity of dyspnea. There is a nonlinear spacing of verbal descriptors of severity that correspond to specific numbers and ratio properties of sensation intensities. The scales go from 0 to 10. Patients are asked to pick the verbal descriptor which best describes their perceived exertion during exercise testing. The Borg scale correlates with physiological parameters of lung disease during exercise.[49] It is usually used in conjunction with an exercise protocol with standardized power output or metabolic loads. When used in this manner, the slope of Borg/time is very reproducible (intraclass correlation $r = 0.8$, $p < 0.001$) and reliable and permits comparisons within individuals and across population groups.[50] Borg measurements of dyspnea during exercise are more stable on repeat testing and more highly correlated with exercise ventilation than VAS dyspnea measurements.[51]

The oxygen cost diagram

The oxygen cost diagram (OCD) is a 10 cm vertical line.[52] Everyday activities are listed along the line at places that correspond to the metabolic equivalence (or oxygen cost) required to perform them. Patients mark the line at the point that they think their breathlessness will not let them go. McGavin et al.[52] found that the distance patients walked correlated with the point marked on the OCD ($r = 0.68$, $p < 0.001$). The OCD correlated significantly with the Baseline Dyspnea Index and the Medical Research Council scale in patients with diverse cardiopulmonary diseases of variable physiological severity.[53] The OCD is one of the scales thought to be most appropriate for statistical comparisons of response to therapy.[53] The scale is of limited use in people who are breathless at rest as it relies heavily on ambulatory activities.

The Medical Research Council Breathlessness Scale

The Medical Research Council Breathlessness Scale is an interview guide or self-report questionnaire with a five-point rating scale. The scale goes from grade 1, where the person is troubled by breathlessness on strenuous exertion, to grade 5, where the person is too breathless to leave the house or after undressing.[54] Content validity,[55] inter-rater reliability,[53] and concurrent validity[56,57] have been established for this instrument.

The scale has been used to define and characterize a patient population. There is emphasis on ambulation; therefore, it might underestimate the consequences of other activities in a debilitated population.

Reading numbers aloud

Reading numbers aloud[58] was designed as an objective measure of the activity-limiting effect of breathlessness in people with cancer who were breathless at very low levels of exertion. The test involves asking subjects to read a grid of numbers as quickly and clearly as possible for 60 seconds. The number of numbers read and the number read per breath are recorded.

In one study, the test showed good test–retest reliability and construct validity; thus, it may prove useful in a debilitated population.[58]

Multidimensional assessment instruments

The Baseline Dyspnea Index

The Baseline Dyspnea Index (BDI) is an interviewer-administered questionnaire.[59] It is a multidimensional assessment instrument that uses a five-point scale (ranging from severe to unimpaired) to quantify functional impairment (the difficulty in performing activities of daily living), magnitude of task (intensity of exertion required to elicit dyspnea), and magnitude of effort (the effort normally exerted). The observer grades the different components of dyspnea, and a baseline total score is obtained by adding the three ratings. The range for scores is 0–12, with a lower score indicating a lower intensity of dyspnea. The BDI has been extensively studied and has demonstrated good psychometric properties for heterogeneous pulmonary and cardiac patients.[60] The instrument has demonstrated inter-rater reliability,[53,59] concurrent validity,[53,57,59,61] construct validity,[53,57,61] and sensitivity.[62]

The Transition Dyspnea Index

The Transition Dyspnea Index (TDI) was developed to measure changes in functional impairment, magnitude of task, and magnitude of effort from the baseline assessment. A transitional focal score is obtained by adding the ratings from each of the three category scales (range of total score −9 to 9, −3 to 3 for individual categories). Inter-rater reliability,[59] concurrent validity,[59] and sensitivity[59,63] are established for this instrument. Eakin et al.[64] report that the TDI is difficult to use in a research protocol as it requires that the interviewer have the patient's baseline scores and a copy of the BDI. They think that the TDI is affected by both rater and patient biases.[64]

The Dyspnea Assessment Questionnaire

The Dyspnea Assessment Questionnaire was developed to measure both qualitative and quantitative components of breathlessness in patients with cancer.[9] This questionnaire includes 43 words divided into 16 categories. A severity score has been assigned for each word. The sum of the severity scores of all words chosen was found to correlate ($r = 0.45$, $p < 0.001$) with the VAS of dyspnea intensity. The total interval score, which takes into account the different number of words in each category, was also significantly correlated ($r = 0.45, p < 0.001$) with the VAS. The questionnaire also included a dyspnea exertion scale, but this was not significantly correlated with the average level of dyspnea over the last 24 hours as measured on the VAS. This questionnaire has some promise, but further work is needed.

The Cancer Dyspnea Scale

The Cancer Dyspnea Scale[65] is a 12-item, three-factor (sense of effort, sense of anxiety, sense of discomfort) scale developed to assess the multidimensional nature of dyspnea in cancer patients. Although further improvements and validation are needed, the Japanese version of the scale has shown some evidence of reliability and validity as a multidimensional instrument. Translation of the scale into an English version was completed, but cross-cultural validation is still required.

Quality-of-life instruments

Measurement of quality of life attempts to provide standardized estimates of the overall impact of the disease or therapeutic efficacy of different types of treatment on the individual. Studies that have looked at the relationship between dyspnea and different components of health-related quality of life show that dyspnea is predominantly related to physical impairment but also to measures of psychosocial dysfunction.[66]

The Chronic Respiratory Disease Questionnaire

The Chronic Respiratory Disease Questionnaire was developed to determine the effect of treatment on the quality of life of patients with COPD. It is a 20-item interview guide with a seven-point rating scale, anchored by "no shortness of breath" and "extremely short of breath." It has four subscales that examine changes in quality of life over a 2-week period in dyspnea, fatigue, emotional function, and the feeling of control over the disease.

The first time this questionnaire is administered it takes 15–25 minutes, subsequently 10–15 minutes.[67] The instrument has demonstrated content and concurrent validity,[68,69] test–retest reliability,[70] and sensitivity.[71] It has also demonstrated good internal consistency and reliability, with Cronbach's α coefficients of 0.76–0.90.[68] This questionnaire has been translated into different languages.[68,72]

One study showed that patients were more likely to seek medical help when their quality of life was affected than by the mere presence of respiratory symptoms or gradually reduced lung function.[72]

The St. George's Respiratory Questionnaire

The St. George's Respiratory Questionnaire[73] is a self-administered questionnaire designed for use in patients with asthma and COPD. It contains 76 items with three sections dealing with the frequency and severity of respiratory symptoms, activities that cause or are limited by breathlessness, and the impact of the respiratory problem on aspects of social and psychosocial function. It takes approximately 10–15 minutes to complete.[67] Concurrent validity,[68,73,74] internal consistency,[68,69] test–retest reliability,[73] and sensitivity to change[73] have been established. In one study, item completion was relatively lower than for other self-administered questionnaires. The authors suggested that there was low comprehensibility and/or that some of the items were irrelevant to the COPD population.[69]

The Seattle Obstructive Lung Disease Questionnaire

The Seattle Obstructive Lung Disease Questionnaire (SOLQ)[75] is a self-administered questionnaire consisting of 29 items measuring four health dimensions: physical function, emotional function, coping skills, and treatment satisfaction. The SOLQ is computer-scannable and useful for monitoring long-term outcomes among large groups of COPD patients.[75] The questionnaire was developed to measure longitudinal differences within persons over time and to discriminate differences between groups of patients with varying disease severity at one point in time. Internal consistency, reliability, validity, and responsiveness have been established.[75]

The Lung Cancer Symptom Scale

The Lung Cancer Symptom Scale (LCSS)[76,77] has nine self-report VASs and an optional six-category observer scale. This instrument addresses the time frame of the past day. Six items measure major symptoms of lung malignancies, and three are related to total symptomatic distress, activity status, and overall quality of life. The LCSS focuses on disease-related factors most affected by treatment and pertinent to the evaluation of therapeutic interventions. There are no therapy-related side effect questions, but it does capture the impact of toxicities.[77] The LCSS is available in three languages. The patient scale requires 8 minutes to administer and the observer scale, 2 minutes.[76] The LCSS Observer Scale was used in a retrospective medical record review to evaluate the benefit of radiotherapy for patients with non-small cell lung cancer.[78] The LCSS has demonstrated high intra-rater and inter-rater reliability,[76] good internal consistency, and test–retest reliability.[77] Content, construct, and criterion-related validity have been established.[76]

The European Organization for Research and Treatment Quality of Life Questionnaire and Lung Cancer Module

The European Organization for Research and Treatment (EORTC) Quality of Life Questionnaire (EORTC-QLQ-C30) includes a 30-item core measure[79] and a 13-item lung cancer module.[80] It is a self-report instrument in which patients are asked to assess the physical role and the emotional, social, and cognitive dimensions of their life over the past week. It includes questions on therapy-related side effects and is available in 17 languages. The EORTC core measure has shown overall reliability of 0.70 or greater in four of nine subscales for pre-treatment scores and eight of nine subscales during treatment.[79] Internal consistency has not been reported for the entire EORTC-QLC-43. The reliability co-efficients for dyspnea and pain subscales for the lung cancer module has been reported, and construct and criterion-related validity have been established.[79,80]

The Functional Assessment of Cancer Therapy—Lung Cancer Quality of Life Instrument

The Functional Assessment of Cancer Therapy—Lung Cancer Quality of Life Instrument (FACT-L, version 3) contains 34 general health items and 10 lung cancer items.[81] This instrument measures five dimensions of quality of life: physical, social and family, emotional and functional well-being, and relationship with physician. It has been translated into eight languages. The FACT-L is a self-report scale, which takes less than 10 minutes to complete.[77] It has established internal consistency, content, and construct validity.[81]

Summary

In summary, dyspnea is a very complex, subjective experience that is multidimensional in nature and involves many factors that modulate both the quality and intensity of its perception. At the present time, there is no single instrument that assesses all components of the sensation of shortness of breath. It is important when assessing dyspnea to choose the appropriate method depending on the setting and the questions to be asked. For the palliative patient, it is also important that the burden be not too onerous and appropriate to the prognosis and stage of disease.

References

1. Guralnik JM, LaCroix AZ, Abbott RD, et al. Maintaining mobility in late life. I. Demographic characteristics and chronic conditions. Am J Epidemiol 1993; 137:845–857.
2. Weber KT. What can we learn from exercise testing beyond the detection of myocardial ischemia? Clin Cardiol 1997; 20:684–696.
3. Dudgeon DJ, Kristjanson L, Sloan JA, et al. Dyspnea in cancer patients: prevalence and associated factors. J Pain Symptom Manage 2001; 21:95–102.
4. Reuben DB, Mor V. Dyspnea in terminally ill cancer patients. Chest 1986; 89: 234–236.
5. Fainsinger R, MacEachern T, Hanson J, et al. Symptom control during the last week of life on a palliative care unit. J Palliat Care 1991; 7:5–11.
6. Twycross RG, Lack SA. Respiratory symptoms. In: Twycross RG, Lack SA, eds. Therapeutics in Terminal Cancer, 2d ed. London: Churchill Livingstone, 1990: 123–136.

7. Curtis EB, Krech R, Walsh TD. Common symptoms in patients with advanced cancer. J Palliat Care 1991; 7:25–29.

8. Heyse-Moore LH, Ross V, Mullee MA. How much of a problem is dyspnea in advanced cancer? Palliat Med 1991; 5:20–26.

9. Heyse-Moore LH. On Dyspnea in Advanced Cancer. Southampton: Southampton University, 1993. Dissertation.

10. Muers MF, Round CE. Palliation of symptoms in non-small cell lung cancer: a study by the Yorkshire Regional Cancer Organization Thoracic Group. Thorax 1993; 48:339–343.

11. Roberts DK, Thorne SE, Pearson C. The experience of dyspnea in late-stage cancer. Patients' and nurses' perspectives. Cancer Nurs 1993; 16:310–320.

12. Brown ML, Carrieri V, Janson-Bjerklie S, et al. Lung cancer and dyspnea: the patient's perception. Oncol Nurs Forum 1986; 13:19–24.

13. Vollmer WM, McCamant LE, Johnson LR, et al. Respiratory symptoms, lung function, and mortality in a screening center cohort. Am J Epidemiol 1989; 129:1157–1169.

14. Reuben DB, Mor V, Hiris J. Clinical symptoms and length of survival in patients with terminal cancer. Arch Intern Med 1988; 148:1586–1591.

15. Higginson I, McCarthy M. Measuring symptoms in terminal cancer: are pain and dyspnoea controlled? J R Soc Med 1989; 82:264–267.

16. Dudgeon D, Harlos M, Clinch JJ. The Edmonton Symptom Assessment Scale (ESAS) as an audit tool. J Palliat Care 1999; 15:14–19.

17. Manning HL, Schwartzstein RM. Mechanisms of dyspnea. In: Mahler D, ed. Dyspnea. New York: Marcel Dekker, 1998:63–95.

18. Manning HL, Schwartzstein RM. Pathophysiology of dyspnea. N Engl J Med 1995; 333:1547–1553.

19. Silvestri GA, Mahler DA. Evaluation of dyspnea in the elderly patient. Clin Chest Med 1993; 14:393–404.

20. Ferrin MS, Tino G. Acute dyspnea. American Association of Critical-Care Nurses Clin Issues 1997; 8:398–410.

21. Gift AG, Plaut SM, Jacox A. Psychologic and physiologic factors related to dyspnea in subjects with chronic obstructive pulmonary disease. Heart Lung 1986; 15:595–601.

22. Cherniack NS, Altose MD. Mechanisms of dyspnea. Clin Chest Med 1987; 8:207–214.

23. Tobin MJ. Dyspnea: pathophysiologic basis, clinical presentation, and management. Arch Intern Med 1990; 150:1604–1613.

24. Burns BH, Howell JBL. Disproportionately severe breathlessness in chronic bronchitis. Q J Med 1969; 38:277–294.

25. Howell J. Behavioral breathlessness. In: Breathlessness. The Campbell Symposium, May 16–19, 1991. Ingelheim: Boehringer-Ingelheim, 1992:149–155.

26. Kellner R, Samet J, Pathak D. Dyspnea, anxiety, and depression in chronic respiratory impairment. Gen Hosp Psychiatry 1992; 14:20–28.

27. Dudgeon D, Lertzman M. Dyspnea in the advanced cancer patient. J Pain Symptom Manage 1998; 16:212–219.

28. Bruera E, Schmitz B, Pither J, et al. The frequency and correlates of dyspnea in patients with advanced cancer. J Pain Symptom Manage 2000; 19:357–362.

29. Simon PM, Schwartzstein RM, Weiss JW, et al. Distinguishable sensations of breathlessness induced in normal volunteers. Am Rev Respir Dis 1989; 140:1021–1027.
30. Simon PM, Schwartzstein RM, Weiss JW, et al. Distinguishable types of dyspnea in patients with shortness of breath. Am Rev Respir Dis 1990; 142:1009–1014.
31. Schwartzstein RM. The language of dyspnea. In: Mahler D, ed. Dyspnea. New York: Marcel Dekker, 1998:35–62.
32. O'Donnell DE, Chau LL, Bertley J, et al. Qualitative aspects of exertional breathlessness in CAL: pathophysiological mechanisms. Am J Respir Crit Care Med 1997; 155:109–115.
33. O'Donnell DE, Chau LKL, Webb KA. Qualitative aspects of exertional dyspnea in interstitial lung disease. J Appl Physiol 1998; 84:2000–2009.
34. D'Arsigny C, Raj S, Abdollah H, et al. Ventilatory assistance improves leg discomfort and exercise endurance in stable congestive heart failure (CHF). Am J Respir Crit Care Med 1998; 157:A451.
35. McFadden ERJ, Kiser R, deGroot WJ. Acute bronchial asthma: relations between clinical and physiologic manifestations. N Engl J Med 1973; 288:221–225.
36. Wilson JR, Rayos G, Yeoh TK, et al. Dissociation between exertional symptoms and circulatory function in patients with heart failure. Circulation 1995; 92:47–53.
37. Gift AG. Clinical measurement of dyspnea. Dimensions Crit Care Nurs 1989; 8:210–216.
38. Stark RD, Gambles SA, Chatterjee SS. An exercise test to assess clinical dyspnea: estimation of reproducibility and sensitivity. Br J Dis Chest 1982; 76:269–278.
39. Dhand R, Kalra S, Malik SK. Use of visual analogue scales for assessment of the severity of asthma. Respiration 1988; 54:255–262.
40. Aitken RCB. Measurement of feelings using visual analogue scales. Proc R Soc Med 1969; 62:989–993.
41. Gift AG. Validation of a vertical visual analogue scale as a measure of clinical dyspnea. Am Rev Respir Dis 1986; 133:A163.
42. Scott J, Huskisson EC. Vertical or horizontal visual analogue scales. Ann Rheum Dis 1979; 38:560.
43. Guyatt GH, Townsend M, Berman LB, et al. A comparison of Likert and visual analogue scales for measuring change in function. J Chronic Dis 1987; 40:1129–1133.
44. Wilcock A, Corcoran R, Tattersfield AE. Safety and efficacy of nebulized lignocaine in patients with cancer and breathlessness. Palliat Med 1994; 8:35–38.
45. van der Molen B. Dyspnea: a study of measurement instruments for the assessment of dyspnoea and their application for patients with advanced cancer. J Adv Nurs 1995; 22:948–956.
46. Killian KJ. Assessment of dyspnea. Eur Respir J 1988; 1:195–197.
47. Borg GAV. Psychophysical basis of perceived exertion. Med Sci Sports Exerc 1982; 14:377–381.
48. Burdon J, Juniper E, Killian K, et al. The perception of breathlessness. Am Rev Respir Dis 1982; 126:825–828.
49. Wolkove N, Dajczman E, Colacone A, et al. The relationship between pulmonary function and dyspnea in obstructive lung disease. Chest 1989; 96:1247–1251.
50. O'Donnell DE, Lam M, Webb KA. Measurement of symptoms, lung hyperinflation, and endurance during exercise in chronic obstructive pulmonary disease. Am J Respir Crit Care Med 1998; 158:1557–1565.

51. Wilson RC, Jones PW. A comparison of the visual analogue scale and modified Borg scale for the measurement of dyspnea during exercise. Clin Sci (Colch) 1989; 76: 277–282.
52. McGavin CR, Artvinli M, Naoe H, et al. Dyspnea, disability and distance walked: comparison of estimates of exercise performance in respiratory disease. BMJ 1978; 2:241–243.
53. Mahler DA, Wells CK. Evaluation of clinical methods for rating dyspnea. Chest 1988; 93:580–586.
54. Fletcher CM, Elmes PC, Wood CH. The significance of respiratory symptoms and the diagnosis of chronic bronchitis in a working population. BMJ 1959; 1: 257–266.
55. Fairbarin A, Wood C, Fletcher C. Variability in answers to a questionnaire on respiratory symptoms. Br J Prev Soc Med 1959; 13:175–193.
56. Mahler DA, Rosiello RA, Harver A, et al. Comparison of clinical dyspnea ratings and psychophysical measurements of respiratory sensation in obstructive airway disease. Am Rev Respir Dis 1987; 135:1229–1233.
57. Mahler DA, Harver A, Rosiello RA, et al. Measurement of respiratory sensation in interstitial lung disease. Chest 1989; 96:767–771.
58. Wilcock A, Crosby V, Clarke D, et al. Reading numbers aloud: a measure of the limiting effect of breathlessness in patients with cancer. Thorax 1999; 54: 1099–1103.
59. Mahler DA, Weinberg DH, Wells CK, et al. The measurement of dyspnea: contents, interobserver agreement, and physiologic correlates of two new clinical indexes. Chest 1984; 85:751–758.
60. McCord M, Cronin-Stubbs D. Operationalizing dyspnea: focus on measurement. Heart Lung 1992; 21:167–179.
61. Mahler DA, Faryniarz K, Tomlinson D, et al. Impact of dyspnea and physiologic function on general health status in patients with chronic obstructive pulmonary disease. Chest 1992; 102:395–401.
62. Mahler DA, Matthay RA, Snyder PE, et al. Sustained-release theophylline reduces dyspnea in nonreversible obstructive airway disease. Am Rev Respir Dis 1985; 131:22–25.
63. Harver A, Mahler DA, Daubenspeck JA. Targeted inspiratory muscle training improves respiratory muscle function and reduces dyspnea in patients with chronic obstructive pulmonary disease. Ann Intern Med 1989; 111:117–124.
64. Eakin EG, Kaplan RM, Ries AL. Measurement of dypsnoea in chronic obstructive pulmonary disease. Qual Life Res 1993; 2:181–191.
65. Tanaka K, Akechi T, Okuyama T, et al. Development and validation of the Cancer Dyspnoea Scale: a multidimensional, brief, self-rating scale. Br J Cancer 2000; 82:800–805.
66. Jones PW. Dyspnea and quality of life in chronic obstructive pulmonary disease. In: Mahler D, ed. Dyspnea. New York: Marcel Dekker, 1998:199–220.
67. Mahler DA, Jones PW. Measurement of dyspnea and quality of life in advanced lung disease. Clin Chest Med 1997; 18:457–469.
68. Hajiro T, Nishimura K, Tsukino M, et al. Comparison of discriminative properties among disease-specific questionnaires for measuring health-related quality of life in patients with chronic obstructive pulmonary disease. Am J Respir Crit Care Med 1998; 157:785–790.

69. Harper R, Brazier JE, Waterhouse JC, et al. Comparison of outcome measures for patients with chronic obstructive pulmonary disease (COPD) in an outpatient setting. Thorax 1997; 52:879–887.

70. Guyatt GH, Berman L, Townsend M, et al. A measure of quality of life for clinical trials in chronic lung disease. Thorax 1987; 42:773–778.

71. Guyatt GH, Townsend M, Pugsley S. Bronchodilators in chronic airflow limitation: effect on airway function, exercise capacity, and quality of life. Am Rev Respir Dis 1987; 135:1069–1074.

72. van den Boom G, Rutten-van Molken MP, Tirimanna PRS, et al. Association between health-related quality of life and consultation for respiratory symptoms: results from the DIMCA program. Eur Respir J 1998; 11:67–72.

73. Jones PW, Quirk FH, Baveystock CM, et al. A self-complete measure of health status for chronic airflow limitation. The St. George's Respiratory Questionnaire. Am Rev Respir Dis 1992; 145:1321–1327.

74. Ferrer M, Alonso J, Morera J, et al. Chronic obstructive pulmonary disease stage and health-related quality of life. The Quality of Life of Chronic Obstructive Pulmonary Disease Study Group. Ann Intern Med 1997; 127:1072–1079.

75. Tu SP, McDonell MB, Spertus JA, et al. A new self-administered questionnaire to monitor health-related quality of life in patients with COPD. Ambulatory Care Quality Improvement Project (ACQUIP) investigators. Chest 1997; 112:614–622.

76. Hollen PJ, Gralla RJ, Kris MG, et al. Quality of life assessment in individuals with lung cancer: testing the Lung Cancer Symptom Scale (LCSS). Eur J Cancer 1993; 29A:S51–S58.

77. Hollen PJ, Gralla RJ. Comparison of instruments for measuring quality of life in patients with lung cancer. Semin Oncol 1996; 23:31–40.

78. Lutz ST, Huang DT, Ferguson CL, et al. A retrospective quality of life analysis using the Lung Cancer Symptom Scale in patients treated with palliative radiotherapy for advanced nonsmall cell lung cancer. Int J Radiat Oncol Biol Phys 1997; 37: 117–122.

79. Aaronson NK, Ahmedzai S, Bergman B. The European Organization for Research and Treatment of Cancer QLQ-C30: a quality-of-life instrument for use in international clinical trials in oncology. J Natl Cancer Inst 1993; 85:365–376.

80. Bergman B, Aaronson NK, Ahmedzai S. The EORTC QLQ-LC13: a modular supplement to the EORTC core quality of life questionnaire (QLQ-C30) for use in lung cancer clinical trials. Eur J Cancer 1994; 30A:635–642.

81. Cella DF, Bonomi AE, Lloyd SR, et al. Reliability and validity of the Functional Assessment of Cancer Therapy—Lung (FACT-L) quality of life instrument. Lung Cancer 1995; 12:199–220.

7

Research into Nonpharmacological Intervention for Respiratory Problems in Palliative Care

JESSICA CORNER

Research into nonpharmacological interventions for respiratory problems in palliative care could not as yet be described as a solid, coherent area of study. It is only comparatively recently that the symptom of breathlessness in the context of life-threatening illness has received significant, or indeed any, attention. In part, this reflects the situation with many symptoms or problems that are difficult or intractable. In general, little research has been conducted that tests or compares approaches to the array of problems experienced by people in palliative care settings. With the exception of pain management, where there is a well-developed research tradition, an accumulation of studies, and strong theoretical work, there are few areas where there is substantial knowledge on symptom management. The palliative care research community has also been slow to acknowledge the prevalence of respiratory problems among patients or that the symptom of breathlessness warrants significant theoretical or clinical attention. There has also been an unconscious sense that little can be done for breathlessness, and few clinicians have a background in respiratory medicine or respiratory physiology and, therefore, may feel ill-equipped to undertake serious research in the area. Fortunately, this situation is changing; there has been an upsurge in interest in the problem of breathlessness, and work into various aspects of its management is beginning.

The term *nonpharmacological intervention* suggests a narrow and tightly defined approach to symptom management that can be tested in clinical trials. Here, I will use it to define a research area that lies beyond that of testing different pharmaceutical preparations on perception of breathlessness and lung function. The notion of nonpharmacological intervention derives from a broader approach to symptom management that suggests not only the need to understand symptoms as the manifestation of disease but also the problems that arise from experiencing symptoms, the meanings symptoms engender, and the facets of life that are lost or interfered with as a result. Approaching symptoms from this perspective entails acknowledging that the problems that arise from illness cannot be neatly packaged or delineated. Advanced disease can cause an array of problems, such as pain, fatigue, anxiety, breathlessness, and more besides; often, these may be manifested as a broad constellation of distressing and interrelated problems, often indistinguishable from each other.[1] Thus, the area I describe is the nature of breathlessness as it is experienced in life-threatening illness, as well as the development and testing of strategies that may assist in alleviation or adaptation. This definition immediately suggests research that may need to straddle a number of disciplines as well as methodological paradigms.

In drawing together "the state of the art" in research, one must identify studies collated from a fragmentary array of work undertaken across a range of respiratory disorders. Some is from research into "normal" respiratory physiology where very significant and careful work exists and yields insight into the problem of breathlessness. Useful studies have also been undertaken outside the context of palliative care, where the goals of research and of intervention are somewhat different.

The Problem of Breathlessness

Little is known about the experience of breathlessness and the precise mechanisms that result in the sensation. A common definition of the symptom is "an uncomfortable awareness of the need to breathe."[2] Physiological studies of healthy volunteers exposed to different stimuli or respiratory loads reveal substantial variation in the level at which individuals experience discomfort and that the sensation of breathlessness does not necessarily result from a simple increase in the rate of ventilation, which in general is well tolerated. The level at which breathlessness is reported tends to be consistent within individuals but varies between them and is not related to physical characteristics.[2] Individuals made breathless by performing different tasks also use different words and phrases to describe the sensation.[3] Further, a large increase in ventilation may go unnoticed; yet if ventilation is already at a high rate, a relatively small increase is noticed and can cause distress.[4] These studies reveal a complex and distressing sensation, uniquely experienced and largely unrelated to physical characteristics or burden of disease.

The results of studies on healthy individuals should not be automatically extrapolated to individuals with cancer or respiratory illness. They do, however, reflect the apparent variability among patients with restricted lung function when reporting breathlessness and that relatively small changes in a patient's condition can render their respiratory problems intolerable even though previously they may have been coping well.

Patients with different respiratory conditions report different types of sensation and use multiple descriptors for their breathlessness simultaneously (Table 7.1).[3,5,6] This suggests that the symptom is caused by multiple factors and may not be explained by a single physiological mechanism; it also may be experienced quite differently among individuals.[3,7]

As well as being experienced by patients with chronic respiratory disorders and cardiopulmonary disease, breathlessness is common among cancer patients. Reuben and Mor's[8] analysis of the U.S. National Hospice Study revealed that over 70% of patients who were terminally ill suffered from breathlessness in the last 6 weeks of life; only eating problems and pain exceeded the incidence of breathlessness. Over 80% of patients with cancer of the lung experience breathlessness at some time.[9] Studies also indicate that breathlessness can be difficult to alleviate and often intractable; for example, a study of the last weeks of life among patients with cancer has shown that, despite the intervention of a specialist palliative care support team, breathlessness worsened as death approached.[10]

There are few data on the nature of breathlessness among patients with cancer; however, a recent study found that cancer in the lungs, anxiety, and reduced maximal inspiratory pressure correlated with a greater reported intensity of breathlessness.[11] In addition to physical influences on the sensation of breathlessness, there may be a variety of other factors that precipitate or exacerbate breathlessness; for example, emotions such as anger and anxiety often accompany the symptom, as do fatigue or tiredness.[12,13]

Studies of patients with chronic pulmonary disease reveal the disability caused by long-term breathlessness: patients experience a gradual decline in their functional ability. Over a prolonged period of time, this results in loss of social roles, isolation, and financial hardship.[14,15] Patients experiencing breathlessness associated with lung cancer report severe limitations in activity, poor concentration, memory loss, fear, anxiety, depression, and social isolation.[12,13] There is also evidence suggesting an important emotional component to breathing disorders and to breathlessness.[16]

Nonpharmacological Interventions for Breathlessness

Interventions for breathlessness have been evaluated, although little work has been conducted within the field of specialist palliative care. In chronic pulmonary disease, nonpharmacolgcial intervention includes pulmonary rehabilitation, changing patterns of breathing, teaching optimal use of bronchodilator therapy, and improving the clearance of bronchial secretions and the use of oxygen.[17] The benefits of pulmonary rehabilitation using exercise therapy have been established.[18] Studies have also evaluated the use of relaxation and psychological support.[19,20] Little information exists about how these techniques might be extrapolated into the palliation of patients with far-advanced disease or

Table 7.1. Respiratory sensations associated with various conditions

Sensation	Chronic obstructive pulmonary disease	Congestive heart failure	Interstitial lung disease	Asthma	Neuromuscular and chest wall disease	Pregnancy	Pulmonary vascular disease
Rapid breathing		X					X
Incomplete exhalation				X			
Shallow breathing				X	X		
Increased work or effort	X		X	X	X		
Feeling of suffocation	X	X					
Air hunger	X	X				X	
Chest tightness				X			
Heavy breathing				X			

Source: Manning and Schwartzstein.[6]

who are dying or about the particular uses of these for patients with advanced cancer.

For patients with advanced cancer, two randomized controlled trials evaluating nursing intervention using an integrated approach of addressing fears and concerns, breathing re-training, and facilitation of adaptation and coping have demonstrated benefits;[21,22] one study evaluated the use of acupuncture,[23] and two studies have compared the use of oxygen with air in alleviating breathlessness.[24,25]

Goals for Research into Nonpharmacological Strategies for Managing Breathlessness

To progress the field of breathlessness management, much research is needed. There is little knowledge about breathlessness as it is experienced in imminently life-limiting conditions such as end-stage respiratory illness, cardiopulmonary disease, or cancer. In keeping with the broad definition of nonpharmacological approaches to the management of breathlessness, the goal for research must firstly be to develop a broad understanding of breathlessness, how it is experienced, and the feelings and problems it engenders. Also, detailed and careful studies of intervention approaches may involve comparisons between people with breathlessness arising from different disorders as well as between different intervention approaches. Goals for future research are shown in Table 7.2.

Research Methods and Approaches

Investigating prevalence

A series of studies have been undertaken to determine the extent of breathlessness among palliative care patients. These include case note reviews and interview studies either of patients themselves or of relatives to recall problems patients had in the weeks or months prior to death. Some studies have been devised with a specific focus on the symptom of breathlessness, and in others breathlessness is one among a checklist of problems under investigation. In general, studies using proxies (relatives or health professionals) to reveal information about symptoms correlate poorly with patients' own reports of symptoms and are therefore considered unreliable.[26–28] Case notes too are known to be a poor record of symptoms since they rely on health professionals consistently asking about symptoms such as breathlessness during patient assessments and accurately recording what was revealed. There is some evidence to suggest that patients do not necessarily report the symptom of breathlessness and that health professionals do not always ask about it routinely.[29] Because of these various results, prospective studies of symptoms experienced by patients are thought to be more reliable.

Table 7.2. Goals for future research into nonpharmacological intervention for breathlessness

---

- Carefully elaborate breathlessness as a problem, including triggers, mechanisms, and psychological, social, and functional sequelae.

- Delineate breathlessness associated with cancer of different sites and stages using techniques employed in research conducted on healthy volunteers and patients with chronic respiratory disorders, to compare similarities and differences.

- Delineate breathlessness in advanced/end-stage chronic respiratory and cardiopulmonary disease, making comparisons with patients who have earlier-stage disease or cancer.

- Evaluate the components of interventions used within pulmonary rehabilitation (for example, diaphragmatic breathing, breathing control, breathing exercises, relaxation, distraction techniques, functional adaptation, energy conservation, anxiety management, psychological support) so that these may be more fully understood and their relative values compared. Information is needed so that more detailed understanding may be developed of the various approaches that may be used and the circumstances where they are effective.

- Examine the use of oxygen therapy for cancer-related breathlessness, comparing oxygen with other techniques such as air, fans, and cold facial stimulation, using limitations to functional ability and costs as measures of outcome as well as ratings of breathlessness. Also, determine the indications for using oxygen therapy in relation to normal, marginal, and low partial pressure of oxygen, as well as in different respiratory disorders in the last weeks or days of life.

- Describe and evaluate psychotherapeutic approaches to the management of breathlessness, identifying patients who might benefit most from such approaches.

Eliciting experiences of breathlessness

Several studies have developed important insights into breathlessness by asking patients directly using qualitative interviews. These have either been tape-recorded, with transcripts analyzed subsequently, or recorded as detailed notes. These data have been used in rather different ways from data of other qualitative studies since it is unusual in qualitative research to acquire information about a physical problem. Qualitative data have been collected as part of studies using a combination of methods, which have allowed researchers to place data from structured outcome measures and lung function scores alongside patient case notes or patients' accounts of their symptom. Williams and Bury[30] for example, presented graded case studies where descriptions of patients' circumstances and illness history, as reported by them, were set against scores from formal measures. This technique reveals consistencies as well as differences between formal measures and patients' own accounts. Accounts from patients also reveal the broader consequences of respiratory illness, such as unemployment, disability, financial hardship, and isolation.

Qualitative studies have used content analysis (for example, O'Driscoll et al.[13]) or a more free-form thematic analysis. Data have also been used to yield important information about the factors that precipitate or exacerbate breathlessness and to develop an understanding of triggers for episodes of breathless-ness and the strategies patients adopt to deal with them. This kind of work suggests an important and fruitful avenue for developing a deeper understanding of the problem in future studies.

Bailey[31] and Plant et al.[32] used qualitative interviews with nurses to elicit information regarding the practice of breathlessness management. Bailey[31] interviewed myself and other nurse research-practitioners after we had spent some years developing a nonpharmacological approach to managing breathlessness in lung cancer, to articulate from an outsider's perspective what the nature of the work was and to examine how as nurses we were being therapeutic with patients. Plant et al.[32] conducted a similar study of specialist nurses who took part in a multicenter evaluation of breathlessness management in lung cancer. Data from the 13 nurses who took part reveal a number of issues about establishing nurse-led care for patients:

- Encountering resistance to innovative nursing practice
- Maintaining uniformity of practice within a diverse group of collaborating researchers
- Measuring well-being in the face of patients' deteriorating condition, the tension between the collaborators' nursing role
- The necessity of an ethically demanding research design as part of undertaking nursing research into using and evaluating nonpharmacological intervention

Selection of subjects

A weakness of studies is a lack of consistency in selecting patients for inclusion. There is no single, or working, definition used to identify whether a patient has breathlessness or not or how severe it is. For studies involving patients with chronic pulmonary disease, the diagnosis itself is most often used as eligibility since it is assumed that breathlessness is an inevitable part of the disease (for example, Gift et al.[19]). This assumption warrants careful exploration.

In studies of patients with cancer, entry criteria have been defined as "any degree of breathlessness or difficulty with breathing reported by the patient."[21,22] In these studies, patients' scores for breathlessness at its worst ranged from 1 to 10 on a 10-point visual analogue scale. Brown et al.[12] relied on patients referred by a physician because of breathlessness. Given the discrepancies between health professionals' assessments of patients' symptom and patients' self-reported symptoms, this seems to be an inadequate means of gathering a representative sample. Roberts et al.[29] relied on nurses to distribute a survey questionnaire designed to identify patients with breathlessness who might agree to take part in interviews. It seemed that nurses were reluctant to distribute the questionnaire and thereby identify patients who would be too unwell to participate; however, there was considerable interest among patients in taking part.

This again reflects the fact that health professionals may not reliably identify patients who may participate in studies since a large number of patients with breathlessness may be excluded for a wide variety of reasons and samples of patients gathered in this way may not be representative. Studies of patients with breathlessness associated with advanced cancer include a significant proportion who also have chronic respiratory illness or cardiac disease (for example, 44% in Booth et al.[25]).

In studies evaluating oxygen therapy for patients with cancer, where the object is to describe patterns of breathlessness severity and occurrence among defined groups, broad entry criteria are appropriate; however, greater specificity is probably warranted for studies testing and comparing interventions. Until more knowledge of the problem of breathlessness among different patient groups is acquired, such specificity will be difficult to determine.

Study designs for evaluating interventions

Evaluating intervention among severely ill or dying patients is difficult, and insufficient is known about the best study designs for use in these situations. Effective studies have been undertaken in laboratory conditions. For example, Booth et al.[25] administered oxygen or air, selected randomly, to consenting patients with cancer who had breathlessness. The gases were administered for 15 minutes from disguised cylinders at the patient's bedside, and assessments were made of the patient's breathlessness using a 100 mm vertical visual analogue scale and the modified Borg scale;[33] arterial oxygen saturation was also assessed using a pulse oximeter with a finger probe transducer. Studies that can be designed to evaluate or compare interventions over a short time scale have many advantages in the palliative care setting since the problem of attrition from the study due to patients deteriorating or dying can be avoided. This kind of study is also relatively undemanding regarding time and the commitment demanded from patients who participate, as well as allowing the researcher a degree of control over extraneous variables. Similar studies testing well-defined and focused questions regarding the management of breathlessness could be designed. It is also noteworthy that the Booth et al.[25] study involved a team of researchers that included expertise in the study of respiratory physiology.

My own research into intervention for breathlessness was more complex since the intervention involved a rehabilitative approach over a period of 4 to 8 weeks with lung cancer patients whose prognosis was poor. Our studies, in contrast to those of Booth et al.,[25] evaluated a management approach which took the form of a nursing clinic, rather than a specific, single intervention. The approach was evaluated using a randomized clinical trial. In the first, a pilot study,[21] patients who consented to take part were allocated to either attend the nursing clinic or to be followed as a control. After randomization and once patients knew which group they had drawn, patients were asked whether they were still happy to take part in the study. Patients attended the clinic, and outcomes were assessed for both intervention and control groups at baseline, 4 weeks, and 3 months. There was considerable attrition from the study, 41% withdrawing due to illness progression or death; however, significant differences were observed in changes in breathlessness scores and in measures of functional ability. The results showed improvements for those who had attended the nursing clinic compared with static or worsening scores for the controls. To overcome the problem of analyzing serial measures in small samples, the data were presented so that scores for key variables for each subject could be scrutinized.

Following the success of the first study, we designed a second study to determine whether these results could be replicated among a larger sample. Nurses established similar clinics in six U.K. centers and evaluated the outcomes for patients. To overcome some of the difficulties of sample attrition, the study was shortened so that outcomes were assessed at 8 weeks, rather than 3 months, and 119 patients were recruited.[22] Again, sample attrition was a problem. Sixteen patients died during the study, and 28 withdrew. Since the major reason for withdrawal was deterioration of the condition, more patients withdrew from the control than the intervention group (13 controls compared to three in the intervention group), and survival was significantly worse in patients withdrawing from the control arm than the intervention arm. All patients who withdrew for reasons other than improvement in their condition were assumed to have a poor outcome relative to all patients, and the data were analyzed using a method recommended by Gould.[34] Patients were allocated a change score that was one more than the maximum (that is worse) of the patients who did not withdraw; similarly, patients who withdrew because they were too well to continue were given a score one less than the minimum score of the patients who did not withdraw. This allowed scores for patients who withdrew to be included in the analysis and reduced bias in the results due to withdrawal. Results from this analysis indicated significantly greater improvement in patients attending for nursing interventions in visual analogue scale scores, World Health Organization performance status, Hospital Anxiety and Depression Scale, depression scores, and physical symptoms scored on the Rotterdam Symptom Checklist. This method of analysis might be valuable in other similar studies conducted with patients in palliative care settings where there is substantial withdrawal and where it might otherwise be difficult to complete meaningful studies.

Single-group, before–after study designs have been used to evaluate nonpharmacological interventions. Filshie et al.[23] evaluated acupuncture by measuring pulse, respiratory rate, oxygen saturation, and patient-rated visual analogue scale scores of breathlessness, pain, anxiety, and depression before and on eight occasions from 5 minutes to 24 hours after acupuncture needle insertion. This study, while intended only as a pilot evaluation, is flawed by the lack of a comparison group and by the fact that a nurse observer remained with the patient for the first 90 minutes following acupuncture, it is difficult to be certain that these substantial reductions in patient-rated breathlessness, pain, and anxiety were recorded, however were due to acupuncture rather than the reassuring presence of the nurse observer.

Table 7.3. Criteria for studies selected for a meta-analysis of respiratory rehabilitation in chronic obstructive pulmonary disease (COPD)

- *Population*: >90% of patients with clinical diagnosis of COPD and a ratio of FEV_1 to FVC of <0.7

- *Rehabilitation program*: inpatient or outpatient therapy of at least 4 weeks' duration that included exercise therapy with any form of education and psychological support for patients with exercise limitation attributable to COPD

- *Primary outcome measures*: maximum or functional exercise capacity, quality of life, or both

- *Methodological criteria*: randomized controlled trials comparing rehabilitation with conventional community care, randomization expected to be concealed and assessment of outcomes blinded

---

Sufficient studies have been conducted into the effectiveness of respiratory rehabilitation in chronic obstructive pulmonary disease to enable Lacasse et al.[18] to conduct a meta-analysis. Criteria for inclusion of the 14 studies into the meta-analysis are shown in Table 7.3. To conduct a meta-analysis, studies need to be sufficiently rigorous and uniform in design to make data pooling and comparison meaningful. These methodological criteria suggest that standard study designs should be adopted in intervention studies of nonpharmacological interventions for breathlessness in the future since, unless there is such uniformity in design, it may be difficult to evaluate the body of work using structured techniques such as meta-analysis.

Measures of outcome

Numerous measures of outcome exist, and studies use a whole array of these. Given that breathlessness is a multifaceted problem to which physical, psychological, functional, and social factors contribute, outcomes should be assessed in each of these domains. Like pain, breathlessness is first and foremost a subjective experience, so self-ratings of perceived severity are important. This is most often assessed using 100 mm visual analogue scales, although these are used in both horizontal and vertical forms and with different verbal descriptors as anchors. Patients do not always find visual analogue scales easy to complete, and this difficulty is occasionally the reason for noncompliance or withdrawal (for example, four patients withdrew from the study of Booth et al.[25] because they were unable to complete study measures). Physiological indices of breathlessness, such as pulmonary function tests [forced expiratory volume in 1 second (FEV_1), forced vital capacity (FVC), etc.] are not closely associated with self-reported measures of breathlessness, nor is oxygen saturation. Although these provide useful information, they are not accurate indicators of symptom perception. Standard measures of function and quality of life have been designed for specific patient groups; for example, the Rotterdam Symptom Checklist and the World Health Organization Performance Status assessment were used by Bredin et al.[22]

These are designed for use with cancer patients. Measures used in the studies included in Lacasse et al.'s[18] meta-analysis include the Profile of Mood State, the chronic respiratory disease questionnaire, the Lubin Depression Adjective Checklist, the Eysenck Personality Questionnaire, and the Bandura Scale of Well-being. The range of measures used suggests a lack of consensus over the best methods of assessing outcomes of intervention.

The Future

Nonpharmacological management of respiratory symptoms is a relatively new field in palliative care; therefore, research is at an early stage of development. Studies to date indicate that intervention may have great potential in assisting patients to cope with the distressing and disabling symptom of breathlessness. Much information is needed to enhance our understanding of breathlessness and how it is manifested among patients with different conditions and at different stages of illness.

References

1. Corner J, Dunlop R. New approaches to care. In: Clark D, Ahmedzai S, Hockley J, eds. New Themes in Palliative Care. Buckingham, UK: Open University Press, 1997.
2. Adams L, Chronos N, Lane R, et al. The measurement of breathlessness induced in normal subjects: validity of two scaling techniques. Clin Sci (Colch) 1985; 69:7–16.
3. Simon P, Schwartzstein R, Weiss J, et al. Distinguishable types of dyspnea in patients with shortness of breath. Am Rev Respir Dis 1990; 2:1009–1014.
4. West D, Ellis C, Campbell E. Ability of man to detect increases in his breathing. J Appl Physiol 1975; 39:372–376.
5. Elliott MW, Adams L, Cockcroft A, et al. The language of breathlessness: use of verbal descriptors by patients with cardiopulmonary disease. Am Rev Respir Dis 1991; 144:826–832.
6. Manning HL, Schwartzstein RM. Pathophysiology of dyspnea. N Engl J Med 1995; 333:1547–1553.
7. Skevington S, Pilaar M, Routh D, et al. On the language of breathlessness. Psychol Health 1996; 12(5):677–689.
8. Reuben D, Mor V. Dyspnea in terminally ill cancer patients. Chest 1986; 89:234–237.
9. Muers M. Palliation of symptoms in non-small cell lung cancer: a study by the Yorkshire Regional Cancer Organization Thoracic Group. Thorax 1993; 48:339–343.
10. Higginson I, McCarthy M. Measuring symptoms in terminal cancer: are pain and dyspnea controlled? J R Soc Med 1989; 82:264–267.
11. Bruera E, Schmitz B, Pither J, et al. The frequency and correlates of dyspnea in patients with advanced cancer. J Pain Symptom Manage 2000; 19:357–362.
12. Brown M, Carrieri V, Janson-Bjerklie S, et al. Lung cancer and dyspnea: the patient's perspective. Oncol Nurs Forum 1986; 13:19–24.

13. O'Driscoll M, Corner J, Bailey C. The experience of breathlessness in lung cancer. Eur J Cancer Care 1999; 8:37–43.

14. Williams S. Chronic Respiratory Illness. London: Routledge, 1993.

15. Skilbeck J, Mott L, Smith D, et al. Nursing care for people dying from chronic obstructive airways disease. Int J Palliat Nurs 1997; 3:100–106.

16. Bass C, Gardner W. Emotional influences on breathing and breathlessness. J Psychosom Res 1985; 29:599–609.

17. Janssens JP, deMuralt B, Titelion V. Management of severe chronic obstructive pulmonary disease. J Pain Symptom Manage 2000; 19:378–392.

18. Lacasse H, Wong E, Guyatt GH, et al. Meta-analysis of respiratory rehabilitation in chronic obstructive pulmonary disease. Lancet 1996; 346:1115–1119.

19. Gift A, Moore T, Soeken K. Relaxation to reduce dyspnea and anxiety in COPD patients. Nurs Res 1992; 41:242–246.

20. Rosser R, Denford J, Heslop A, et al. Breathlessness and psychiatric morbidity in chronic bronchitis and emphysema: a study of psychotherapeutic management. Psychol Med 1983; 13:93–110.

21. Corner J. Non-pharmacological intervention for breathlessness in lung cancer. Palliat Med 1996; 10:299–305.

22. Bredin M, Corner J, Krishnasamy M, et al. Multicentre randomised controlled trial of nursing intervention for breathlessness in patients with lung cancer. BMJ 1999; 318:901–904.

23. Filshie J, Penn K, Ashley S, et al. Acupuncture for the relief of cancer-related breathlessness. Palliat Med 1996; 10:145–150.

24. Bruera E, de Stoutz N, Velasco-Leiva A, et al. Effects of oxygen on dyspnoea in hypoxaemic terminal-cancer patients. Lancet 1993; 342:13–14.

25. Booth S, Kelly M, Cox N, et al. Does oxygen help dyspnea in patients with cancer? Am J Respir Crit Care Med 1996; 153:1515–1518.

26. Jennings BM, Muhlempkemp AF. Systematic misperception: oncology patients' self-reported affective states and their care-givers' perceptions. Cancer Nurs 1981; 6:485–489.

27. Hinton J. How reliable are relatives' retrospective reports of terminal illness? Patients' and relatives' accounts compared. Soc Sci Med 1996; 43:1229–1236.

28. Holmes S, Edburn E. Patients' and nurses' perceptions of symptom distress in cancer. J Adv Nurs 1989; 14:840–846.

29. Roberts D, Thorne S, Pearson C. The experience of dyspnea in late stage cancer. Cancer Nurs 1993; 16:310–320.

30. Williams S, Bury M. "Breathtaking:" the consequences of chronic respiratory disorder. Int Disabil Stud 1989; 11:114–120.

31. Bailey C. Nursing as therapy in the management of breathlessness in lung cancer. Eur J Cancer Care 1995; 4:184–190.

32. Plant H, Bredin M, Corner J. Working with resistance, tension and objectivity: conducting a randomised controlled trial of a nursing intervention for breathlessness. Nursing Times Research 2000; 5:426–433.

33. Burdon JWW, Juniper EF, Killian KJ, et al. The perception of breathlessness in asthma. Am Rev Respir Dis 1982; 137:1285–1288.

34. Gould AL. A new approach to the analysis of clinical drug trials with withdrawals. Biometrics 1980; 36:721–727.

IV

RESEARCH IN
FATIGUE/ASTHENIA

8

Studying Nonpharmacological Interventions for Fatigue

SIMON C. WESSELY

Many doctors are frustrated by the problem of chronic fatigue. Over the years, numerous attempts have been made to measure it,[1,2] but this has always proved elusive. There are certain circumstances, such as myasthenia gravis, in which our pathological understanding of the nature of fatigue might well be reflected directly in patient complaints (although I am unaware if even this has been formally tested); but in general, this is not the case. At the risk of overgeneralizing, fatigue is better conceptualized as a subjective feeling, with only weak correlations with objective measures of muscle or neuropsychological function but stronger links to measures of affect, inactivity, and general psychological distress.[2] "Feeling tired does not necessarily correlate with physiological impairment, nor with reduced efficiency in work output or other kinds of human performance,"[3] while "level of physical disability cannot be objectively predicted from any putative measure of fatigue."[4] Recent work in the cancer field[5,6] confirms what has been established in many other settings: measures of neuromuscular or neuropsychological fatigability provide only limited information on subjective fatigue and can mislead as often as inform. Although there may be some exceptions, such as the suggestion of a specific interferon-α induced neuromuscular fatigue,[7] the overall picture of fatigue in cancer is multidimensional,[8,9] with effects on physical, cognitive, and emotional function.[2] Other contributors to this volume will discuss in more detail the measurement of subjective fatigue.

Why Is Fatigue Important?

It would be tedious to document all of the studies that draw attention to the high prevalence of fatigue in patients with cancer and/or terminal illness; it would be easier to point out that I know of no exceptions. Even when self-reported fatigue is apparently not a prominent complaint, this may be because patients have come to regard it as "normal."[10] It would be equally tedious to list all of the studies that document the impact fatigue has on quality of life and enjoyment.[11]

Nevertheless, even if patients are in little doubt about the importance of fatigue, the same is not always the case of their doctors. Outside the cancer literature, there is a discrepancy between the importance placed by doctors and patients on the symptom of fatigue. Dohrenwend and Crandell[12] used instruments derived from the Midtown Manhattan study, a classic piece of psychiatric epidemiology, to study professional and nonprofessional attitudes to common symptoms. Doctors and patients were found to regard different symptoms with differing degrees of concern. "Feeling weak all over for much of the time" was regarded as "very serious" by only 6% of psychiatrists and 9% of physicians, making it one of the least important of 43 listed symptoms.[12] In contrast, the same symptom was one of the most important listed by nonprofessional samples. These differences are understandable: doctors, aware of the nonspecificity of fatigue, focus more on specific complaints, such as hemoptysis or self-harm. However, patients experience it as disabling, distressing, and perhaps of sinister significance.

Something similar has been shown in the cancer literature: oncologists rate pain as of more significance than fatigue, but patients were substantially more likely to report the converse.[13] Even families may underestimate the impact of fatigue,[14] although again the literature is a little conflicting on this issue.[15] The fact that, as others have noted, the majority of papers on fatigue in cancer are contained in the nursing literature may be an indicator of the relative lack of importance traditionally ascribed to the topic by doctors.[8] It may be for this reason that in practice most patients receive little if any intervention with the sole purpose of reducing fatigue. Only one-quarter of a representative sample of cancer patients in the United States reported that their oncologists had recommended any treatment for fatigue.[13]

However, the good news is that this situation is changing. "A consensus is emerging among patients, caregivers, and oncologists that cancer-related fatigue is the most important untreated symptom in cancer today."[16]

How Do We Understand Fatigue?

A series of studies on a variety of illnesses confirm that fatigue in physical illness not only is a multidimensional concept but it also has multifactorial causes.[17] The editors of this volume would rebel if I listed the number of reviews that point out the multifactorial nature of fatigue in cancer and palliative care. I will take it for granted that the readership already acknowledges the contributions made by adrenal insufficiency, anemia, malnutrition, chemotherapy, depression, cytokines, immobility, pain, sleep deprivation, and so on. Even apparently simple links, such as those between anemia and fatigue, are, in practice, less straight-forward. For example, as one might predict, there is a link between hemoglobin levels and measures of subjective energy during acute chemotherapy,[18] but this has not been found in the general population and perhaps postchemotherapy patients.[19]

Fatigue thus occurs because of factors related to the person who has the cancer, the cancer itself, and the treatment given for that cancer.[17] In general, treatment effects, like so much else, are rather nonspecific. Numerous studies attest to the importance of fatigue during acute treatment, such as radiotherapy.[20–22] However, what do we make of the long-term outcome in terms of symptoms after the end of active treatment? Controlled studies clearly document that fatigue remains a problem even many years later, as in the survivors of childhood malignancy.[23,24] The Tampa group has published a series of carefully controlled studies of women with breast cancer an average of 16 to 22 months after the end of treatment. The results confirm the contribution to fatigue made by bone marrow transplantation[25] and chemotherapy[26] but, perhaps surprisingly, not radiotherapy.[27] Indeed, recent studies that incorporate population controls show that fatigue in cancer patients postradiotherapy does not differ to any substantial degree, either quantitatively or qualitatively, from fatigue in the normal population,[28] although there are dissenting opinions.[29] This does not, however, downplay the importance of fatigue in cancer patients; instead, it draws further attention to the public health impact of fatigue in both cancer and noncancer populations.[2]

Causes of Fatigue in Cancer Patients

I will also assume that most people accept that not only are there several causes of fatigue in cancer patients (Table 8.1) but that these also interact. We have recently suggested that a general model can be developed to understand fatigue in physical illness and that, as a rule, unique mechanisms for fatigue, which have

Table 8.1. Causes of fatigue in cancer patients

Anemia
Anxiety
Chemotherapy
Cytokines
Depression
Emesis
Inactivity
Malnutrition
Radiotherapy
Sleep disturbance

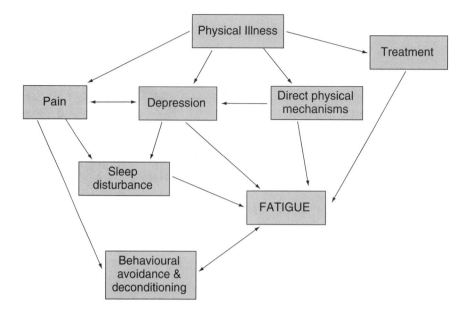

Figure 8.1. Integrated scheme of potential mechanisms between physical illness and fatigue (From Wessely et al.[2] with permission).

been proposed for various conditions such as cholestasis, multiple sclerosis, Parkinson's disease, and many others, are less important than general, multifactorial models. The predictors of fatigue among the many physical illnesses in which it has been studied show more overlaps than differences (Fig. 8.1).[2] For example, rather than stating the number of studies that show a strong association between fatigue and depression, again, it is simpler to state that I know of no exceptions, whether in physically ill or well subjects. Hence, depression is an association of fatigue irrespective of context.

Is there something special about fatigue in cancer and palliative care? If this were true, then we would be unable to generalize or learn from either the considerable literature on fatigue in other physical disorders[2] or the rapidly expanding literature on "pure" fatigue syndromes.[2] However, at the risk of simplification, I believe that there is much to learn from the noncancer data. Just as there is little that fundamentally distinguishes how we understand, and in an ideal world how we treat, malignant and nonmalignant pain,[30] I suspect the same is true of chronic fatigue; and evidence is steadily accumulating in support of this proposition.[24,28] There are specific processes involved, for example, anemia, which can be reversed by the administration of erythropoietin with consequent benefits for fatigue. However, these must be seen in the context of the multifactorial nature of chronic fatigue, in which threads common to both cancer-related and non-cancer-related fatigue can be discerned. Note the emphasis placed on *chronic*: everything that we know about fatigue points to the important distinction between acute and chronic fatigue. Some of the discrepancies between, for example, my interpretation of our knowledge on the nature and management of fatigue and that of Portenoy (see Chapter 10) may be understood by my emphasis on the treatment of chronic fatigue, fatigue that persists after the original stimulus has ended, and his on acute fatigue as may emerge during palliative care.

Why Do We Need Nonpharmacological Treatments?

There are already general interventions used to manage fatigue, the treatment of anemia or malnutrition, for example. High-dose steroids are frequently used to provide symptomatic improvement of fatigue. Also, specific antifatigue interventions may be developed. If fatigue is indeed related to levels of certain cytokines, such as interleukin-1, then targeted interventions to reduce those cytokines could be of benefit. However, this is for the future. At present, management of fatigue is more likely to be general than specific. In particular, nonpharmacological management of fatigue revolves around the treatment of inactivity and/or mood disorder.

What Kind of Interventions Are We Talking About, and Do They Work?

Nondirective psychotherapies

Nondirective psychotherapies covers any nonbehavioral, nondirective psychotherapies, such as interpersonal, psychodynamic, and counseling approaches, sometimes lumped together as the "talking therapies." All are intended to improve emotional distress. Some, such as psychoanalytic psychotherapy, are based on a complex model of emotional functioning, albeit unproven, while others, such as nondirective counseling, are rather less theoretical.

There are now several well-known studies on the efficacy of the newer psychotherapies in the management of psychological distress in cancer. These are well known and, as they are principally concerned with general psychological well-being and depression, outside the scope of this chapter. However, given the interactive model that we propose and the reciprocal link between depression and fatigue, one would predict that any intervention which improves depression would have a positive effect on fatigue or vigor as well; indeed, this proves to be the case in some,[31,32] but not all,[33] studies. Similarly, a study using a broad range of cognitive and behavioral interventions delivered via group therapy reported improvement in both mood and fatigue,[34] while a study of relaxation per se, rather than as part of a cognitive behavioral therapy package, found that it caused greater improvement of fatigue than education and counseling.[35]

Information, education, and support

The field of psycho-oncology is well ahead of many others in the provision of specific packages to patients including education and information about their illness, treatments, side effects, and other practical or supportive issues. Although there is ample evidence that cancer patients continue to lack adequate information about fatigue, there is little evidence about the utility of such measures at reducing fatigue.[36] One recent trial showed a significant impact of routine care and support from a breast care nurse on overall somatic distress, which includes fatigue.[37] Similar packages have been used to reduce anxiety and physical symptoms after operative procedures. Hann and colleagues[38] suggested that their empirical finding that fatigue after radiotherapy for breast cancer is no different in quantity or quality from "normal" fatigue might be incorporated into one such education program, as others have suggested for simple education packages designed to overcome the general expectation, not borne out by evidence, that major surgery inevitably leads to substantial fatigue.[39] Nevertheless, there is little compelling evidence that broad supportive, educational, or counseling interventions are effective at reducing fatigue in malignant disease and little theoretical reason to suspect that they should. Supportive therapy alone had no effect on measures of fatigue in one previously cited study of cancer patients.[34]

Exercise

When experiencing fatigue, nearly all patients, including those with cancer, make some attempt to deal with the symptom. This can take a variety of forms, such as taking a nutritional supplement, but most often involves some form of activity management. Recent surveys of patients undergoing chemotherapy or radiotherapy report that by far the most common strategy to deal with fatigue involves an alteration in activity and rest patterns, most usually rest, sleeping, or reducing activity levels.[22,40] The most common treatment option reported by American oncologists was "rest and relaxation," suggested by 68% of oncologists who reported any fatigue treatment option, in contrast to only 7% promoting exercise.[13]

Is this the best option? Almost certainly not. There is not the space to go into the adverse effects of rest as a way of coping with chronic fatigue. The physiological consequences on cardiac and neuromuscular function are too well known to bear repetition, as are the psychological effects, which include increased depression, helplessness, anxiety, increased sense of effort, and increased reluctance to engage in activity. Outside the cancer field, there is widespread acceptance of the dangers of promoting rest as a principle coping strategy for chronic fatigue.[41] The authors of the report finding that many oncologists recommend rest for chronic fatigue associated with cancer cautiously conclude that advising rest may be "problematic."[13] This author would abandon such caution.

Given that inactivity is such a potent cause of chronic fatigue, there is an overwhelming case for suggesting the opposite, exercise. In our review of the wider subject of fatigue in physical illness, we concluded that "apart from the overtraining syndrome and a few rare neuromuscular disorders, regular exercise is nearly always associated with improvements in fatigue."[2] In pure chronic fatigue syndrome, new trials have confirmed earlier reports on the benefits of exercise as effective, but there are problems with engagement and compliance.[42,43] What can we say about the cancer literature?

Assessing the evidence for the efficacy of exercise has been made easier by a recent systematic review that located 11 studies, of which nine were available for review.[44] All were restricted to breast cancer patients only. The results suggested improvements in physical functioning, physiological measures of fitness, and general measures of symptomatic fatigue and well-being. However, sample sizes were generally low, and only one included a comprehensive assessment of both physical and psychological measures.

Since publication of the systematic review, the literature has been expanded. Promising results were reported from a small randomized controlled trial of exercise in patients with early breast cancer.[45] A nonrandomized study suggested that aerobic exercise significantly improved physical performance of cancer patients after bone marrow transplantation.[46] The same group then reported a nonrandomized study of 16 patients who had completed high-dose chemotherapy.[47] Four out of 40 refused, but only 16 actually entered the trial because of problems of distance; those who lived too far away became the nonrandom controls. The intervention was pure exercise in the form of walking on a treadmill. There was a greater reduction in fatigue in the intervention group. No direct measures were made of physical fitness after therapy, but it is interesting that measures based on maximum heart rate achieved during exercise showed no change. Finally, the same group, who clearly do not show any evidence of research fatigue, performed a randomized (method of randomization not stated) study in which the cases were patients with solid tumors receiving high-dose chemotherapy followed by autologous peripheral blood stem cell transplantation and the intervention was use of an exercise bicycle.[48] Fatigue and psychological distress were significantly reduced.[49] The authors also reported fewer infection-related side effects in the intervention group and reduced use of analgesics. Again, the improvement was not related to simple measures of physical conditioning (maximum heart rate).[49]

Are there contraindications to exercise? In the above studies, the authors routinely screened for cardiac problems, such as an abnormal electrocardiogram, and excluded the occasional patient as a consequence. It is not clear whether this was because of the greater restrictions that operate in many clinical trials or a genuine concern. If the latter, this was probably misplaced. Even in the presence of active heart disease, modest exercise is not contraindicated; a seminal clinical trial clearly established its benefits even in uncontrolled heart failure.[50]

Thus far I have emphasized the similarities between fatigue associated with cancer and fatigue in other contexts. However, a possible difference between the chronic fatigue and cancer literatures lies in the relationship between exercise and fatigue. When chronically fatigued patients attending chronic fatigue syndrome (CFS) clinics attempt exercise, they often report a distinct lack of success. In the CFS literature, what is striking is how many patients report that exercise is one, if not the main, precipitant of their symptoms. Achieving compliance in exercise programs can be difficult[43] except in very controlled and monitored situations.[42] However, the reactions of cancer patients who chose to use exercise are different: cancer patients who report using exercise as a coping strategy for fatigue also report that it is effective,[51] and there are few reports from the controlled trials of any problems with compliance.

The lack of any clear correlation between actual physiological changes in exercise parameters and clinical improvement is not surprising. First, the amount of exercise prescribed in all of the studies was probably insufficient to promote a substantial change in physical fitness. Second, the authors report only a weak correlation between fatigue and maximal physical performance, in contrast to the strong correlation between fatigue and measures of depression, somatization, and anxiety;[6] the literature on fatigue and other physical illnesses is scattered with similar conclusions.[2] In the previously cited controlled trial of exercise in CFS, measures of physical fitness were not associated with overall outcome.[42] Some of the comments made by participants in one exercise study clearly suggest that at least part of the efficacy of treatment is related to increased self-esteem, control, and confidence: "I feel fit and proud of myself to be doing something positive. It helped show that I was not made useless by this disease or its treatment."[52]

Cognitive and behavioral therapies

If the benefits of exercise come not from its effect on measures of physical fitness but more via the agency of improved self-efficacy and confidence and decreased anxiety, might not the same effect be obtained without the necessity of a formal exercise program? Such is the aim of what is loosely labeled *cognitive behavioral therapy* (CBT), which in practice covers a range of interventions linked by underlying shared themes.

Cognitive behavioral therapies are popular, one might almost say trendy, psychologically based interventions focused on changing specific thoughts and/or behaviors linked with learning improved coping skills. It is a very broad area, ranging from purely cognitive interventions with proven efficacy in the management of depression, behavioral interventions that are the treatments of choice for phobias, and something in between which is rapidly becoming widely accepted as effective in the treatment of chronic pain and CFS.

The success of CBT depends on understanding the differences between factors that originally caused the symptom and those now responsible for its perpetuation. Treatment is directed at perpetuating, rather than precipitating, factors. It is also assumed that there are links between a patient's beliefs about the causes and nature of their symptoms and what they do in response. Thus, a patient may be avoiding activity because of fear that activity-induced symptoms mean physical harm. Finally, it is assumed that individuals are capable of active change and should be involved in collaborative approaches in which the emphasis is on changing thoughts, feelings, and behaviors. Treatment would look at alternative ways of managing symptoms in a collaborative and empirical fashion.

Contrary to the idea in certain circles, CBT is not restricted to, or even particularly effective in, illnesses with a "psychological" basis, whatever that may be, but instead simply assume that the level of functioning of the individual is not as good as it might be, given the context of their condition. Likewise, CBT does not involve suggesting that a patient's problems are psychological as opposed to physical; that would be not only impractical and inaccurate[52] but also unnecessary.[54]

Elements of CBT can be found in several of the interventions described whose primary objective is to improve psychological functioning; hence, Fawzy and colleagues[32] included not only stress management but also a package designed to enhance coping skills.

Another cognitive distortion is called *catastrophic thinking* or *catastrophizing*, a particular cognitive style that might be defined as "always thinking the very worst." Hence, a person with chronic low back pain who experiences further pain may be worried that this indicates a risk of permanent damage or have a mental image of a person in a wheelchair. This in turn provides justification for further avoidance of activity because of fear of further injury.[55] It has been linked with greater degrees of pain and greater disability in a variety of illnesses associated with chronic pain. Catastrophizing is also seen in CFS, where it is linked to disability.[56] None of this is particularly surprising, given that we already know from classic experimental manipulation studies that expectancy is a powerful predictor of fatigue in normal subjects.[2,3]

What about cancer? We already know that women with breast cancer whose chosen method of coping involves disengaging from their life situation, usually by behavioral but also cognitive avoidance, experience greater distress.[57] What about fatigue? Jacobsen and colleagues studied women with breast cancer[58] and developed a special inventory to measure cognitions relevant to fatigue ("I find myself expecting the worst when I am fatigued"). Greater use of catastrophizing was associated with fatigue that was more persistent and intense, as well as generally worse psychological symptoms and lower quality of life, as shown in chronic pain subjects. Indeed, the authors estimated that fatigue intensity was 2.6-fold higher in women scoring high on the measure.[58] Another interesting finding was that catastrophizing was commoner in younger patients, although this has not been found in low back pain samples.[55] Catastrophic cognitions are thus linked to behavioral disengagement, which in turn predicts greater fatigue both cross-sectionally and prospectively.[59] Catastrophic cognitions are a classic focus for cognitive therapy.

The importance of the cognitive dimension is again well illustrated in the CFS literature, and suggests a limitation to the scope of exercise interventions. In CFS, we know from both theory and controlled trials that exercise is beneficial;[42,60] however, the anecdotal and first-person literature is littered with accounts describing the exact opposite, and persuading patients to actually join or complete exercise programs is difficult.[43] The reason may be that exercise is associated with symptoms, particularly in anyone who undertakes it after a period of ill health or inactivity. These symptoms are physiological, rather than pathological; but if they are interpreted as evidence of ongoing illness, with potentially devastating consequences (a classic catastrophic cognition), one can understand the reluctance of sufferers to engage in activity. In a prospective study, Ray and colleagues[59] showed how some sufferers learn to cope and accept their illness by withdrawing from activity to guard against short-term exacerbation of symptoms. These sufferers also described how they generally felt unable to alter the course of their illness or affect illness outcome, a situation which means that "coping is likely to be undertaken without expectation of real or long-term benefit." [59]

In the CFS literature, controlled trials have demonstrated that CBT is effective and provides better symptomatic and functional outcomes than either standard medical care[61] or an equivalent number of sessions of relaxation[62] and can be delivered by general psychologists.[63] The data suggest that CBT has a direct effect on chronic fatigue, independent of either nonspecific effects of treatment or improvements in mood. New studies also have made direct links between the long-term fatigue experienced in cancer patients now disease-free and that found in CFS.[24] There are as yet no trials of CBT in the cancer literature directed at reducing fatigue rather than emotional distress. Clearly, they are needed.

Practical Issues

There is a strong case for undertaking trials of CBT to reduce symptomatic distress in patients with cancer; indeed, such trials are at last under way. When these are performed, one or two points need to be borne in mind. First, one can expect that the task will be easier in the cancer setting than in the CFS clinic. In noncancer settings, considerable difficulties can be experienced in attempting to "sell" these treatments to patients with unexplained fatigue because of the ever-present fear of having one's symptoms labeled as being "all in the mind" and consequently dismissed. Fortunately, this is rarely a problem in the cancer setting. Although the models of fatigue that we have proposed in both CFS and physical illness have considerable overlap and both depend on the distinction between precipitating and perpetuating factors, in the real world the fact that cancer patients have an established, clear-cut, and noncontroversial diagnosis firmly rooted in a physical model of disease means that paradoxically one can anticipate far less problem in engaging patients in treatments that appear to be more ambiguous in their nature. In contrast, the grey area of CFS makes this task more difficult.

Second, there are also some factors that may limit the application of CBT to the cancer field. Trials of CBT for chronic fatigue show that this is not a short-term solution; indeed, one of the most striking findings is that treatment benefits are not maximal at the end of active therapy but continue during follow-up, with the maximum benefit not achieved until some 6 months after the end of treatment. This is because the samples studied were unusually chronic (5 years of illness prior to treatment was the mean) and because the tertiary care nature of the subjects studied and the social and even political dimensions of CFS meant that unusual time and care had to be devoted to reassurance, explanation and support. A study using an intervention of only six sessions was less satisfactory.[64]

For reasons that will be obvious, such medium-term therapy may not be applicable to the palliative care setting. Instead, skilled interventions such as CBT are best applied to the circumstances of a patient who has completed active treatment, be it chemotherapy or radiotherapy, but who remains symptomatic. Those in whom there is a continuing and documented contribution to symptoms from advanced cachexia, severe anemia, and so on, may well not be the best subjects for this intervention, given that the fundamental rationale behind CBT is that whatever the trigger for symptoms, the original trigger no longer plays an active and progressive part in continuing symptomatology. It is, however, possible that in the appropriate population less intensive interventions than those required for CFS encountered in the specialist clinic may be effective. When we studied a group of chronically fatigued patients in primary care, most of whom did not carry the label, whether self-diagnosed or otherwise, of CFS, even a simple self-help book had a measurable benefit on chronic fatigue.[65]

Conclusions

Chronic fatigue is common, and almost ubiquitous, in cancer and palliative care. Other than for acute, short-term fatigue, the associations of fatigue are more general than specific and not unique to cancer care. For those who have completed active treatment, the original trigger for symptoms may not be the cause of persistent fatigue. Inactivity may play a part, but the links between patient beliefs about the cause of symptoms and subsequent behavior in response to symptoms may play an important role. Any intervention that reduces emotional distress in cancer patients will probably indirectly reduce fatigue as well, but fatigue and depression, though correlated, are certainly not the same thing.[66] Hence, more direct interventions may produce better results. Exercise is safe and effective, but its benefits are not simply due to improved physical fitness. Newer rehabilitation approaches, chiefly CBT, in which attention is paid to maintaining rather than triggering factors and there is an explicit attempt to work with patients' own beliefs about the causes of symptoms and their consequences, are of proven efficacy in the noncancer literature and are now being studied in the palliative care field.

References

1. Muscio B. Is a fatigue test possible? Br J Psychol 1921; 12:31–46.
2. Wessely S, Hotopf M, Sharpe M. Chronic Fatigue and its Syndromes. Oxford: Oxford University Press, 1998.
3. Holding D. Fatigue. In: Hockey G, ed. Stress and Fatigue in Human Performance. Chichester: John Wiley and Sons, 1983:145–167.
4. Potempa K. Chronic fatigue. Annu Rev Nurs Res 1993; 11:57–76.
5. Cull A, Hay C, Love S, et al. What do cancer patients mean when they complain of concentration and memory problems? Br J Cancer 1996; 74:1674–1679.
6. Dimeo F, Stieglitz R, Novelli-Fischer U, et al. Correlation between physical performance and fatigue in cancer patients. Ann Oncol 1997; 8:1251–1255.
7. Dalakas M, Mock V, Hawkins M. Fatigue: definitions, mechanisms and paradigms for study. Semin Oncol 1998; 25(Suppl 1):48–53.
8. Smets EM, Garssen B, Schuster Uitterhoeve AL, et al. Fatigue in cancer patients. Br J Cancer 1993; 68:220–224.
9. Smets E, Visser M, Garssen B, et al. Understanding the level of fatigue in cancer patients undergoing radiotherapy. J Psychosom Med 1998; 45:277–294.
10 Breetvelt I, Van Dam F. Under-reporting by cancer patients: the case of response-shift. Soc Sci Med 1991; 32:981–987.
11. Curt G, Breitbart W, Cella D, et al. Impact of cancer-related fatigue on the lives of patients: new findings from the Fatigue Coalition. Oncologist 2000; 5:353–360.
12. Dohrenwend B, Crandell D. Psychiatric symptoms in community, clinic and mental hospital groups. Am J Psychiatry 1970; 126:1611–1621.
13. Vogelzang N, Breitbart W, Cella D, et al. Patient, caregiver, and oncologist perception of cancer-related fatigue: results of a tripart assessment survey. Semin Hematol 1997; 34(Suppl 2):4–12.
14. Sneeuw KC, Aaronson NK, Osoba D, et al. The use of significant others as proxy raters of the quality of life of patients with brain cancer. Med Care 1997; 35:490–506.
15. Kurtz M, Kurtz J, Given C, et al. Concordance of cancer patient and caregiver symptom reports. Cancer Pract 1996; 4:185–190.
16. Curt G. Fatigue in cancer. BMJ 2001; 322:1560.
17. Richardson A. Fatigue in cancer patients: a review of the literature. Eur J Cancer Care 1995; 4:20–32.
18. Glaspy J, Bukowski R, Steinberg D, et al. Impact of therapy with epoetin alfa on clinical outcomes in patients with nonmyeloid malignancies during cancer chemotherapy in community oncology practice. J Clin Oncol 1997; 15:1218–1234.
19. Lennartsson J, Bengtsson C, Halberg L, et al. Characteristics of anemic women: the population study of women in Goteborg 1968–69. Scand J Hematol 1979; 22:17–24.

20. Hughson A, Cooper A, McArdle C, et al. Psychosocial effects of radiotherapy after mastectomy. BMJ 1987; 294:1515–1516.

21. Irvine D, Vincent L, Graydon JE, et al. The prevalence and correlates of fatigue in patients receiving treatment with chemotherapy and radiotherapy. A comparison with the fatigue experienced by healthy individuals. Cancer Nurs 1994; 17: 367–378.

22. Irvine D, Vincent L, Graydon J, et al. Fatigue in women with breast cancer receiving radiation therapy. Cancer Nurs 1998; 21:127–135.

23. Zeltzer LK, Chen E, Weiss R, et al. Comparison of psychologic outcome in adult survivors of childhood acute lymphoblastic leukemia versus sibling controls: a cooperative Children's Cancer Group and National Institutes of Health study. J Clin Oncol 1997; 15:547–556.

24. Servaes P, Van Der Wert S, Prins J, et al. Fatigue in disease-free cancer patients compared with fatigue in patients with chronic fatigue syndrome. Support Care Cancer 2001; 9:11–17.

25. Hann D, Jacobsen P, Martin S. Fatigue in women treated with bone marrow transplantation for breast cancer: a comparison with women with no history of cancer. Support Care Cancer 1997; 5:44–52.

26. Broeckel J, Jacobsen P, Balducci L, et al. Characteristics of correlates of fatigue after adjuvant chemotherapy for breast cancer. J Clin Oncol 1998; 16:1689–1696.

27. Hann DG, Garovoy N, Finkelstein B, Jacobsen PB, et al. Fatigue and quality of life in breast cancer patients undergoing autologous stem cell transplantation: a longitudinal comparative study. J Pain Symptom Manage 1999; 5:311–319.

28. Smets E, Visser M, Willems-Groot A, et al. Fatigue and radiotherapy: (B) experience in patients 9 months following treatment. Br J Cancer 2002 (in press).

29. Holley S. Cancer-related fatigue—suffering a different fatigue. Cancer Pract 2000; 8:87–95.

30. Turk D, Fernandez E. On the putative uniqueness of cancer pain. Behav Res Ther 1990; 28:1–13.

31. Speigel D, Bloom J, Yalom I. Group support for patients with metastatic cancer. Arch Gen Psychiatry 1981; 38:527–533.

32. Fawzy F, Cousins N, Fawzy N, et al. A structured psychiatric intervention for cancer patients: I. Changes over time in methods of coping and affective disturbance. Arch Gen Psychiatry 1990; 47:720–725.

33. Greer S, Moorey S, Baruch J, et al. Adjuvant psychological therapy for patients with cancer: a prospective randomised trial. BMJ 1992; 304:675–680.

34. Telch C, Telch M. Group coping skills instructions and supportive group therapy for cancer patients: a comparison of strategies. J Consult Clin Psychol 1986; 54: 802–808.

35. Decker T, Elsen J, Gallagher M. Relaxation therapy as an adjunct in radiation oncology. J Clin Psychol 1992; 48:388–393.

36. Stone P, Richards M, Hardy J. Fatigue in patients with cancer. Eur J Cancer 1998; 34:1670–1676.

37. McArdle J, George W, McArdle C, et al. Psychological support for patients undergoing breast cancer surgery: a randomised study. BMJ 1996; 312:813–817.

38. Hann D, Jacobsen P, Martin S, et al. Fatigue and quality of life following radiotherapy for breast cancer: a comparative study. J Clin Psychol Med Settings 1998; 5:19–33.

39. Salmon P, Hall G. A theory of postoperative fatigue. J R Soc Med 1997; 90:661–664.
40. Richardson A, Ream E. Self-care behaviors initiated by chemotherapy patients in response to fatigue. Int J Nurs Stud 1997; 34:35–43.
41. Sharpe M, Wessely S. Putting the rest cure to rest. BMJ 1998; 316:796.
42. Fulcher K, White P. Randomised controlled trial of graded exercise in patients with chronic fatigue syndrome. BMJ 1997; 314:1647–1652.
43. Wearden A, Morriss R, Mullis R, et al. A double-blind, placebo controlled treatment trial of fluoxetine and a graded exercise program for chronic fatigue syndrome. Br J Psychiatry 1998; 172:485–490.
44. Friendenreich CM, Courneya KS. Exercise as rehabilitation for cancer patients. Clin J Sport Med 1996; 6:237–244.
45. Mock V, Dow K, Meares C, et al. Effects of exercise on fatigue, physical functioning, and emotional distress during radiation therapy for breast cancer. Oncol Nurs Forum 1997; 24:991–1000.
46. Dimeo F, Berzt H, Finke J, et al. An aerobic training program for patients with haematological malignancies after bone marrow transplantation. Bone Marrow Transplant 1996; 18:1157–1160.
47. Dimeo F, Tilmann M, Bertz H, et al. Aerobic exercise in the rehabilitation of cancer patients after high dose chemotherapy and autologous peripheral stem cell transplanation. Cancer 1997; 79:1717–1722.
48. Dimeo F, Fetscher S, Lange W, et al. Effects of aerobic exercise on the physical performance and incidence of treatment-related complications after high-dose chemotherapy. Blood 1997; 90:3390–3394.
49. Dimeo F, Stieglitz R, Novelli-Fischer U, et al. Effects of physical activity on the fatigue and psychologic status of cancer patients during chemotherapy. Cancer 1999; 85:2273–2277.
50. Coats A, Adamopoulos A, Meyer T, et al. Effects of physical training in chronic heart failure. Lancet 1990; 335:63–66.
51. Graydon JE, Bubela N, Irvine D, et al. Fatigue-reducing strategies used by patients receiving treatment for cancer. Cancer Nurs 1995; 18:23–28.
52. Mock V, Burke M, Sheehan P, et al. A nursing rehabilitation program for women with breast cancer receiving adjuvant chemotherapy. Oncol Nurs Forum 1994; 21: 899–907.
53. Watts F. Attributional aspects of medicine. In: Antaki C, Brewin C, eds. Attributions and Psychological Change. London: Academic Press, 1982:135–155.
54. Deale A, Chalder T, Wessely S. Illness beliefs and treatment outcome in chronic fatigue syndrome. J Psychosom Res 1998; 45:77–83.
55. Vlaeyen J, Kole-Snijders A, Boeren R, et al. Fear of movement/(re)injury in chronic low back pain and its relation to behavioral performance. Pain 1995; 62:363–372.
56. Petrie K, Moss-Morris R, Weinman J. The impact of catastrophic beliefs on functioning in chronic fatigue syndrome. J Psychosom Res 1995; 39:31–37.
57. Dunkel-Schetter C, Feinstein L, Taylor S, et al. Patterns of coping with cancer. Health Psychol 1992; 11:79–87.
58. Jacobsen PB, Azzarello LM, Hann DM. Relation of catastrophizing to fatigue severity in women with breast cancer. Cancer Research, Therapy and Control 1999; 8:155–164.
59. Ray C, Jefferies S, Weir W. Coping and other predictors of outcome in chronic fatigue syndrome: a 1-year follow-up. J Psychosom Res 1997; 43:405–415.

60. Powell P, Bentall R, Nye F, et al. Randomized controlled trial of patient education to encourage graded exercise in chronic fatigue syndrome. BMJ 2001; 322: 387–390.
61. Sharpe M, Hawton K, Simkin S, et al. Cognitive behavior therapy for chronic fatigue syndrome; a randomized controlled trial. BMJ 1996; 312:22–26.
62. Deale A, Chalder T, Marks I, et al. A randomized controlled trial of cognitive behaviour versus relaxation therapy for chronic fatigue syndrome. Am J Psychiatry 1997; 154:408–414.
63. Prins J, Bleijenberg G, Bazelmans E, et al. Cognitive behavior therapy for chronic fatigue syndrome: a multicenter randomized controlled trial. Lancet 2001; 357: 841–847.
64. Lloyd A, Hickie I, Brockman A, et al. Immunologic and psychological therapy for patients with chronic fatigue syndrome. Am J Med 1993; 94:197–203.
65. Chalder T, Wallace P, Wessely S. Self-help treatment of chronic fatigue in the community: a randomised controlled trial. Br J Health Psychol 1997; 2:189–197.
66. Visser M, Smets E. Fatigue, depression and quality of life in cancer patients: how are they related? Support Care Cancer 1998; 6:101–108.

9

Evaluating the Relationship of Fatigue to Depression and Anxiety in Cancer Patients

PAUL B. JACOBSEN AND MICHAEL A. WEITZNER

There is a growing recognition among oncology professionals that fatigue is one of the most common and distressing symptoms experienced by cancer patients.[1,2] In seeking to learn more about the etiology and treatment of fatigue, clinicians and researchers alike have been challenged to understand how fatigue may be related to depression and anxiety in patients with cancer. The need to understand this relationship stems from two basic facts: (1) fatigue, in addition to being a symptom of cancer and its treatment, is a symptom of certain mood and anxiety disorders[3] and (2) depression and anxiety, like fatigue, are relatively common among cancer patients.[4] To clarify the relationship of fatigue to depression and anxiety in cancer patients, we have identified four questions that are of particular importance and will serve to organize this chapter. First, what are the conceptual similarities and differences between fatigue, on the one hand, and depression and anxiety, on the other hand? Second, to what extent do depression and anxiety co-occur with fatigue, and how might they be distinguished? Third, what are the possible causal relationships between fatigue and depression and between fatigue and anxiety? Fourth, what are the treatment implications of the relationship of fatigue to depression and anxiety?

Any attempt to answer these questions should be based on empirical findings, and whenever possible, we have done so. However, given the limited amount of research on fatigue in cancer patients, there is relatively little empirical evidence to answer several of our questions. We hope that, by identifying areas where evidence is lacking, this chapter will stimulate additional and much needed research into the relationship of fatigue to depression and anxiety in patients with cancer.

What Are the Similarities and Differences Between Fatigue, Depression, and Anxiety?

To understand the conceptual similarities and differences between fatigue, depression, and anxiety, it is necessary to consider how these concepts have been defined. Our approach to this issue focuses on the different ways in which fatigue, depression, and anxiety have been assessed in cancer patients. Three distinct approaches to the assessment of depression and anxiety can be identified: the single-symptom approach, the symptom-cluster approach, and the clinical syndrome approach.

The *single-symptom approach* refers to assessment methods that focus specifically on measuring depressed mood or anxious mood. These symptoms can be measured as continuous variables (for example, visual analogue scales measuring severity of depressed or anxious mood) or categorical variables (for example, clinical interview items measuring presence/absence of depressed or anxious mood).

The *symptom-cluster approach* refers to assessment methods that focus on measuring multiple symptoms of depression or anxiety. A common approach to measuring depressive symptomatology in cancer patients has been to administer a multi-item self-report scale, such as the Beck Depression Inventory (BDI)[5] or the Center for Epidemiologic Studies Depression Scale (CES-D).[6] Both instruments assess a constellation of symptoms (depressed mood, loss of appetite, and difficulty concentrating) that are theorized to reflect the construct of depression. Since fatigue is generally regarded as one of the core symptoms of a depressive disorder,[3] it is not surprising to find that many depressive symptomatology measures include at least one item assessing fatigue-related phenomena. For example, the BDI asks respondents to choose among alternatives ranging from "I don't get more tired than usual" to "I am too tired to do anything." Similarly, on the CES-D, respondents are asked to rate the extent to which they "could not get going" from "rarely or none of the time" to "most or all of the time."

Multi-item self-report scales are also frequently used to assess symptoms of anxiety in cancer patients. Among the most widely used measures is the State-Trait Anxiety Inventory (STAI).[7] As with measures of depressive symptomatology, these instruments assess a constellation of symptoms (anxious mood, restlessness, and difficulty concentrating) that are theorized to represent the construct of anxiety. Since sleep disturbance and being easily fatigued are features of several anxiety disorders,[3] it is not surprising to find these symptoms represented on a number of measures of anxiety symptomatology. For example, the STAI includes items asking respondents to rate the extent to which they "tire easily" and "feel rested" (the latter item being reverse-coded prior to scoring).

The *clinical syndrome approach* refers to assessment methods that focus on detecting the presence of a mood disorder, such as major depressive disorder, or an anxiety disorder, such as generalized anxiety disorder. As defined in the fourth edition of the American Psychiatric Association's *Diagnostic and Statistical*

Manual of Mental Disorders (DSM-IV),[3] a diagnosis of major depressive disorder requires the presence of four or more depressive symptoms during the same 2-week period besides depressed mood or loss of interest or pleasure in usual activities. Among the other symptoms whose presence counts toward the criterion of four or more symptoms is "fatigue or loss of energy." As defined in the same volume, a diagnosis of generalized anxiety disorder requires that feelings of anxiety or worry over a 6-month period be accompanied by three or more additional symptoms of anxiety during the same time period. Among the other symptoms whose presence counts toward the criterion of three or more symptoms is "being easily fatigued." Accordingly, items assessing fatigue are a standard feature of structured interviews designed to diagnose major depressive disorder and generalized anxiety disorder.[8]

Fatigue can also be assessed as a single symptom, a cluster of symptoms, or a clinical syndrome. The single-symptom approach refers to assessment methods in which fatigue is conceptualized as a unidimensional phenomenon. Measures of fatigue severity, such as the Profile of Mood States Fatigue Scale (POMS-F),[9] exemplify this approach. Overlap can be identified between the single-symptom approach to measuring fatigue and both the symptom-cluster and clinical syndrome approaches to measuring depression and anxiety. As described above, instruments used to measure depressive and anxiety symptomatology and to diagnose major depressive disorder and generalized anxiety disorder typically include one or more items assessing fatigue-related phenomena.

The symptom-cluster approach refers to assessment methods in which fatigue has been conceptualized as a multidimensional phenomenon. Although the specific dimensions that characterize fatigue in cancer patients remain a topic of debate,[1,2] at least two teams of investigators[10,11] have identified similar clusters of symptoms, including general symptoms (for example, tiredness), physical symptoms (for example, feelings of weakness or heaviness), and mental symptoms (for example, difficulty concentrating). Self-report measures reflecting this conceptualization of fatigue include the Multidimensional Fatigue Inventory (MFI)[10] and the Multidimensional Fatigue Symptom Inventory (MFSI).[11] Overlap can be identified between this approach to measuring fatigue and both the symptom-cluster and clinical syndrome approaches to measuring depression and anxiety. For example, both multidimensional fatigue measures referred to above assess a general symptom of fatigue (such as tiredness) and a mental symptom of fatigue (such as difficulty concentrating) that are also included in instruments used to measure depressive and anxiety symptomatology and to diagnose major depressive disorder and generalized anxiety disorder.

The clinical syndrome approach represents a relatively new method of assessing fatigue in cancer patients. Recognizing the need for a standard case definition, a group of investigators[12] has proposed a set of criteria for the diagnosis of "cancer-related fatigue." These diagnostic criteria (see Table 9.1) have been submitted for inclusion in the tenth edition of the International Classification of Diseases (ICD-10). Examination of the criteria indicates that overlap exists

Table 9.1. International Classification of Diseases criteria for cancer-related fatigue

A. Six (or more) of the following symptoms have been present every day or nearly every day during the same 2-week period in the past month and at least one of the symptoms is significant fatigue.

- Significant fatigue, diminished energy, or increased need to rest, disproportionate to any recent change in activity level
- Complaints of generalized weakness or limb heaviness
- Diminished concentration or attention
- Decreased motivation or interest in usual activities
- Insomnia or hypersomnia
- Experience of sleep as unrefreshing or nonrestorative
- Perceived need to struggle to overcome inactivity
- Marked emotional reactivity (sadness, frustration, or irritability) to feeling fatigued
- Difficulty completing daily tasks attributed to feeling fatigued
- Perceived problems with short-term memory
- Postexertional malaise lasting several hours

B. The symptoms cause clinically significant distress or impairment in social, occupational, or other important areas of functioning.

C. There is evidence from the history, physical examination, or laboratory findings that the symptoms are a consequence of cancer or cancer therapy.

D. The symptoms are not primarily a consequence of co-morbid psychiatric disorders such as major depression, somatization disorder, somatoform disorder, or delirium.

between this approach to measuring fatigue and both the symptom-cluster and clinical syndrome approaches to measuring depression and anxiety. As shown in Table 9.1, a diagnosis of cancer-related fatigue requires the presence of six or more symptoms listed under criterion A. Several of the symptoms listed (fatigue, sleep disturbance, diminished concentration, and decreased interest in usual activities) are also present in measures of depressive and anxiety symptomatology and included in diagnostic criteria for major depressive disorder and generalized anxiety disorder.

Although similarities are present in approaches to measuring fatigue, depression, and anxiety, important differences can also be identified. Symptom-cluster and clinical syndrome conceptualizations of depression and anxiety generally include a number of symptoms that are not consistent with symptom-cluster and clinical syndrome conceptualizations of fatigue. These include changes in appetite or weight, muscle tension, irritability, recurrent thoughts of death, feelings of worthlessness or excessive guilt, and psychomotor agitation or retardation. Likewise, symptom-cluster and clinical syndrome conceptualizations of fatigue include a number of symptoms that are not consistent with symptom-cluster and clinical syndrome conceptualizations of depression and anxiety. These include generalized feelings of weakness or heaviness, postexertional malaise, and difficulty completing daily tasks due to fatigue. Moreover, clinical syndrome approaches to measuring fatigue, depression, and anxiety include criteria that seek to differentiate cancer-related fatigue from mood and anxiety disorders. For example, criterion D for cancer-related fatigue (in Table 9.1) states that this syndrome is not diagnosed if symptoms of fatigue are considered to be the primary consequence of a co-morbid psychiatric disorder. Similarly, the DSM-IV criteria[3] specify that major depressive disorder and generalized anxiety are not diagnosed if the symptoms present (including fatigue) are considered to be the direct physiological effects of substance use or a general medical condition such as cancer.

In summary, a review of measurement approaches indicates that overlap is present between all three approaches to measuring fatigue and both the symptom-cluster and clinical syndrome approaches to measuring depression and anxiety. This overlap is consistent with the fact that the symptom of fatigue is encompassed within current conceptualizations of depressive and anxiety symptomatology as well as major depressive disorder and generalized anxiety disorder. Overlap also reflects the fact that several symptoms commonly associated with depression and anxiety (such as tiredness, diminished attention, and sleep disturbance) are encompassed within symptom-cluster and clinical syndrome approaches to measuring fatigue in cancer patients. Based on these considerations, one would expect empirical studies to show that depression and anxiety frequently co-occur with fatigue in cancer patients.

To What Extent Do Depression and Anxiety Co-occur with Fatigue and How Might They Be Distinguished?

One way to determine the extent to which depression and anxiety co-occur with fatigue in cancer patients is to examine the magnitude of correlations between measures of fatigue and depression and measures of fatigue and anxiety administered concurrently. Toward this end, a Medline search was conducted using the keywords *fatigue* and *cancer*. This search identified 23 studies that reported correlations between measures of fatigue and depression and 15 studies that reported correlations between measures of fatigue and anxiety.

As shown in Table 9.2, depression was usually assessed in these studies using measures of depressive symptomatology, such as the CES-D, the BDI, or the depression subscale of the Hospital Anxiety and Depression Scale (HADS). Exceptions include three studies[13-15] that used the POMS Depression Scale, a measure that reflects primarily depressed mood, and one study[16] that included only mood items from the CES-D. No studies were identified that assessed mood disorders and fatigue concurrently in cancer patients. Fatigue was usually assessed in these studies using measures of general fatigue severity, such as the POMS Fatigue Scale or the MFI General Scale. Five studies were identified[10,11,15,17,18] in which measures of general, mental, and physical symptoms of fatigue were administered to the same patients as part of a multidimensional approach. No studies were identified that assessed the clinical syndrome of cancer-related fatigue concurrent with depression.

Table 9.2. Studies assessing fatigue and depression concurrently in cancer patients

Study	Cancer diagnoses	No.	Treatment modality/focus	Depression measure	Fatigue measure	r
Andrykowski et al., 1998[68]	Breast	88	Mixed	CES-D CES-D CES-D CES-D	ChFS Total PFS Total Weakness rating Tiredness rating	0.68 0.68 0.47 0.63
Blesch et al., 1991[13]	Breast, lung	77	Mixed	POMS Depression	VAS Fatigue	0.46
Dimeo et al., 1997[14]	Mixed	78	Transplantation	POMS Depression SCL-90 Depression	POMS Fatigue POMS Fatigue	0.61 0.68
Gaston-Johansson et al., 1999[69]	Breast	127	Chemotherapy	BDI	VAS Fatigue	0.58
Hann et al., 1997[70]	Breast	43	Transplantation	CES-D	POMS Fatigue	0.80
Hann et al., 1998[71]	Breast	45	Radiation	CES-D CES-D	FSI Severity FSI Interference	0.68 0.73
Hann et al., 1999[20]	Breast	31	Transplantation	CES-D	POMS Fatigue	0.77
Howell et al., 2000[17]	Hematologic	66	Mixed	HADS-D	MFI General MFI Mental MFI Physical	0.64 0.46 0.57
Loge et al., 2000[72]	Lymphoma	421	Mixed	HADS-D	FQ Total FQ Mental FQ Physical	0.49 0.39 0.55
Meek et al., 2000[15]	Mixed	212	Mixed	POMS Depression	POMS Fatigue MAF MAF Interference LFS Fatigue MFI General MFI Mental MFI Physical	0.53 0.53 0.37 0.41 0.30 0.37 0.37
Miaskowski et al., 1999[73]	Mixed	24	Radiation	CES-D CES-D (minus 3 items)	LF S Severity LFS Severity	0.48 0.52
Mock et al., 1997[59]	Breast	46	Radiation	VAS Depression	VAS Fatigue	0.61

Study	Cancer type	Treatment	N	Depression measure	Fatigue measure	r
Okuyama et al., 2000[74]	Breast	Mixed	134	HADS-D	CFS Total	0.63
					CFS Physical	0.49
					CFS Affective	0.42
					CFS Cognitive	0.24
Okuyama et al., 2000[75]	Mixed	Unknown	218	HADS-D	CFS Total	0.69
					CFS Physical	0.59
					CFS Affective	0.54
					CFS Cognitive	0.47
Pickard-Holley, 1991[76]	Ovarian	Chemotherapy	12	BDI	RFS	0.20
Schneider, 1998[18]	Mixed	Mixed	54	BDI	MFI General	0.56
				BDI	MFI Mental	0.55
				BDI	MFI Physical	0.61
Smets et al., 1996[10]	Mixed	Radiation	116	HADS-D	MFI General	0.77
				HADS-D	MFI Mental	0.61
				HADS-D	MFI Physical	0.67
				HADS-D (minus item 8)	MFI General	0.67
				HADS-D (minus item 8)	MFI Mental	0.58
				HADS-D (minus item 8)	MFI Physical	0.56
Smets et al., 1998[77]	Mixed	Radiation	250	CES-D	MFI General	0.43
Smets et al., 1998[78]	Mixed	Radiation	154	CES-D	MFI General	0.49
Stein et al., 1998[11]	Breast	Mixed	326	CES-D	MFSI General	0.68
				CES-D	MFSI Mental	0.64
				CES-D	MFSI Physical	0.61
Stone et al., 1999[79]	Mixed	Unknown	95	HADS-D (minus item 8)	FSS	0.16
Stone et al., 2000[19]	Prostate	Hormone therapy	60	HADS-D	FSS	0.55
				HADS-D (minus item 8)	FSS	0.46
Visser and Smets, 1998[16]	Mixed	Radiation	250	CES-D (mood only) time 1	MFI General	0.35
				CES-D (mood only) time 2	MFI General	0.43
				CES-D (mood only) time 3	MFI General	0.48
				CES-D (mood only) time 1	MFI Physical	0.37
				CES-D (mood only) time 2	MFI Physical	0.50
				CES-D (mood only) time 3	MFI Physical	0.46

r, correlation coefficient; BDI, Beck Depression Inventory; CES-D, Center for Epidemiologic Studies Depression Inventory; CFS, Cancer Fatigue Scale; ChFS, Chalder Fatigue Scale; FSI, Fatigue Symptom Inventory; FSS, Fatigue Severity Scale; FQ, Fatigue Questionnaire; HADS-D, Hospital Anxiety and Depression Scale–Depression Subscale; LFS, Lee Fatigue Scale; MAF, Multidimensional Assessment of Fatigue; MFI, Multidimensional Fatigue Inventory; MFSI, Multidimensional Fatigue Symptom Inventory; PFS, Piper Fatigue Scale; POMS, Profile of Mood States; RFS, Rhoten Fatigue Scale; SCL-90, Symptom Checklist 90; VAS, visual analogue scale.

Correlations between measures of fatigue and depression reported in the studies listed in Table 9.2 were positive and ranged from a low of 0.16 to a high of 0.80. The average correlation between fatigue and depression across studies was 0.53. Thus, on average, measures of fatigue and depression administered concurrently to cancer patients shared approximately 28% of their variance. There was little evidence that the individual dimensions of fatigue were differentially related to depression. Specifically, in those studies that used a multidimensional approach,[10,11,15,17,18] the average correlations between depression and general fatigue (0.59), mental fatigue (0.53), and physical fatigue (0.57) were quite similar.

As noted above, four studies used measures of depression that focused specifically on depressed mood. There was no evidence to suggest that limiting the assessment of depression to its mood component substantially diminished correlations with fatigue. Correlations between depression and fatigue in these studies averaged 0.44.

One of the studies listed in Table 9.2 included analyses designed specifically to examine the effects of overlap on correlations between measures of fatigue and depression. In this study,[10] the MFI and the depression subscale of the HADS were administered concurrently to cancer patients undergoing radiotherapy. The latter measure includes one item ("I feel as if I am slowed down") that would appear to overlap with fatigue. Correlations were computed between the MFI and both the original version of the HADS depression subscale and a version that excluded this item. Although correlations between depression and fatigue declined in size after exclusion of the item, the magnitude of the change was relatively modest. The average correlation between MFSI subscales and the HADS depression subscale was 0.68 before exclusion of the item and 0.60 after exclusion of the item. A similarly modest decline was evident in another study[19] in which correlations were reported between the Fatigue Severity Scale and the HADS depression subscale before and after exclusion of the same item.

Studies reporting correlations between measures of anxiety and fatigue administered concurrently to cancer patients are listed in Table 9.3. Anxiety was usually assessed in these studies using measures of anxiety symptomatology, such as the STAI or the anxiety subscale of the HADS. Exceptions include two studies[13,15] that used the POMS Anxiety Scale, a measure that reflects primarily anxious mood. No studies were identified that assessed anxiety disorders and fatigue concurrently in cancer patients. Similar to the studies described above, fatigue was usually assessed using measures of general fatigue severity, such as the POMS Fatigue Scale, the MFI General Scale, or visual analogue scale measures of fatigue. Three studies were identified[10,11,15] in which measures of general, mental, and physical symptoms of fatigue were administered to the same patients as part of a multidimensional approach. No studies were identified that assessed the clinical syndrome of cancer-related fatigue concurrent with anxiety.

Correlations between measures of fatigue and anxiety reported in the studies listed in Table 9.3 were positive and ranged from a low of 0.16 to a high of 0.69.

The average correlation between fatigue and anxiety across studies was 0.48. Thus, on average, measures of fatigue and anxiety administered concurrently to cancer patients shared approximately 23% of their variance. As with depression, there was little evidence that the individual dimensions of fatigue were differentially related to anxiety. Specifically, in those studies that used a multidimensional approach,[10,11,15] the average correlations between anxiety and general fatigue (0.49), mental fatigue (0.49), and physical fatigue (0.44) were quite similar.

As noted above, two studies used measures of anxiety that focused specifically on anxious mood. There was no evidence to suggest that limiting the assessment of anxiety to its mood component substantially diminished correlations with fatigue. Correlations between anxiety and fatigue in these studies averaged 0.43.

Fifteen of the studies listed in both Tables 9.2 and 9.3 reported correlations between measures of fatigue, depression, and anxiety administered concurrently to the same patients. A comparison of these correlations provides a rough index of the relative magnitude of relationships between fatigue and depression and between fatigue and anxiety in cancer patients. Across the 15 studies, the average correlation between measures of depression and fatigue was 0.54 and that between measures of anxiety and fatigue was 0.47. The relative magnitude of these correlations can also be evaluated by directly comparing the 35 pairs of fatigue–depression and fatigue–anxiety correlations reported in the 15 studies. In 26 instances, correlations between and fatigue and depression were greater than correlations between fatigue and anxiety. In only nine instances were correlations between fatigue and anxiety equal to or greater than those between fatigue and depression. These observations suggest that, among cancer patients, fatigue and depression may be more closely related than fatigue and anxiety.

In summary, empirical studies yield consistent evidence of a relatively high degree of correspondence between levels of fatigue and levels of depression and anxiety in patients with cancer. This state of affairs is not particularly surprising considering the overlap present in many current approaches to assessing these constructs. There is evidence to suggest, however, that the degree of correspondence is not solely a function of overlap in assessment approaches. First, correlations between fatigue and depression remained relatively high even when items reflecting phenomena associated with fatigue were removed from measures of depressive symptomatology.[10] Second, relatively high correlations have been observed between measures of fatigue and measures focusing specifically on depressed mood and anxious mood.[13–16]

Taken together, findings from these empirical studies suggest that the two fatigue-measurement approaches currently in use (the single-symptom approach and the symptom-cluster approach) are of limited usefulness in attempts to distinguish fatigue from depression and anxiety. One measurement strategy that has yet to be investigated for its ability to distinguish these constructs is the clinical syndrome approach. As noted earlier, criteria have been proposed for diagnosing a clinical syndrome of cancer-related fatigue.[12] With the advent of these criteria,

Table 9.3. Studies assessing fatigue and anxiety concurrently in cancer patients

Study	Cancer diagnoses	No.	Treatment modality focus	Anxiety measure	Fatigue measure	r
Blesch et al., 1991[13]	Breast, lung	77	Mixed	POMS Anxiety	VAS Fatigue	0.40
Dimeo et al., 1997[14]	Mixed	78	Transplantation	SCL-90 Anxiety	POMS Fatigue	0.63
Hann et al., 1997[69]	Breast	43	Transplantation	STAI-State	POMS Fatigue	0.65
				STAI-Trait	POMS Fatigue	0.69
Hann et al., 1998[70]	Breast	45	Radiation	STAI-State	FSI Severity	0.56
				STAI-State	FSI Interference	0.58
				STAI-Trait	FSI Severity	0.46
				STAI-Trait	FSI Interference	0.48
Hann et al., 1999[20]	Breast	31	Transplantation	STAI	POMS Fatigue	0.52
Howell et al., 2000[17]	Hematologic	66	Mixed	HADS-A	MFI General	0.47
					MFI Mental	0.52
Loge et al., 2000[70]	Lymphoma	421	Mixed	HADS-A	FQ Total	0.44
					FQ Mental	0.38
					FQ Physical	0.40
Meek et al., 2000[15]	Mixed	212	Mixed	POMS Anxiety	POMS Fatigue	0.57
					MAF	0.52
					MAF Interference	0.29
					LFS Fatigue	0.47
					MFI General	0.37
					MFI Mental	0.41
					MFI Physical	0.37

Study	Cancer type	Treatment	N	Anxiety measure	Fatigue measure	r
Mock et al., 1997[59]	Breast	Radiation	46	VAS Anxiety	VAS Fatigue	0.60
Okuyama et al., 2000[72]	Breast	Mixed	134	HADS-A	CFS Total	0.52
					CFS Physical	0.44
					CFS Affective	0.23
					CFS Cognitive	0.43
Okuyama et al., 2000[73]	Mixed	Unknown	218	HADS-A	CFS Total	0.69
					CFS Physical	0.52
					CFS Affective	0.32
					CFS Cognitive	0.44
Smets et al., 1996[10]	Mixed	Radiation	116	HADS-A	MFI General	0.51
					MFI Mental	0.52
					MFI Physical	0.45
Stein et al., 1998[11]	Breast	Mixed	326	STAI	MFSI General	0.58
					MFSI Mental	0.54
					MFSI Physical	0.51
Stone et al., 1999[77]	Mixed	Unknown	95	HADS-A	FSS	0.16
Stone et al., 2000[19]	Prostate	Hormone therapy	60	HADS-A	FSS	0.52

r, correlation coefficient; CFS, Cancer Fatigue Scale; FSI, Fatigue Symptom Inventory; FSS, Fatigue Severity Scale; FQ, Fatigue Questionnaire; HADS-A, Hospital Anxiety and Depression Scale–Anxiety Subscale; LFS, Lee Fatigue Scale; MAF, Multidimensional Assessment of Fatigue; MFI, Multidimensional Fatigue Inventory; MFSI, Multidimensional Fatigue Symptom Inventory; POMS, Profile of Mood States; SCL-90, Symptom Checklist 90; STAI, State Trait Anxiety Inventory; VAS, visual analogue scale.

there is a need for research in which clinical syndrome measures of fatigue, depression, and anxiety are administered concurrently to cancer patients. The results of this research would indicate the extent to which it is possible to distinguish fatigue associated with cancer and its treatment from fatigue associated with a mood or anxiety disorder. Likewise, this research would indicate the extent to which it is possible to distinguish whether certain depressive or anxiety symptoms of (such as loss of concentration) are a reflection of an underlying mood or anxiety disorder or are part of a cancer-related fatigue syndrome. The ability to distinguish clinical syndromes of fatigue from clinical syndromes of depression and anxiety may be particularly important as studies are initiated that seek to determine the efficacy of psychotropic medications at relieving fatigue in cancer patients.

What Are the Causal Relationships Between Fatigue and Depression and Between Fatigue and Anxiety?

As noted earlier, there is considerable evidence that levels of fatigue, depression, and anxiety correspond in cancer patients. At least three different causal relationships can be theorized to explain this correspondence. One possibility is that the fatigue produced by cancer and its treatment may result in patients becoming depressed or anxious. A second possibility is that fatigue may develop in cancer patients as a consequence of their being depressed or anxious. A third possibility is that no causal relationship exists; instead, the correspondence may reflect the presence of a third factor that is the cause of both fatigue and depression or anxiety in patients with cancer. As will be shown, there is evidence to suggest the existence of each of these mechanisms.

Two lines of research provide support for the view that cancer patients can become depressed or anxious as a consequence of experiencing disease-related or treatment-related fatigue. One line of research consists of reports indicating that patients perceive disease-related or treatment-related fatigue as having adverse effects on their mood. For example, women undergoing transplantation for breast cancer report more severe fatigue and greater interference of fatigue with their mood than a comparison group of women with no history of cancer.[20] Differences between groups on these measures were evident only after the breast cancer patients had started treatment. A second line of evidence consists of research examining whether, over the course of cancer treatment, fatigue predicts subsequent depression better than depression predicts subsequent fatigue. Of particular relevance is a study in which fatigue and depression were assessed before the start of radiotherapy treatment and, again, 2 weeks after treatment completion.[16] Pretreatment fatigue severity accounted for 11% of the variability in subsequent depressed mood, whereas pretreatment depressed mood accounted for only 4% of the variability in subsequent fatigue severity. Additional supportive evidence comes from a study that examined relations between psychiatric disorder (mood, anxiety, and adjustment disorders) and fatigue in women previously treated with adjuvant chemotherapy for breast cancer.[21] The presence of a psychiatric disorder prior to cancer diagnosis was not related to fatigue severity following chemotherapy treatment; in contrast, more severe fatigue following chemotherapy treatment was related to the concurrent presence of a psychiatric disorder.

The possibility that cancer patients may develop fatigue as a consequence of being depressed or anxious is intuitively obvious. Actually demonstrating this relationship represents a methodological challenge since most cancer patients can also develop fatigue as a consequence of their disease or its treatment. There is, however, indirect evidence to support the possibility that fatigue in cancer patients may occur as a consequence of depression. Research has shown that patients with a prior history of depression are more likely to develop mood disorders following the diagnosis of cancer.[22] Evidence indicating that these patients also experience worse fatigue than patients without mood disorders would be consistent with the possibility that fatigue can occur as a consequence of depression. Likewise, patients with a prior history of anxiety disorder may experience a worsening of their anxiety symptoms, including fatigue, following cancer diagnosis. Another indirect piece of evidence consists of reports indicating that reliance on specific forms of coping characteristic of depressed individuals is related to fatigue severity in cancer patients. For example, among women with breast cancer previously treated with chemotherapy, greater reliance on *catastrophizing* (a coping strategy characterized by negative self-statements and overly negative thoughts about the future) was associated with more severe fatigue.[21] Greater reliance on this coping strategy also has been related to higher levels of depressive symptomatology in breast cancer patients.[23]

There is considerable evidence to suggest that a correspondence between fatigue and depression in cancer patients may be due to their causal relationship to a third factor. Along these lines, attention has focused on certain cancers that are believed to cause depressive symptoms. Pancreatic cancer is one neoplasm that appears to display these characteristics. The prevalence of depression-related disorders among patients with pancreatic cancer is estimated to be as high as 71%.[24] Moreover, numerous reports have documented the presence of depressive symptoms in patients before their pancreatic cancer was diagnosed.[25–27] Recent physiological findings provide further evidence of a causal link between pancreatic cancer and depression. Pancreatic tumors secrete various neuropeptides and neurohormones, such as corticotropin and cortisol.[28–29] These findings are consistent with a wealth of data showing that hypercortisolemia, as evidenced by nonsuppression of cortisol after dexamethasone administration, is associated with major depressive disorder.[30] Pancreatic tumors also secrete calcitonin. These secretions can result in hypercalcemia,[31,32] a condition characterized by prominent symptoms of lethargy and fatigue.[33] In addition, there is evidence that pancreatic tumors also secrete growth hormone,[34,35] another substance associated with increased depressive symptoms.[30]

Similarly, there is evidence to suggest that a correspondence between fatigue and anxiety in cancer patients may be due to their causal relationship to a third factor. Just as some neoplasms can secrete factors that cause depressive symptoms, other neoplasms (for example, neuroendocrine tumors) can secrete neurotransmitters or other neuropeptides that induce anxiety symptoms, such as panic attacks and generalized feelings of anxiety. For example, pheochromocytoma, a malignancy of the adrenal gland medulla, can be associated with both panic attacks and generalized anxiety. This particular malignancy secretes norepinephrine and epinephrine, two neurotransmitters involved in the generation of anxiety.[36] Carcinoid tumors, particularly involving the pulmonary system, are also associated with panic attacks due to their secretion of norepinephrine and serotonin. As mentioned above, small cell lung cancer secretes corticotropin, an ectopic secretion that stimulates cortisol production, causing hypercortisolemia and the generation of anxiety.[37] In each instance, the fatigue and anxiety observed in patients may be due to a common underlying biological mechanism.

Certain forms of cancer treatment may also be a direct cause of both fatigue and depression. Along these lines, attention has focused on biological response modifiers, such as the interferons and the interleukins. These agents are used increasingly to treat a variety of cancers, including renal cell cancer and melanoma, and to control chronic myelogenous leukemia. Administration of supraphysiological doses of these substances has been associated with prominent depressive symptoms, including fatigue.[38-40] The occurrence of these psychiatric side effects is consistent with research showing that elevated levels of both interferons and interleukins are present in psychiatric patients with major depressive disorder.[41-45] Similar findings have been described for the impact of cytokines (interferon and interleukin-2) on anxiety. Studies have documented the generation of anxiety symptoms by administration of interferon with or without interleukin-2.[46,47]

What Are the Treatment Implications of the Relationship of Fatigue to Depression and Anxiety?

In the previous section, we reviewed evidence suggesting the existence of three different causal relationships between fatigue and depression or anxiety in cancer patients. One possibility suggested by prior research is that patients experience fatigue as part of an underlying mood or anxiety disorder. A second possibility is that patients develop symptoms of depression or anxiety as a result of experiencing disease-related or treatment-related fatigue. A third possibility is that the correspondence between fatigue and depression or anxiety in cancer patients is due to a third factor, such as high-dose interferon therapy. In this section, we examine how these causal mechanisms may have implications for the management of fatigue.

The situation in which fatigue is part of a mood or anxiety disorder is perhaps the easiest to manage since therapy will revolve around treatment of the underlying primary psychiatric disorder. Treatment of major depressive disorder in cancer patients typically involves both pharmacological and nonpharmacological therapies.[48] The selection of a specific antidepressant is likely to be guided by the symptom presentation. For example, if sleep disturbance were one of the chief presenting symptoms of depression, an antidepressant with sedating properties (such as amitriptyline) would be preferred. If, however, the patient's depression were accompanied by problems with diarrhea, as with several gastrointestinal cancers, then an antidepressant with constipating properties (such as paroxetine) would be preferred. By and large, research indicates that serotonin-selective reuptake inhibitors (SSRIs, e.g., paroxetine, sertraline, and citalopram) and medications that inhibit primarily norepinephrine reuptake (SNRIs, such as venlafaxine, bupropion, and the tricyclic antidepressants) are equally efficacious in the treatment of major depressive disorder.[49–51] As depressed mood improves, the associated fatigue can also be expected to resolve. Similarly, the treatment of anxiety disorders is focused on the use of high-dose SSRI or SNRI medications.[52,53] The choice of medication is also guided by the symptom presentation. Patients with increased ruminations and worries are started preferentially on an SNRI, such as venlafaxine. Those with more of a panic presentation are started on an SSRI. Both classes of antidepressants are activating and can help to improve the fatigue that is part of the particular anxiety syndrome. Low-dose benzodiazepines (such as alprazolam, lorazepam, and clonazepam) may be used in the beginning phase of treatment until the antidepressant takes full effect. Although these medications are also effective for anxiety disorders,[54] they are not recommended for long-term use since they can increase the patient's perception of fatigue, largely due to their sedating properties.[55,56]

The management of disease-related or treatment-related fatigue accompanied by depressive symptoms or anxiety symptoms is more complex. This situation reflects, in part, the relative lack of empirically supported interventions for fatigue in cancer patients. In the absence of a strong body of empirical evidence, several authors[12,57] have proposed preliminary guidelines for the management of fatigue based largely on clinical experience with cancer patients and research with other patient populations (Fig. 9.1). According to these guidelines, efforts to manage fatigue should focus on correcting potential etiologies as well as relieving symptoms. Potentially correctable etiologies, besides depression and anxiety, include anemia, infection, other symptoms (such as pain), and centrally acting medications (such as opioids). Symptomatic therapies may include pharmacological as well as nonpharmacological interventions. Several of the proposed symptomatic therapies for fatigue (physical exercise, psychostimulant medications, and antidepressant medications) also have antidepressant and/or anxiolytic properties.

A growing body of evidence indicates that exercise may be effective at relieving fatigue in patients who are undergoing or recovering from cancer treatment.[58] Positive changes in mood are a likely consequence of regular exercise. At least one study[59] has documented that reductions in treatment-related fatigue

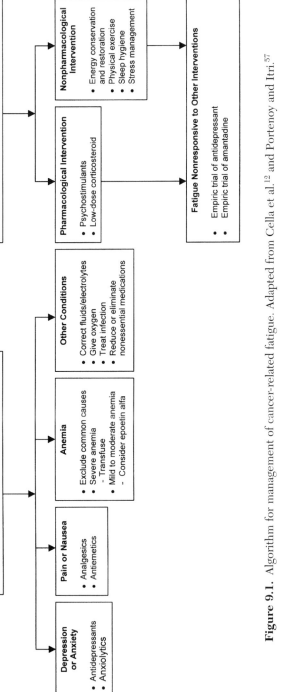

Figure 9.1. Algorithm for management of cancer-related fatigue. Adapted from Cella et al.[12] and Portenoy and Itri.[57]

among regular exercisers were accompanied by corresponding reductions in anxiety and, to a lesser extent, depressed mood. These findings suggest that the beneficial effects of exercise on fatigue in cancer patients may be due, in part, to the mood-enhancing properties of exercise.

There is evidence that psychostimulants (such as methylphenidate, dextroamphetamine, and pemoline) may be useful in relieving fatigue related to opioid-induced somnolence,[60] neurobehavioral slowing,[61,62] and depression[63] in cancer patients. Clinical experience suggests that these agents are also useful in relieving disease-related or treatment-related fatigue in cancer patients. For those patients with significant anxiety and fatigue, the traditional stimulants may worsen perceived anxiety due to their potential to induce tremulousness. A newer medication, modafinil, may be useful with these patients since it appears to increase alertness without causing or accentuating anxiety.[64] The mechanisms by which psychostimulants relieve disease-related or treatment-related fatigue have yet to be identified. In particular, it is unclear whether the effects of psychostimulants on fatigue are related to or distinct from their mood-enhancing properties.

Recommendations regarding the use of antidepressant medications to relieve fatigue in cancer patients are based largely on clinical observations that these agents can produce increases in energy disproportionate to any changes in mood.[56] Accordingly, these agents may be indicated for patients who are not depressed or anxious but are experiencing disease-related or treatment-related fatigue. Controlled trials are needed to identify the specific antidepressant agents that are effective at relieving fatigue. Two agents that appear to merit study are venlafaxine and bupropion. This suggestion is based on clinical observations that these two agents have particularly energizing effects.[65] Both agents appear to function similarly to psychostimulants in that their use is associated with increased synaptic levels of norepinephrine.[66] These findings are consistent with animal and human studies suggesting that increased levels of norepinephrine and/or dopamine are associated with increased levels of cortical arousal.[67] As with the psychostimulants, it will be important to clarify whether any observed effects of these agents on fatigue are related to or distinct from their mood-enhancing effects.

The guidelines described above[12,56] are also applicable to the management of fatigue and depression or anxiety related to a third factor. To the extent that the etiology of these symptoms is identifiable and correctable, efforts should focus on correcting the underlying cause(s). Often, correction of the underlying etiology is not practical or feasible. For example, it may be inadvisable to discontinue interferon even though a patient has become severely fatigued and depressed during the course of therapy. Under these circumstances, management efforts should focus on symptomatic relief. In the absence of a strong body of empirical evidence, clinical experience suggests the use of agents that are likely to have beneficial effects on both fatigue and mood symptoms ("activating" antidepressants or psychostimulants). Clearly, this is an area in which controlled outcome studies are needed.

Conclusions

In this chapter, we addressed four issues regarding the relationship of fatigue to depression and anxiety in cancer patients. First, we identified conceptual similarities and differences between fatigue, on the one hand, and depression and anxiety, on the other hand. As noted previously, fatigue, depression, and anxiety can each be assessed as a single symptom, a cluster of symptoms, or a clinical syndrome. Overlap was present between all three of these approaches to measuring fatigue and both the symptom-cluster and clinical syndrome approaches to measuring depression and anxiety. This overlap reflects the inclusion of fatigue within symptom-cluster and clinical syndrome approaches to measuring depression and anxiety and the inclusion of certain symptoms of depression and anxiety (such as difficulty concentrating) within symptom-cluster and clinical syndrome approaches to measuring fatigue. Important conceptual differences were also identified. Certain symptoms (such as recurrent thoughts of death and muscle tension) generally appear only in measures of depression or anxiety, whereas other symptoms (such as postexertional malaise) generally appear only in measures of fatigue. Moreover, the clinical syndrome measurement approaches include criteria intended to differentiate cancer-related fatigue from mood and anxiety disorders.

A second aim of this chapter was to determine the extent to which fatigue co-occurs with depression and anxiety in cancer patients. A review of the literature indicated that research on this topic has been limited to the use of either single-symptom or symptom-cluster measurement approaches. The average correlations observed across studies between fatigue and depression (0.53) and fatigue and anxiety (0.48) were relatively high. In those studies in which measures of fatigue, depression, and anxiety were administered concurrently to patients, there was a slightly greater correspondence of fatigue with depression (0.54) than with anxiety (0.47). The magnitude of these correlations is consistent with the previously noted overlap between measures of fatigue and measures of depression and anxiety. There is evidence, however, that this correspondence is not solely a function of overlap in measurement approaches. For example, correlations between measures of fatigue and depression remained relatively high even when items reflecting phenomena associated with fatigue were removed from measures of depressive symptomatology. These findings suggest that the two measurement approaches currently in use (the single-symptom and symptom-cluster approaches) are of limited usefulness in attempts to distinguish fatigue from depression and anxiety. Clinical syndrome approaches to measuring fatigue, depression, and anxiety may be better suited to this task and merit further study.

A third aim of the chapter was to explore the causal relationships between fatigue and depression and between fatigue and anxiety in cancer patients. A review of the literature suggested the existence of three different causal mechanisms. First, there is evidence consistent with the view that cancer patients may become depressed or anxious as a consequence of experiencing disease-related or treatment-related fatigue. Second, there is evidence suggesting that fatigue may develop in cancer patients as a consequence of their becoming depressed or anxious. Third, there is evidence indicating that the correspondence of fatigue with depression or anxiety may be due to the presence of a common third factor. Examples of such a third factor include certain neoplasms (pancreatic cancer) and certain forms of cancer treatment (interferon therapy) that appear to be a direct cause of both fatigue and depression or anxiety. The specific mechanisms by which these neoplasms and treatments give rise to both fatigue and depression or anxiety are not well understood and need to be investigated further.

The fourth and final aim was to consider the treatment implications of the relationship between fatigue and depression in cancer patients. When evidence suggests that fatigue is the consequence of a psychiatric disorder, efforts to manage the fatigue typically focus on treatment of the underlying psychiatric disorder. Management of fatigue that is disease-related or treatment-related and accompanied by depression or anxiety is more complex, owing in part to the relative lack of empirically validated interventions. Current guidelines,[12,56] based largely on clinical experience and research with other patient populations, suggest that efforts to manage fatigue under these circumstances should focus on correcting potential etiologies and relieving symptoms. Several of the proposed symptomatic therapies (physical exercise, psychostimulant medications, and antidepressant medications) have antidepressant or anxiolytic properties. These therapies may be particularly useful in managing fatigue accompanied by depression or anxiety as well as fatigue and depression or anxiety attributable to a common third factor. Evaluating the efficacy of these therapies and understanding their mechanisms of action in relieving fatigue should be considered high priorities for future research.

References

1. Richardson A. Fatigue in cancer patients: a review of the literature. Eur J Cancer Care 1995; 4:20–32.
2. Winningham ML, Nail LM, Burke MB, et al. Fatigue and the cancer experience: the state of the knowledge. Oncol Nurs Forum 1994; 21:23–36.
3. American Psychiatric Association. Diagnostic and Statistical Manual of Mental Disorders, 4th ed. Washington DC: American Psychiatric Association, 1994.
4. Bottomley A. Depression in cancer patients: a literature review. Eur J Cancer Care 1998; 7:181–191.
5. Beck AT, Ward CH, Mendelson M, et al. An inventory for measuring depression. Arch Gen Psychiatry 1961; 4:53–63.
6. Radloff LS. The CES-D scale: a self-report depression scale for research in the general population. Appl Psychol Measures 1977; 1:385–401.
7. Spielberger CD, Gorsuch RL, Lushene RD. STAI Manual for the State-Trait Anxiety Inventory. Palo Alto, CA: Consulting Psychologists Press, 1970.
8. First MB, Gibbon M, Spitzer RL, et al. User's Guide for the Structured Clinical Interview for DSM-IV Disorders. New York: Biometrics Research, 1996.

9. McNair DM, Lorr M, Droppleman LF. Profile of Mood States Manual. San Diego: Educational and Industrial Testing Service, 1971.

10. Smets EMA, Garssen B, Cull A, et al. Application of the multidimensional fatigue inventory (MFI-20) in cancer patients receiving radiotherapy. Br J Cancer 1996; 73: 241–245.

11. Stein KD, Martin SC, Hann DM , et al. A multidimensional measure of fatigue for use with cancer patients. Cancer Pract 1998; 6:143–152.

12. Cella D, Peterman A, Passik S, et al. Progress toward guidelines for the management of fatigue. Oncology 1998; 12:369–377.

13. Blesch KS, Paice JA, Wickham R, et al. Correlates of fatigue in people with breast or lung cancer. Oncol Nurs Forum 1991; 18:81–87.

14. Dimeo F, Stieglitz RD, Novelli-Fischer U, et al. Correlation between physical performance and fatigue in cancer patients. Ann Oncol 1997; 8:1251–1255.

15. Meek PM, Nail LM, Barsevick A, et al. Psychometric testing of fatigue instruments for use with cancer patients. Nurs Res 2000; 49:181–190.

16. Visser MRM, Smets EMA. Fatigue, depression and quality of life in cancer patients: how are they related? Support Care Cancer 1998; 6:101–108.

17. Howell SJ, Radford JA, Smets EM, et al. Fatigue, sexual function and mood following treatment of haemotological malignancy: the impact of mild Leydig cell dysfunction. Br J Cancer 2000; 82:789–793.

18. Schneider RA. Concurrent validity of the Beck Depression Inventory and the Multidimensional Fatigue Inventory-20 in assessing fatigue among cancer patients. Psychol Rep 1998; 82:883–886.

19. Stone P, Hardy J, Huddart R, et al. Fatigue in patients with prostate cancer receiving hormone therapy. Eur J Cancer 2000; 36:1134–1141.

20. Hann DM, Garovoy N, Finkelstein B, et al. Fatigue and quality of life in breast cancer patients undergoing autologous stem cell transplantation: a longitudinal comparative study. J Pain Symptom Manage 1999; 17:311–319.

21. Broeckel JA, Jacobsen PB, Horton J, et al. Characteristics and correlates of fatigue after adjuvant chemotherapy for breast cancer. J Clin Oncol 1998; 16:1689–1696.

22. Leopold KA, Ahles TA, Walch S, et al. Prevalence of mood disorders and utility of the prime-MD in patients undergoing radiation therapy. Int J Radiat Oncol Biol Phys 1998; 42:1105–1112.

23. Jacobsen PB, Azzarello LM, Hann DM. Relation of catastrophizing to fatigue severity in women with breast cancer. Cancer Res Ther Control 1999; 8:155–164.

24. Green AI, Austin CP. Psychopathology of pancreatic cancer: a psychobiologic probe. Psychosomatics 1993; 34:208–221.

25. Joffe R, Rubinow D, Demicoff K, et al. Depression and carcinoma of the pancreas. Gen Hosp Psychiatry 1986; 8:241–245.

26. Holland JC, Korzun A, Tross S, et al. Comparative psychological disturbance in patients with pancreatic and gastric cancer. Am J Psychiatry 1986; 143:982–986.

27. Kelsen D, Portenoy RK, Thaler H, et al. Pain and depression in patients with newly diagnosed pancreas cancer. J Clin Oncol 1995; 13:748–755.

28. Raddatz D, Horstmann O, Basenau D, et al. Cushing's syndrome due to ectopic adrenocorticotropic hormone production by a non-metastatic gastrinoma after long-term conservative treatment of Zollinger-Ellison syndrome. Ital J Gastroenterol Hepatol 1998; 30:636–640.

29. Drake WM, Perry LA, Hinds CJ, et al. Emergency and prolonged use of intravenous etomidate to control hypercortisolemia in a patient with Cushing's syndrome and peritonitis. J Clin Endocrinol Metab 1998; 83:3542–3544.
30. Geffken GR, Ward HE, Staab JP, et al. Psychiatric morbidity in endocrine disorders. Psychiatr Clin North Am 1998; 21:473–489.
31. Sugimoto F, Sekiya T, Saito M, et al. Calcitonin-producing pancreatic somatostatin-oma: report of a case. Surg Today 1998; 28:1279–1282.
32. Fleury A, Flejou JF, Sauvanet A, et al. Calcitonin-secreting tumors of the pancreas: about six cases. Pancreas 1998; 16:545–550.
33. Hutto B. Subtle psychiatric presentations of endocrine diseases. Psychiatr Clin North Am 1998; 21:905–916.
34. Kawa S, Ueno T, Iijima A, et al. Growth hormone–releasing hormone (GRH)–producing pancreatic tumor with no evidence of multiple endocrine neoplasia type 1. Dig Dis Sci 1997; 42:1480–1485.
35. Losa M, von Werder K. Pathophysiology and clinical aspects of the ectopic GH-releasing hormone syndrome. Clin Endocrinol (Oxf) 1997; 47:123–135.
36. Sandur S, Dasgupta A, Shapiro JL, et al. Thoracic involvement with pheochromocytoma: a review. Chest 1999; 115:511–521.
37. Freda PU, Wardlaw SL, Bruce JN, et al. Differential diagnosis in Cushing's syndrome: use of corticotropin-releasing hormone. Medicine 1995; 74:74–82.
38. Valentine AD, Meyers CA, Kling MA, et al. Mood and cognitive side effects of interferon-alpha therapy. Semin Oncol 1998; 25(Suppl 1):39–47.
39. Licinio J, Kling MA, Hauser P. Cytokines and brain function: relevance to interferon-alpha-induced mood and cognitive changes. Semin Oncol 1998; 25(Suppl 1): 30–38.
40. Meyers CA. Mood and cognitive disorders in cancer patients receiving cytokine therapy. Adv Exp Med Biol 1999; 461:75–81.
41. Anforth HR, Bluthe RM, Bristow A, et al. Biological activity and brain actions of recombinant rat interleukin-1-alpha and interleukin-1-beta. Eur Cytokine Netw 1998; 9:279–288.
42. Anisman H, Ravindran AV, Griffiths J, et al. Endocrine and cytokine correlates of major depression and dysthymia with typical or atypical features. Mol Psychiatry 1999; 4:182–188.
43. Licinio J, Wong ML. The role of inflammatory mediators in the biology of major depression: central nervous system cytokines modulate the biological substrate of depressive symptoms, regulate stress-responsive systems, and contribute to neurotoxicity and neuroprotection. Mol Psychiatry 1999; 4:317–327.
44. Maes M, Bosmans E, Meltzer HY. Immunoendocrine aspects of major depression. Relationships between plasma interleukin-6 and soluble interleukin-2 receptor, prolactin and cortisol. Eur Arch Psychiatry Clin Neurosci 1995; 245: 172–178.
45. Maes M, Meltzer HY, Bosmans E, et al. Increased plasma concentrations of interleukin-6, soluble interleukin-6, soluble interleukin-2 and transferrin receptor in major depression. J Affect Disord 1995; 34:301–309.
46. Caraceni A, Gangeri L, Martini C, et al. Neurotoxicity of interferon-alpha in melanoma therapy: results from a randomized controlled trial. Cancer 1998; 83: 482–489.

47. Capuron L, Ravaud A, Dantzer R. Early depressive symptoms in cancer patients receiving interleukin-2 and/or interferon alfa-2b therapy. J Clin Oncol 2000; 18: 2143–2151.
48. Pirl WF, Roth AJ. Diagnosis and treatment of depression in cancer patients. Oncology 1999; 13:1293–1301.
49. Feighner J, Cohn J, Fabre L, et al. A study comparing paroxetine, placebo, and imipramine in depressed patients. J Affect Disord 1993; 28:71–79.
50. Moller H, Berzewski H, Eckmann F, et al. Double-blind multicenter study of paroxetine and amitriptyline in depressed inpatients. Pharmacopsychiatry 1993; 26: 75–78.
51. Stuppaeck CH, Geretsegger C, Whitwirth AB, et al. A multicenter double-blind trial of paroxetine versus amitriptyline in depressed inpatients. J Clin Psychopharmacol 1994; 14:241–246.
52. Rickels K, Pollack MH, Sheehan DV, et al. Efficacy of extended-release venlafaxine in nondepressed outpatients with generalized anxiety disorder. Am J Psychiatry 2000; 157:968–974.
53. Ballenger JC, Wheadon DE, Steiner M, et al. Double-blind, fixed-dose, placebo-controlled study of paroxetine in the treatment of panic disorder. Am J Psychiatry 1998; 155:36–42.
54. Tesar GE, Rosenbaum JF, Pollack HM, et al. Double-blind, placebo-controlled comparison of clonazepam and alprazolam for panic disorder. J Clin Psychiatry 1991; 52:69–76.
55. Rickels K, Schweizer E, DeMartinis N, et al. Gepirone and diazepam in generalized anxiety disorder: a placebo-controlled trial. J Clin Psychopharmacol 1997; 17: 272–277.
56. Lechin F, van der Dijs B, Benaim M. Benzodiazepines: tolerability in elderly patients. Psychother Psychosom 1996; 65:171–182.
57. Portenoy RK, Itri LM. Cancer-related fatigue: guidelines for evaluation and management. Oncologist 1999; 4:1–10.
58. Courneya KS, Friedenreich CM. Physical exercise and quality of life following cancer diagnosis: a literature review. Ann Behav Med 1999; 21:171–179.
59. Mock V, Dow KH, Meares CJ, et al. Effects of exercise on fatigue, physical functioning, and emotional distress during radiation therapy for breast cancer. Oncol Nurs Forum 1997; 24:991–1000.
60. Bruera E, Brenneis C, Paterson AH, et al. Use of methylphenidate as an adjuvant to narcotic analgesics in patients with advanced cancer. J Pain Symptom Manage 1989; 4:3–6.
61. Weitzner MA, Meyers CA, Valentine AD. Methylphenidate in the treatment of neurobehavioral slowing associated with cancer and cancer treatment. J Neuropsychiatry Clin Neurosci 1995; 7:347–350.
62. Meyers CA, Weitzner MA, Valentine AD, et al. Methylphenidate therapy improves cognition, mood, and function in brain tumor patients. J Clin Oncol 1998; 16: 2522–2527.
63. Breitbart W, Mermelstein H. An alternative psychostimulant for the management of depressive disorders in cancer patients. Psychosomatics 1992; 33:352–356.
64. Ferraro L, Antonelli T, Tanganelli S, et al. The vigilance promoting drug modafinil increases extracellular glutamate levels in the medial preoptic area and the posterior

hypothalamus of the conscious rat: prevention by local $GABA_A$ receptor blockade. Neuropsychopharmacology 1999; 20:346–356.

65. Marin RS. Apathy: concept, syndrome, neural mechanisms, and treatment. Semin Neuropsychiatry 1996; 1:304–314.

66. Popper CW. Pharmacologic alternatives to psychostimulants for the treatment of attention-deficit/hyperactivity disorder. Child Adolesc Psychiatr Clin North Am 2000; 9:605–646.

67. Duffy JD. The neural substrates of motivation. Psychiatr Ann 1997; 27:24–29.

68. Andrykowski MA, Curran SL, Lightner R. Off-treatment fatigue in breast cancer survivors: a controlled comparison. J Behav Med 1998; 21:1–18.

69. Gaston-Johansson F, Fall-Dickson JM, Bakos A, et al. Fatigue, pain, and depression in pre-autotransplant breast cancer patients. Cancer Pract 1999; 7:240–247.

70. Hann DM, Jacobsen PB, Martin SC, et al. Fatigue in women treated with bone marrow transplantation for breast cancer: a comparison with women with no history of cancer. Support Care Cancer 1997; 5:44–52.

71. Hann DM, Jacobsen PB, Martin S, et al. Fatigue and quality of life following radiotherapy for breast cancer: a comparative study. J Clin Psychol Med Settings 1998; 5:19–33.

72. Loge JH, Abrahamsen AF, Ekeberg O, et al. Fatigue and psychiatric morbidity among Hodgkin's disease survivors. J Pain Symptom Manage 2000; 9:91–99.

73. Miaskowski C, Lee KA. Pain, fatigue, and sleep disturbances in oncology outpatients receiving radiation therapy for bone metastasis: a pilot study. J Pain Symptom Manage 1999; 17:320–332.

74. Okuyama T, Akechi T, Kugaya A, et al. Factors correlated with fatigue in disease-free breast cancer patients: application of the Cancer Fatigue Scale. Support Care Cancer 2000; 8:215–222.

75. Okuyama T, Akechi T, Kugaya A, et al. Development and validation of the Cancer Fatigue Scale: a brief, three-dimensional, self-rating scale for assessment of fatigue in cancer patients. J Pain Symptom Manage 2000; 19:5–14.

76. Pickard-Holley S. Fatigue in cancer patients. Cancer Nurs 1991; 14:13–19.

77. Smets EM, Visser MR, Willems-Grott AF, et al. Fatigue and radiotherapy: (A) experience in patients undergoing treatment. Br J Cancer 1998; 78:899–906.

78. Smets EM, Visser MR, Willems-Grott AF, et al. Fatigue and radiotherapy: (B) experience in patients 9 months following treatment. Br J Cancer 1998; 78:907–912.

79. Stone P, Hardy J, Broadley K, et al. Fatigue in advanced cancer: a prospective controlled cross-sectional study. Br J Cancer 1999; 79:1479–1486.

10

Fatigue in Medical Illness:
Research Issues

RUSSELL K. PORTENOY

Fatigue is a highly prevalent and complex symptom in populations with chronic illness.[1] Although there have been significant advances in the methodologies to measure fatigue, few scientific investigations have focused on the nature of the problem and its management in clinical settings. In many ways, fatigue research is now at a point similar to pain research a quarter-century ago. Valid and reliable measurement is possible, and a growing number of epidemiological studies have established the seriousness of the clinical problem. The field is primed for studies that may illuminate the pathophysiology of the disorder in varied patient populations and provide an evidence base for treatment selection.

The Nature of the Problem

Epidemiology

The management of fatigue in serious medical illness can be subsumed under the therapeutic model of palliative care. To optimize palliative care, clinicians must ensure that physical comfort is a priority, practical needs are addressed, psychosocial and spiritual distress is managed, values and decisions are respected, and opportunities become available for growth and closure. Although the need for palliative care intensifies as death approaches, fatigue and other concerns are addressed by this model throughout the course of a life-threatening illness.

Fatigue is common in the general population, and the first step in clarifying the nature of the problem in the medically ill is to distinguish a disorder, or group of disorders, that may be characterized as pathological fatigue. The prevalence rates highlight the distinction. The base rate for fatigue in the general population is less than 20%.[2,3] A recent population-based survey observed that 78% of cancer patients had experienced significant fatigue,[4] and other surveys confirm that more than 75% of patients with metastatic neoplasms report clinically significant fatigue.[5-10] In the cancer population, prevalence rates are even higher following some types of chemotherapy, radiation therapy, and treatment with biological response modifiers such as the interferons and interleukins.[11-18] Fatigue associated with progressive disease or persistent co-morbidities can be prolonged, and several studies also have documented the potential for chronic fatigue in long-term cancer survivors.[19-24]

The pathological nature of disease-related and treatment-related fatigue in the cancer population is suggested by its correlation with phenomena related to impaired quality of life. Studies evaluating these relationships have shown that fatigue is associated with negative mood, diminished performance status, and sleep disturbance.

Epidemiological data in other patient populations are more limited. The prevalence of fatigue has varied between 44% and 85% in surveys of populations with human immunodeficiency virus,[25] chronic obstructive pulmonary disease,[26] multiple sclerosis,[27] Parkinson's disease,[28] systemic lupus erythematosis,[29,30] and primary biliary sclerosis.[31] Fatigue in these populations is also associated with impaired performance and poor mood.

Definition and clinical variability

As a symptom, like pain and dyspnea, fatigue can be validly ascertained only through patient report. Although objective measurements, such as exercise tolerance, can be informative, fatigue itself is inherently subjective. For this reason, case ascertainment and measurement rely on the use of valid and reliable questionnaires.

The development of a well-accepted nomenclature for pathological fatigue would help to guide measurement strategies. A definition of cancer-related fatigue developed for the International Classification of Diseases (10th Revision, Clinical Modification)[32] is undergoing validation (Table 10.1). This definition explicitly notes the multidimensional nature of fatigue. Like all symptoms, this multidimensionality relates, in part, to the personal experience of intensity, timing (for example, fluctuation and course), and quality.

Based on clinical observation, the quality of fatigue may be relevant to an understanding of its pathophysiology and management. Patients may describe fatigue in terms that denote a global lack of energy, cognitive impairment, sleepiness, muscle weakness, mood disturbance, or some combination of these descriptors (Table 10.2). This variability suggests the existence of fatigue subtypes, each of which may have distinct mechanisms. In this way, fatigue may be similar to pain, subtypes of which based on inferred mechanisms (somatic, visceral, and neuropathic) are used clinically in treatment planning. Studies are needed that better define fatigue subtypes and the syndromes with which they

Table 10.1. Proposed critera for cancer-related fatigue

1. The following symptoms have been present every day or nearly every day during the same 2-week period in the past month:

    Significant fatigue, diminished energy, or increased need to rest, disproportionate to any recent change in activity level

2. Plus five (or more) of the following:

    Complaints of generalized weakness or limb heaviness
    Diminished concentration or attention
    Decreased motivation or interest in engaging in usual activities
    Insomnia or hypersomnia
    Experience of sleep as unrefreshing or nonrestorative
    Perceived need to struggle to overcome inactivity
    Marked emotional reactivity (sadness, frustration, or irritability) to feeling fatigued
    Difficulty completing daily tasks attributed to feeling fatigued
    Perceived problems with short-term memory
    Postexertional malaise lasting several hours

3. The symptoms cause clinically significant distress or impairment in social, occupational, or other important areas of functioning.

4. There is evidence from the history, physical examination, or laboratory findings that the symptoms are the consequence of cancer or cancer-related therapy.

5. The symptoms are not primarily a consequence of comorbid psychiatric disorders such as major depression, somatization disorder, somatoform disorder, or delirium.

may be linked. The pathophysiologies of fatigue should be explored in relation to these phenomenological subtypes.

One of the challenges of fatigue assessment is to capture the multidimensionality of the experience. Although fatigue can be assessed as a dichotomous variable (present or absent, according to some criterion definition) or unidimensionally (for example, by an intensity measurement alone), the simplicity of these approaches must be balanced by the missed opportunity to capture information about the other dimensions, including qualitative differences that could potentially distinguish clinically meaningful fatigue subtypes. The use of more sophisticated assessment methodologies can yield far more information (see below).

Mechanisms

The likelihood of fatigue subtypes gains credence from the proposed diversity of mechanisms, and this diversity poses other opportunities for research. Theoretically, fatigue could be related to changes in energy metabolism associated with increased requirement (due to disease-related metabolic activity, infection or fever, or tissue injury), decreased availability of metabolic requirements (due to anemia, hypoxemia, or poor nutrition), or the production of substances that impair metabolism or normal muscle function (cytokines or

Table 10.2. Descriptors applied to fatigue

Related to a sense of energy or vitality	Related to sleep
Fatigue	Somnolent
Lack of energy	Nonrestorative sleep
Lethargy	**Related to strength**
Tiredness	Weakness
Exhaustion	Fatigability of muscles
Related to cognitive change	Postexertional breathlessness or exhaustion
Cloudedness or confusion	**Related to mood**
Apathy	Irritability
Inattentiveness	Lability
Poor concentration	Depression
Poor memory	

antibodies). Other proposed mechanisms link fatigue to the pathophysiology of sleep disorders or major depression.

Research Questions

In contrast to the epidemiology of cancer-related fatigue, which has been explored in many surveys, including several large population-based studies,[33,34] there are few data on other populations of seriously ill patients. Additional epidemiological surveys are needed to better clarify the nature of fatigue (including prevalence, severity, time course, and phenomenology), to identify syndromes, and to document impact. These surveys promise to yield a strong foundation for clinical trials and studies of fatigue mechanisms.

There have been very few studies of treatments for fatigue in medically ill patients. At the present time, treatment strategies derive largely from clinical observation.[35] This experience suggests numerous targets for research.

The initial approach to the management of fatigue typically involves efforts to correct potential etiologies, if possible and appropriate given the goals of care. This may include elimination of nonessential drugs, treatment of a sleep disorder, reversal of anemia or other metabolic abnormalities, improvement in nutrition, or management of major depression. None of these interventions has been systematically studied in any population with fatigue. Surveys and controlled clinical trials are needed to address the many clinical questions suggested by these approaches.

Studies of treatment for anemia exemplify the issues. Combined data from three randomized, placebo-controlled trials of epoetin alfa, the recombinant form of human erythropoietin, revealed an association between increased hematocrit and improvement in overall quality of life.[36] Three large, prospective, nonrandomized, multicenter community trials (combined $n > 6000$) similarly observed that patients who experienced a rise in hemoglobin following treatment with epoetin alfa reported significant improvements in energy level, activity level, functional status, and overall quality of life.[37-39] These outcomes were independent of antitumor response. Controlled studies that use fatigue as the primary end point and evaluate the effect of hemoglobin change are clearly justified by these data.

Fatigue that cannot be satisfactorily controlled following treatment for a probable etiology may benefit from symptomatic therapy. Symptomatic therapies may be pharmacological or nonpharmacological. Very few of these interventions have been evaluated in controlled clinical trials.

Psychostimulants, such as methylphenidate, pemoline, and dextroamphetamine, have been studied as treatments for opioid-related somnolence and cognitive impairment[40] as well as depression.[41] Modafinil, a newer psychostimulant, is also being used for fatigue. Studies are needed to confirm efficacy and safety, clarify impact on functional outcomes and quality of life, compare the various drugs, and assess the dose–response relationship and the duration of effect.

Limited data from controlled trials[42,43] also support the use of low-dose corticosteroids, such as prednisone and dexamethasone. Studies are needed to assess the efficacy of these drugs in other diseases, determine the relationship between dose and response, clarify the risks and benefits of different steroids, and compare this class against others.

Anecdotal observation suggests that some antidepressant drugs may be effective for fatigue even in patients without clinical depression. Specifically, the selective serotonin-reuptake inhibitors, secondary amine tricyclics (such as nortriptyline and desipramine), and bupropion sometimes appear to yield increased energy disproportionate to mood change. Studies are needed to evaluate their efficacy as primary therapy for fatigue.

There is evidence from controlled trials that patient education[44] and exercise[45] can be helpful interventions for cancer-related fatigue. Other nonpharmacological approaches are supported by favorable anecdotal experience. Many of these interventions, such as instruction in so-called sleep hygiene principles and cognitive therapies like relaxation, guided imagery, or hypnosis, deserve further study. Additional studies are needed to clarify the most appropriate populations and protocols for exercise.

Fatigue Assessment

In the clinical setting, fatigue assessment may involve comprehensive evaluation of the symptom itself and a broad range of associated physical and psychosocial factors. Measurement of fatigue intensity or other specific characteristics is an essential aspect of this comprehensive assessment. Measurement can apply to any dimension that can be validly scaled, including severity, other common descriptors (such as duration), related elements within the larger experience (such as sleep quality, muscle strength, or mood), and impact on functioning (such as the ability to work or socialize).

Given the many aspects of fatigue that could be specifically measured, researchers must thoughtfully consider the aims of a study and select an assessment strategy that provides sufficient information about the characteristics of the symptom, the co-morbidities, and the clinical context to enhance the interpretability and generalizability of the data.

Unidimensional fatigue measurement

Fatigue measurement using simple unidimensional scales typically focuses on severity (Table 10.3). The most common are four- or five-point verbal rating scales, numeric scales, and visual analogue scales (also called linear analogue scale assessment). The psychometrics of a linear analogue and a numeric scale have been evaluated in a population with end-stage renal disease.[46] Verbal rating

Table 10.3. Examples of unidimensional measures of fatigue severity

---

Four-point verbal rating scale

| None | Mild | Moderate | Severe |

Five-point verbal rating scale

| None | Mild | Moderate | Severe | Very Severe |

Eleven-point numeric scale

On a 0–10 scale, where 0 equals no fatigue and 10 equals the worst fatigue imaginable, how severe has fatigue been, on average, during the past week

Four-point numeric scale (Common Toxicity Criteria of the National Cancer Institute)

	0	**1**	**2**	**3**	**4**
Fatigue (lethargy, malaise, asthenia)	None	Increased fatigue over baseline but not altering normal activities	Moderate (decrease in performance status by 1 ECOG level *or* 20% Karnofsky or Lansky) *or* causing difficulty performing some activities	Severe (decrease in performance status by ≥2 ECOG levels *or* 40% Karnofsky or Lansky) *or* loss of ability to perform some activities	Bedridden

10 cm visual analogue scale

| | |
| No Fatigue | Worst Possible Fatigue |

---

scales and numeric scales have been incorporated into a number of symptom checklists.[47–49]

Several other unidimensional approaches have been used to acquire a global measure of fatigue severity. The widely translated and validated quality-of-life measure created for the European Organization for Research and Treatment of Cancer (EORTC), the EORTC QLQ-C30, has a subscale for fatigue that may be used apart from the rest of the instrument.[50] This subscale has three items: Were you tired?, Have you felt weak?, Did you need a rest? Each is graded on a four-point verbal rating scale. The nine-item Fatigue Severity Scale[27] and the vigor/fatigue subscale of the Profile of Mood States[51] similarly reflect global fatigue severity. An older scale, the Pearson-Byars Fatigue Checklist, has been used in studies of cancer patients but was validated in a healthy population and has been supplanted by newer measures.[52]

Multidimensional fatigue measurement

Multidimensional fatigue questionnaires complement the measurement of fatigue severity with information about other characteristics or the impact of fatigue on different types of functioning.[53] Efforts to measure multiple dimensions of fatigue began three decades ago in nonmedically ill populations[54,55] and have advanced significantly since then. There are now many validated instruments of this type (Table 10.4).[14,27,56–64]

There are advantages and disadvantages in selecting a multidimensional assessment instrument in a study of fatigue. The most important advantage is that multidimensional assessment allows analyses that potentially clarify the nature of a fatigue syndrome or the type of response that occurs following an intervention. For example, a multidimensional instrument could clarify the extent to which an intervention such as epoetin alfa affects fatigue in general, the cognitive component of fatigue, or mood.

There also may be disadvantages, however. All of the validated multidimensional assessment questionnaires have been developed in the cancer population,

Table 10.4. Multidimensional fatigue questionnaires

Piper Fatigue Scale[56]
Lee Fatigue Scale[57]
Fatigue Assessment Questionnaire[58]
Functional Assessment of Cancer Therapy–Anemia/Fatigue[59]
Fatigue Symptom Inventory[60]
Brief Fatigue Inventory[61]
Cancer Fatigue Scale[62]
Schwartz Cancer Fatigue Scale[63]
Multidimensional Fatigue Inventory[64]

---

and there has been no cross-validation to populations with other serious illnesses. There also have been no studies to determine the extent to which the different instruments measure similar constructs in the same population. For this reason, the information collected during a study may not be reliable or valid for the population in question or may not be fully relevant to address the specific aims of the study.

The investigator considering the use of a specific multidimensional questionnaire should be familiar with the supporting literature and carefully review the items to determine whether they cover the domains and characteristics of interest. The investigator may discover that the questionnaire most suited for the study still lacks important items. For example, many questionnaires do not adequately assess the varied qualities of fatigue discussed previously (for example, sleep disturbance, mood disturbance, or cognitive impairment). Some, but not others, assess fatigue-associated distress, temporal characteristics (such as onset, duration, fluctuation, and course), or factors that worsen or relieve the fatigue.

To complement a multidimensional questionnaire, specific items can be developed or additional validated questionnaires can be added to the questionnaire packet. The use of single items is simpler but must be recognized as face-valid only. If the investigator has a particular interest in depression, for example, either a single item on depressed mood (numeric or visual analogue scale) or a brief and validated depression inventory could be added. The use of a validated measure provides more confidence in the information but may compromise efforts to keep the questionnaire packet brief.

Other elements in fatigue assessment

The goals of some studies justify the addition of ancillary measurements. For example, a study that evaluated changes in sleep patterns among fatigued patients undergoing radiation therapy used a noninvasive technique of wrist actigraphy to measure hours of sleep, sleep efficiency, and number of awakenings.[65] Studies of therapies for fatigue that could have strong effects on cognitive dysfunction, such as a new psychostimulant, might justify the addition of a neuropsychological assessment as a secondary outcome.

Some objective tests may be used to provide data that can complement the measurement of subjective outcomes. For example, a randomized trial of an exercise program in women with fatigue following radiotherapy[45] incorporated a 12-minute walk test, in which the distance in feet that can be traveled in 12 minutes is measured.[66] This type of test correlates highly with results from laboratory measurements of oxygen consumption during exercise,[67] which also could be used as such an ancillary measure.

Assessment also can focus on any of the numerous potential etiologies and relevant co-morbidities of fatigue (Table 10.5). Formal approaches to the assessment of medical co-morbidities have been developed using either chart review[68] or patient interview.[69] Alternatively, a checklist can be developed that can codify

Table 10.5. Potential etiologies and relevant co-morbidities considered for measurement in studies of fatigue

Variable	Types	Examples of measurements
Medical/Physical		
Primary disease severity	Extent of disease	Stage (cancer)
	Degree of organ failure	Ejection fraction (heart failure)
		FEV_1 (lung disease)
Primary therapy	Chemotherapy	Type and timing
	Surgery	Type and timing
Metabolic disorders	Anemia	Hemoglobin
	Electrolyte disturbances	Electrolytes, calcium
	Malnutrition	Weight, calorie count, skinfold thickness
Presence of infection	—	Record diagnosis and severity
Cardiopulmonary disorders	Co-morbid CHF, COPD	Record diagnosis
		Po_2, pulse oximetry, ejection fraction, FEV_1
Renal disorders	Co-morbid renal insufficiency	Record diagnosis
		Creatinine clearance
Hepatic disorders	Co-morbid insufficiency	Record diagnosis
		Albumin, bilirubin, liver function tests
Neuromuscular disorders	Neuropathy	Record diagnosis
	Myopathy	Dynomometry
		Electrodiagnostic studies
Centrally acting drugs	Opioids	Medication diary
	Sedative/hypnotics	
Sleep disorder	—	Sleep questionnaire
Other symptoms	Pain	Symptom questionnaire
	Dyspnea	
Deconditioning	—	Performance status or function questionnaire
		50-foot or 12-minute walk test
Psychological/social		
Mood disorder	Depression	Psychological distress, depression, or anxiety questionnaire

FEV_1, forced expiratory volume in 1 second; CHF, congestive heart failure; COPD, chronic obstructive pulmonary disease; Po_2, partial pressure of oxygen.

the existence of the most important of these phenomena. The checklist can be completed using information from the medical record (such as recent hemoglobin level), patient history and physical examination (such as degree of physical inactivity), or brief screening tools that are added to the questionnaire packet (such as a depression screen).

Additional relevant information can be obtained from a minimally burdensome intervention, such as pulse oximetry or blood sampling to measure hemoglobin or electrolytes. Other information is obtainable only with more elaborate testing, such as pulmonary function tests or electrodiagnostic studies. Respondent burden must be balanced against the anticipated value of the data when designing the assessment protocol for a study.

Assessment of related constructs

An assessment of fatigue also may consider broader concerns, such as global quality of life and symptom distress. Some of the fatigue scales, such as the unidimensional three-item scale of the EORTC QLQ-C30 and the multidimensional fatigue subscale of the Functional Assessment of Cancer Therapy, are themselves modules of well-validated quality-of-life instruments. In other cases, fatigue measurement is included in scales that assess multiple other symptoms or global symptom distress. If the broader construct is of key interest, the larger scales may be most relevant. Alternatively, a separate quality-of-life or symptom-assessment questionnaire can be added to accomplish the same goal.

Issues in Designing Fatigue Surveys

Well-conducted surveys can generate hypotheses about the biological underpinnings of the symptom, characterize fatigue syndromes in different populations of medically ill patients, and clarify the relationships among fatigue characteristics and various etiologies or comorbidities. The relationships between fatigue qualities (possible subtypes), demographic disease-related or treatment-related variables, and objective indicators of disease (specific metabolic disturbances such as cytokine levels) can be illuminated by this research. Surveys also can potentially clarify responses to therapy and guide the development of subsequent trials.

Case definition

Case definition for fatigue must be carefully considered when designing a study. Cases may be defined simply by the descriptor *fatigue* or some other related label (such as *lack of energy* or *weakness*). Presumably, this approach will yield the largest number of cases and a broad range of symptom severity. In survey research, this broad distribution of severity may allow more robust multivariate analyses of factors associated with fatigue.

The potential benefits in using a simple term to define cases for study are balanced by the possibility of a skewed distribution, with a large majority of cases reflecting mild fatigue or even possibly, fatigue that is not "pathological." If this occurs, it could complicate the interpretation of the data or lead to questions about the generalizability of the results.

To address the latter concern, a case of fatigue may be identified by specific eligibility criteria. For example, eligibility for a survey may be established by a question about fatigue impact (an affirmative response to an item such as "Have you experienced fatigue severe enough to impair your ability to function during the past week?") or severity (for example, score ≥5 on the item "How would you rate your fatigue, on average during the past week, using a 0 to 10 scale, where 0 is no fatigue at all and 10 is the worst fatigue that you can imagine?"). Even the use of a simple descriptor, such as *debilitating* or *significant*, should lead to the capture of a more clinically relevant sample.

Specific criteria are valuable to more precisely define the cases under study and provide a sample more likely to reflect clinically important pathological fatigue. The investigator must realize, however, that a poorly chosen criterion could lead to exclusion of a large proportion of those with milder fatigue. Depending on the population and the study questions, the sample may be skewed and poorly representative.

Clearly, there is no one best approach to case definition in surveys of fatigue. For each study, the investigator must make some informed guesses about the type of sample that will provide information on the key aims. In this process, discussion with a biostatistician is important and may clarify the types of analysis to which the data will ultimately be subjected.

Data collection

The data collected during fatigue surveys usually include details concerning the characteristics of the symptom and information about demographics, the disease and its treatments, and drug therapies. Additional information about potential etiologies or relevant co-morbidities, which may be obtained from the medical record, questionnaire or interview, or specific tests, should be pursued if it can clarify the nature of the clinical problem or the population studied and will not impose excessive respondent burden.

Data-collection methodologies can be prospective or retrospective. Prospective data collection from the patient is the "gold standard" for surveys of subjective phenomena. The challenge in these surveys is to design a questionnaire packet and an assessment protocol that will yield high recruitment and completion rates and will adequately address the specific aims of the study.

Retrospective data typically are gleaned from the medical record. Given the reality of poor clinical assessment of subjective outcomes and limitations in record keeping, this information is credible only if the symptom was systematically evaluated as an integral aspect of clinical practice. For example, routine administration of a symptom assessment scale to all patients admitted to a hospital unit might yield interpretable information captured through a retrospective review.

The timing of data collection is a critical element in the survey process. A cross-sectional survey, in which patients are recruited to complete a questionnaire battery on one occasion, is simple and far less costly to perform than a longitudinal study. A longitudinal approach, however, is capable of providing important information about time course and variability and may allow more precise hypotheses to be developed about causal links among variables. Changes over time can be assessed using a methodology that repeatedly evaluates a specific patient sample over time or different samples from a defined population over time.

Whether the survey is cross-sectional or longitudinal, the specific questions must define a time period of assessment. Recall bias becomes a problem if queries relate back to periods beyond a few days or a week. The *response shift*, or change in perception of past events due to shifting contexts, is similarly a concern when assessing a subjective phenomenon that commonly changes over time. To reduce these concerns and assess fatigue prevalence in a population at any point in time (*point prevalence*), the inquiry must define a relatively brief period of assessment. This can be done by assessing "fatigue right now" or "fatigue during the past day (or week)." Some surveys query a longer interval that attempts to cue the patient by linking to a specific event (for instance, "since radiation or chemotherapy was given"). The latter may be better understood as a so-called period prevalence, rather than point prevalence.

Maximizing completion

Questionnaire packets should be as brief as possible to reduce the refusal rate for participation in the study, the dropout rate among those who initially agree to participate, and the rate of missing data. A variety of factors may influence the decision concerning the length of the packet. Use of a relatively brief questionnaire (15–20 minutes to complete) would be reasonable if there is no access to a dedicated data collector, if the questionnaire must be completed in one sitting and there is no one to help read it to the patient, or if the population has a large proportion of patients with significant medical or psychiatric co-morbidities. A longer questionnaire packet (more than 20 minutes) becomes feasible if there is a dedicated data collector, if an option is given to complete the packet over two or three contacts or at home, if the data collector or some other investigator is available to read the questions to the patient (in person or over the phone), or if medical or psychiatric co-morbidities are minimal.

In the absence of prior experience with the questionnaire packet in the study population, it is usually prudent to build into a survey a pilot phase during which the questionnaire packet is given to a small number of representative patients (usually about 10–20). Patients who participate in the pilot can be asked for feedback about the questionnaires. Length can be adjusted and specific questions deleted or changed on the basis of this information.

Given the inevitability of missing data, it is appropriate to establish guidelines for the handling of this eventuality. There is no one best approach. If there are important subscales, such as for depression or sleep, it is appropriate to stipulate the number of missing items from the scale that would lead to deletion of the subscale score. This usually depends on the number of items in the scale. For the questionnaire overall, it may be appropriate to designate 15% missing data as the threshold for withdrawing the patient from the totals.

Issues in Designing Fatigue Intervention Trials

Selecting a design

Intervention trials may be designed with a greater or lesser degree of control. It is helpful to consider the options as a hierarchy of progressive controls, each of which is intended to further reduce the risk of systematic bias that could lead to erroneous results.

Quasi-experimental studies

The least control, and hence the greatest doubt about validity of the findings, is available when an intervention is administered openly to a series of patients without comparison data. This type of survey can provide information about safety and some information about efficacy but must be interpreted cautiously because of potentially powerful influences on response. These include the placebo effect and a tendency for subjects entering a clinical trial to "regress to the mean." In surveys of fatigue, the latter effect presumably occurs because many subjects agree to participate when the problem is relatively severe and the desire for help is greatest.

Evaluation of many therapies begins with simple studies of this type. Although all conclusions should be considered tentative, some results may be particularly meaningful. For example, the inability to demonstrate any positive outcomes would suggest that the specific intervention is unlikely to be effective.

Quasi-experimental designs that collect "pre/post" data can be enhanced in several ways. Entry criteria should be carefully stipulated to identify a sample that is best suited to show the effects of the intervention, and the timing and duration of data collection should be selected to maximize the likelihood of capturing effects and illuminating the time course, if this is of interest. For example, in a study of an intervention for fatigue following radiation therapy for early-stage breast carcinoma, all patients undergoing radiation would become candidates for weekly screening questions, the purpose of which is to identify those patients who develop a level of fatigue appropriate for the study. Patients who experience a criterion level of fatigue (for instance, fatigue severe enough to interfere with functioning during the past week) would be asked to complete a baseline assessment. In most cases, this would occur before the radiation is completed. After this point, assessments might be planned for intervals that would likely capture additional weeks on therapy and a period of 1–2 months after radiation is completed.

The addition of a comparison group(s) can provide more information, even if the design is nonrandomized and open-label. Comparison groups can be retrospective or prospective. Prospectively assessed patients who are similar to those who receive the study intervention and undergo identical assessment yield much more credible data. In all cases, the comparison group must be similar to the study group or distinct from the study group in some systematic way that can be statistically controlled after the data are collected. It is often worthwhile to match the study and comparison groups on one or more key variables, such as age and gender, or specific fatigue-related or disease-related variables.

Use of multiple comparison groups may illuminate the effect of more than one key variable. For example, a study of an exercise protocol in patients with metastatic cancer may yield interesting "pre/post" information about energy level, mental clarity, and potential adverse effects. Collection of data from similar but untreated patients would be the comparison of first priority. If feasible, however, additional comparisons, such as the effect of the exercise protocol on fatigued patients following curative resection of the same disease, would be informative.

In quasi-experimental studies, decisions about sample size often consider both the primary outcome, usually fatigue intensity, and the potential for covariate analyses. Some of these analyses relate specifically to the fatigue assessment. If this assessment has included multidimensional data, such as information about cognitive impairment, sleep, and depressed mood, it is possible to control for these phenomena when determining the impact of the intervention on fatigue intensity or to analyze the effect of the intervention on the different dimensions. If the sample size is large enough and information about potential etiologies and relevant comorbidities is carefully collected, it may be possible to explore the extent to which various other elements, such as low hemoglobin levels or physical deconditioning, influence the effect of the intervention on fatigue. Multivariate statistical models require numerous subjects for each variable assessed (10 or more). Consultation with a biostatistician while designing the study can clarify the types of analysis that might be undertaken and, in turn, determine the optimal sample size.

Controlled trials

The most valid methodologies to determine the efficacy of a treatment randomly assign patients to receive either the treatment or some alternate intervention for comparison. Random assignment minimizes the risk of systematic bias by distributing variables that may influence outcome between the study groups.

Random assignment does not, however, eliminate the possibility that the outcomes observed are related to placebo effects. To establish the efficacy of an intervention distinct from a nonspecific placebo effect, the intervention must be compared directly with placebo. If feasible, a study design that incorporates randomization, double-blinding of treatments, and a placebo control is most likely to provide evidence that either confirms or refutes efficacy.

A placebo control is not possible with most nonpharmacological interventions, such as exercise or cognitive therapies. In these studies, patients are usually randomly assigned to receive the study intervention or a control selected to reduce some sources of bias. For example, contact with the investigator is a potential source of bias (through nonspecific positive effects that lessen symptom distress), and a useful control group may include some degree of investigator contact without access to the study intervention. More than one control group of this type can be created, to further clarify the intervention effect. For example, a study of a cognitive therapy (such as hypnosis) may incorporate a control group that receives some educational materials related to the problem of fatigue and another control group that is allowed to make an appointment with the investigator but will receive no intervention (so-called waiting list control).

If the efficacy of a drug therapy is established, future trials may directly compare the proposed treatment to this established approach. In such studies, the established therapy becomes an active control. There may be advantages to this type of study (such as greater clinical relevance), but the investigator must recognize the potential problem in a finding of "no difference" between treatments. In two-arm studies that compare potentially active therapies, the finding of "no difference" has two potential interpretations: (*1*) the two treatments are therapeutically equivalent or (*2*) the study methodology was insufficiently sensitive to identify important differences. This methodology, therefore, can yield a meaningless outcome even if randomization, double-blinding and other controls are in place.

To ensure the interpretability of comparative studies, it is best to include treatment arms that can directly evaluate the sensitivity of the methods. In drug studies, for example, this may be done by including both a placebo and the active control (the established treatment) or by testing two or more doses of the active control. If the study cannot identify a difference between the placebo and the active control or cannot identify a dose–response relationship for the effective drug, then the sensitivity of the methods is in question and a finding of no difference between the study drug and the comparator cannot be viewed as evidence of therapeutic equivalence.

In comparative studies of nonpharmacological therapies, it may not be possible to assess the method's sensitivity. In some cases, however, treatment arms may be created that vary in the intensity of an established approach and accomplish this. For example, a study comparing aerobic exercise, an established treatment for cancer-related fatigue, with another nonpharmacological approach could randomly assign patients to two different levels of exercise.

In controlled clinical trials, it is important to establish a primary end point at the outset. The end point is defined by both the primary outcome variable and the primary time point for analysis. This information is used in sample size calculations.

The primary end point is chosen based on the existing literature, clinical experience, or theoretical considerations related to the likely effects of an intervention. For example, the primary end point in a study of a psychostimulant drug for chronic cancer-related fatigue might be the change in average daily fatigue measurable after 1 week of treatment. A study of the same drug in patients undergoing curative radiation therapy might select the same variable (change in average daily fatigue) but would miss the relevant timing of the effect unless the primary end point was designated to be 3–6 weeks after treatment started.

Selecting study procedures

The implementation of successful intervention trials requires intensive planning and management of innumerable details. Procedures must be developed to identify and recruit patients, obtain informed consent, organize the study treatments, and collect and manage data. Most decisions about these procedures require an assessment of trade-offs. Simplicity, ease of administration, and limited respondent burden must be balanced against the need for careful controls to maintain quality, allow interpretability, and enhance the scope of the information ultimately available from the trial. Each decision also has cost implications, and the availability of funds may strongly influence sample size (the number of treatment arms possible) and the specific procedures used.

Given the limited experience in the practical administration of controlled drug trials for fatigue, there can be no firm guidelines for specific study approaches (for example, the use of crossover versus parallel groups, the use of placebo and active controls, the techniques to assay study sensitivity). It is reasonable to consider the experience gained in pain research when making these decisions.[70]

Inclusion and exclusion criteria should be selected to yield a study sample that is relevant to the research question, willing to participate, likely to complete the study's tasks, and unlikely to present complications that would undermine the validity of the data collected. The inclusion criteria for fatigue must consider case definition, as discussed previously. In most situations, a fatigue duration of 1 or 2 weeks is sufficient to consider the symptom significant enough to study.

To systematically implement the intervention under study, the investigator must ensure reliable procedures and adequate quality control. Studies of nonpharmcological interventions may require a written resource guide and detailed training of researchers, followed by testing to establish uniformity in the intervention across individuals. Controlled drug trials also rely on investigator training and typically require a research pharmacist, who prepares the study and comparator drugs and dispenses these to a researcher based on a predetermined randomization protocol.

The protocol stipulates the methods and timing of data collection. The usual desire to collect as much data as possible must be tempered by the risk of excessive respondent burden. Perceived or actual respondent burden can result in poor recruitment and patient dropout. In the absence of any meaningful experience from which to judge the capabilities of the population, it is prudent to build a pilot phase into the study.

If the population from which the study sample is recruited has a high prevalence of fatigue, patients can be screened with a brief verbal item about fatigue to determine eligibility. Eligible patients can then be recruited directly, sign consent, and be given the baseline assessment questionnaire packet. In some populations, such as those with fatigue that evolves after a treatment, the protocol may need to stipulate repeated verbal screening of cases to identify those who become eligible as fatigue develops.

In studies that randomly assign treatments, randomization typically occurs prior to baseline data collection. The protocol must be very specific in defining the procedures for implementation of the study treatments and the data collection that occurs in tandem. The intervention may require weeks and involve titration (gradual dose adjustment, increasing exercise, or other). Repeated data collection should be timed to provide relevant information about time course or accruing effects, as well as information about maximum effect.

In drug trials, there are considerable advantages to the linkage of an open-label extension trial to a controlled study. It can provide information about the durability of the effects and the safety of the treatment on prolonged exposure. Because treatment mimics clinical practice, the extension phase can help assess the overall utility of therapy to the patient in a way that the more intensive exposure during the controlled trial cannot. Finally, it is likely that access to a long treatment period after the study enhances recruitment.

Issues in data analysis

The analytic approaches adopted for analgesic trials can be extrapolated for fatigue research. Change scores, which can be summarized by subtracting the baseline data from subsequent data points, are informative outcomes because they take the baseline level of fatigue into account. An alternative approach that also allows interpretable group comparisons is to control for baseline fatigue by entering it into an appropriate covariate analysis. Exploratory post-hoc multivariate analyses also should be considered, to clarify the relationships among fatigue characterisics and other variables. There is so much yet to learn about fatigue that this type of analysis is justified and could potentially identify associations that were obscure and suggest future lines of research.

Conclusion

Studies are needed to clarify the mechanisms that underlie various types of fatigue, understand the epidemiology of the symptom, and provide an evidence base for management decisions. There have been important advances in fatigue-assessment methodologies during the past decade, and there are now opportunities to advance fatigue-related research and provide new tools to benefit the quality of life of medically ill patients.

References

1. Portenoy RK, Miaskowski C. Assessment and management of cancer-related fatigue. In: Berger A, Weissman D, Portenoy RK, eds. Principles and Practice of Supportive Oncology. Philadelphia: JB Lippincott, 1998:109–118.
2. Pawlikowska T, Chalder T, Hirsch SR, et al. Population-based study of fatigue and psychological distress. BMJ 1994; 308:763–766.
3. Loge JH, Ekeberg O, Kaasa S. Fatigue in the general Norwegian population: normative data and associations. J Psychosom Res 1998; 45:53–65.
4. Vogelzang N, Breitbart W, Cella D, et al. Patient, caregiver, and oncologist perceptions of cancer-related fatigue: results of a tripart assessment survey. Semin Hematol 1997; 34(Suppl 2):4–12.
5. Curtis EB, Kretch R, Walsh TD. Common symptoms in patients with advanced cancer. J Palliat Care 1991; 7:25–29.
6. Dunphy KP, Amesbury BDW. A comparison of hospice and homecare patients: patterns of referral, patient characteristics and predictors of place of death. Palliat Med 1990; 4:105–111.
7. Dunlop GM. A study of the relative frequency and importance of gastrointestinal symptoms and weakness in patients with far-advanced cancer: student paper. Palliat Med 1989; 4:37–43.
8. Portenoy RK, Thaler HT, Kornblith AB, et al. Symptom prevalence, characteristics, and distress in a cancer population. Qual Life Res 1994; 3:183–189.
9. Ventafridda V, DeConno F, Ripamonti C, et al. Quality of life assessment during a palliative care program. Ann Oncol 1990; 1:415–420.
10. Vainio A, Auvinen A, and members of the Symptom Prevalence Group. Prevalence of symptoms among patients with advanced cancer: an international collaborative study. J Pain Symptom Manage 1996; 12:3–10.
11. Greenberg DB, Sawicka J, Eisenthal S, et al. Fatigue syndrome due to localized radiation. J Pain Symptom Manage 1992; 7:38–45.
12. Haylock PJ, Hart LK. Fatigue in patients receiving localized radiation. Cancer Nurs 1979; 2:461–467.
13. Hickok JT, Morrow GR, McDonald S, et al. Frequency and correlates of fatigue in lung cancer patients receiving radiation therapy. J Pain Symptom Manage 1996; 11:370–377.
14. Smets EMA, Garssen B, Cull A, et al. Application of the Multidimensional Fatigue Inventory (MFI-20) in cancer patients receiving radiotherapy. Br J Cancer 1996; 73:241–245.
15. Irvine DM, Vincent L, Bubela N, et al. A critical appraisal of the research literature investigating fatigue in the individual with cancer. Cancer Nurs 1991; 14:188–199.
16. Irvine D, Vincent L, Graydon JE, et al. The prevalence and correlates of fatigue in patients receiving treatment with chemotherapy and radiotherapy: a comparison with the fatigue experienced by healthy individuals. Cancer Nurs 1994; 17: 367–378.

17. Dean GE, Spears L, Ferrell B, et al. Fatigue in patients with cancer receiving interferon alpha. Cancer Pract 1995; 3:164–171.
18. Pickard-Holley S. Fatigue in cancer patients: a descriptive study. Cancer Nurs 1991; 14:13–19.
19. Fobair P, Hoppe RT, Bloom J, et al. Psychosocial problems among survivors of Hodgkin's disease. J Clin Oncol 1986; 4:805–814.
20. Joly F, Henry-Amar M, Arveux P, et al. Late psychosocial sequelae in Hodgkin's disease survivors: a French population-based case-control study. J Clin Oncol 1996; 14:2444–2453.
21. Berglund G, Bolund C, Fornander T, et al. Late effects of adjuvant chemotherapy and postoperative radiotherapy on quality of life among breast cancer patients. Eur J Cancer 1991; 27:1075–1081.
22. Okuyama T, Akechi T, Kugaya A, et al. Factors correlated with fatigue in disease-free breast cancer patients: application of the Cancer Fatigue Scale. Support Care Cancer 2000; 8:215–222.
23. Loge JH, Abrahamsen AF, Ekeberg O, et al. Hodgkin's disease survivors more fatigued than the general population. J Clin Oncol 1999; 17:253–261.
24. Loge JH, Abrahamsen AR, Ekeberg O, et al. Fatigue and psychiatric morbidity among Hodgkin's disease survivors. J Pain Symptom Manage 2000; 19: 91–99.
25. Vogl D, Rosenfeld B, Breitbart W, et al. Symptom prevalence, characteristics, and distress in AIDS outpatients. J Pain Symptom Manage 1999; 18:253–262.
26. Bradley J, Dempster M, Wallace E, et al. The adaptations of a quality of life questionnaire for routine use in clinical practice: the Chronic Respiratory Disease Questionnaire in cystic fibrosis. Qual Life Res 1999; 8:65–71.
27. Krupp LB, LaRocca NG, Muir-Nash J, et al. The fatigue severity scale: application to patients with multiple sclerosis and systemic lupus erythematosis. Arch Neurol 1989; 46:1121–1123.
28. Karlsen K, Larsen JP, Tandberg E, et al. Fatigue in patients with Parkinson's disease. Mov Disord 1999; 14:237–241.
29. Wysenbeck AJ, Leibovici L, Weinberger A, et al. Fatigue in systemic lupus erythematosis: prevalence and relation to disease expression. Br J Rheumatol 1993; 32: 633–635.
30. Bruce IN, Mak VC, Hallett DC, et al. Factors associated with fatigue in patients with systemic lupus erythematosis. Ann Rheumat Dis 1999; 58:379–381.
31. Huet PM, Deslauriers J, Tran A, et al. Impact of fatigue in primary biliary sclerosis. Am J Gastroenterol 2000; 95:760–767.
32. Cella D, Peterman A, Passik S, et al. Progress toward guidelines for the management of fatigue. Oncology 1998; 12:1–9.
33. Vogelzang NJ, Breitbart W, Cella D, et al. Patient, caregiver, and oncologist perceptions of cancer-related fatigue: results of a tripart assessment survey. The Fatigue Coalition. Semin Hematol 1997; 34(Suppl 2):4–12.
34. Curt GA, Breitbart W, Cella D, et al. Impact of cancer-related fatigue on the lives of patients: new findings from the fatigue coalition. Oncologist 2000; 5:353–360.
35. Portenoy RK, Itri LM. Cancer-related fatigue: guidelines for evaluation and management. Oncologist. 1999; 4:1–10.
36. Abels RI, Larholt KM, Drantz KD, et al. Recombinant human erythropoietin (r-HuEPO) for the treatment of the anemia of cancer. In: Murphy MJ, ed. Blood Cell Growth Factors: Their Present and Future Use in Hematology and Oncology. Dayton, OH: AlphaMed Press, 1992:121–141.

37. Demetri GD, Kris M, Wade J, et al. Quality-of-life benefit in chemotherapy patients treated with epoetin alfa is independent of disease response or tumor type: results from a prospective community oncology study. J Clin Oncol 1998; 16: 3412–3425.

38. Glaspy J, Bukowski R, Steinberg D, et al. The impact of therapy with epoetin alfa on clinical outcomes during cancer chemotherapy in community oncology practice. J Clin Oncol 1997; 15:1218–1234.

39. Gabrilove J. Overview: erythropoiesis, anemia, and the impact of erythropoietin. Semin Hematol 2000; 37:1–3.

40. Bruera E, Brenneis C, Paterson AH, et al. Use of methylphenidate as an adjuvant to narcotic analgesics in patients with advanced cancer. J Pain Symptom Manage 1989; 4:3–6.

41. Breitbart W, Mermelstein H. An alternative psychostimulant for the management of depressive disorders in cancer patients. Psychosomatics 1992; 33:352–356.

42. Bruera E, Roca E, Cedaro L, et al. Action of oral methylprednisolone in terminal cancer patients: a prospective randomized double-blind study. Cancer Treat Rep 1985; 69:751–754.

43. Tannock I, Gospodarowicz M, Meakin W, et al. Treatment of metastatic prostatic cancer with low-dose prednisone: evaluation of pain and quality of life as pragmatic indices of response. J Clin Oncol 1989; 7:590–597.

44. Fortin F, Kirouac S. A randomized controlled trial of preoperative patient education. Int J Nurs Stud 1976; 13:11–24.

45. Mock V, Dow KH, Meares CJ, et al. Effects of exercise on fatigue, physical functioning, and emotional distress during radiation therapy for breast cancer. Oncol Nurs Forum 1997; 24:991–1000.

46. Brunier G, Graydon J. A comparison of two methods of measuring fatigue in patients on chronic haemodialysis: visual analogue vs Likert scale. Int J Nurs Stud 1996; 33:338–348.

47. de Haes JCJM, van Kippenberg FCE, Neijt JP. Measuring psychological and physical distress in cancer patients: structure and application of the Rotterdam Symptom Checklist. Br J Cancer 1990; 62:1034–1038.

48. McCorkle R, Young K. Development of a symptom distress scale. Cancer Nurs 1978; 1:373–378.

49. Portenoy RK, Thaler HT, Kornblith AB, et al. The Memorial Symptom Assessment Scale: an instrument for the evaluation of symptom prevalence, characteristics, and distress. Eur J Cancer 1994; 30A:1326–1336.

50. Aaronson NK, Ahmedzai S, Bergman B, et al. The European Organization for Research and Treatment of Cancer QLQ-C30: a quality-of-life instrument for use in international clinical trials in oncology. J Natl Cancer Inst 1993; 85:365–376.

51. Cella DF, Jacobsen PB, Orav EJ, et al. A brief POMS measure of distress for cancer patients. J Chronic Dis 1987; 40:939–942.

52. Pearson P, Byars G. The Development and Validation of a Checklist Measuring Subjective Fatigue (report no. 56-115). Randolph Air Force Base, TX: School of Aviation, 1956.

53. Richardson A. Measuring fatigue in patients with cancer. Support Care Cancer 1998; 6:94–100.

54. Kogi K, Saito Y, Mitsuhashi T. Validity of three components of subjective fatigue feelings. J Sci Labour 1970; 46:251–270.

55. Yoshitake H. Relations between the symptoms and the feeling of fatigue. Ergonomics 1971; 14:175–186.
56. Piper BF, Dibble SL, Dodd MJ, et al. The revised Piper Fatigue Scale: psychometric evaluation in women in breast cancer. Oncol Nurs Forum 1998; 25:677–684.
57. Lee KA, Hicks G, Nino-Murcia G. Validity and reliability of a scale to assess fatigue. Psychiatry Res 1991; 36:291–298.
58. Glaus A. Fatigue in patients with cancer—analysis and assessment. Recent Results Cancer Res 1998; 145:1–172.
59. Yellen SB, Cella DF, Webster MA, et al. Measuring fatigue and other anemia-related symptoms with the Functional Assessment of Cancer Therapy (FACT) measurement system. J Pain Symptom Manage 1997; 13:63–74.
60. Hann DM, Jacobsen PB, Azzarello LM, et al. Measurement of fatigue in cancer patients: development and validation of the Fatigue Symptom Inventory. Qual Life Res 1998; 7:301–310.
61. Mendoza TR, Wang XS, Cleeland CS, et al. The rapid assessment of fatigue severity in cancer patients: use of the Brief Fatigue Inventory. Cancer 1999; 85:1186–1196.
62. Okuyama, T, Akechi T, Kugaya A, et al. Development and validation of the Cancer Fatigue Scale: a brief, three-dimensional, self-rating scale for assessment of fatigue in cancer patients. J Pain Symptom Management 2000; 19:5–14.
63. Schwartz AL. The Schwartz Cancer Fatigue scale: testing reliability and validity. Oncol Nurs Forum 1998; 25:711–717.
64. Smets E, Garssen B, Bonke B, et al. The Multidimensional Fatigue Inventory: psychometric qualities of an instrument to assess fatigue. J Psychosom Res 1995; 39:315–329.
65. Miaskowski C, Lee KA. Pain, fatigue, and sleep disturbances in oncology outpatients receiving radiation therapy for bone metastases: a pilot study. J Pain Symptom Manage 1999; 17:320–332.
66. Larson JL, Covey MK, Vitalo CA, et al. Reliability and validity of the 12-minute distance walk in patients with chronic obstructive pulmonary disease. Nurs Res 1996; 45:203–210.
67. McGavin CR, Gupta SP, McHardy GJR. Twelve minute walking test for assessing disability in chronic bronchitis. BMJ 1976; 1:822–823.
68. Charlson ME, Pompei P, Ales KL, et al. A new method of classifying prognostic comorbidity in longitudinal studies: development and validation. J Chronic Dis 1987; 40:373–383.
69. Katz JN, Chang LC, Sangha O, et al. Can cormorbidity be measured by questionnaire rather than medical record review. Med Care 1996; 34:73–84.
70. Max MB. Pain. In: Max MB, Lynn J, eds. Interactive Textbook on Clinical Symptom Research. www.symptomresearch.com, 2001.

11

Methodological Considerations
in the Treatment of Fatigue

LYNNE I. WAGNER, DAVID CELLA,
AND AMY H. PETERMAN

Due to recent medical advances, the life expectancy of people with chronic medical illness has been increasing. Fatigue is a symptom commonly associated with medical illness and has a high prevalence in palliative care settings. Fatigue is multidimensional in clinical expression and manifest in physical, emotional, and cognitive impairments. Fatigue is one of the most prevalent symptoms reported by patients with cancer,[1–3] acquired immunodeficiency syndrome (AIDS),[4] and multiple sclerosis.[5] The presence of fatigue has been associated with functional limitations and impaired quality of life among chronically ill populations, including cancer patients[6–8] and AIDS patients,[4,9] and has been found to interfere with adherence to cancer treatment.[10] Effective strategies for the clinical management of fatigue would reduce the overall symptom burden of many chronic illnesses.

State-of-the-Art Research on Fatigue Management

The pathophysiology of fatigue is poorly understood, and its causes vary based on the presence and severity of medical conditions. Few basic research studies have been conducted to investigate the mechanism of fatigue.[11] Identifying the etiological factors that contribute to fatigue often proves to be complicated as multiple causes typically coexist. Some of the more common causes of fatigue are listed in Table 11.1.

Among cancer patients, fatigue can be one of the first indicators of the presence or recurrence of cancer, and it tends to increase with the progression of cancer and cancer treatment.[12–14] Moderate to severe fatigue is commonly reported by patients receiving interferon therapy, of whom 70%–100% report fa-

Table 11.1. Causes of fatigue

Physiological factors
    Direct effects of illness
        Cancer
        Human immunodeficiency virus/acquired immunodeficiency syndrome
        Multiple sclerosis
        Chronic obstructive pulmonary disease
        Congestive heart failure
    Treatment effects
        Medication side effects
        Chemotherapy
        Radiotherapy
        Surgery
    Co-morbid medical conditions
        Anemia
        Infection
        Pulmonary disorders
        Thyroid dysfunction
        Malnutrition
    Exacerbating factors
        Chronic pain
        Sleep disturbances
        Deconditioning
Psychosocial factors
    Coping with chronic illness
    Anxiety
    Depression

Sources: Portenoy and Itri,[34] Atkinson et al.,[44] Cella et al.[54]

tigue.[15,16] Morrow and colleagues[17] present four hypotheses for the development of cancer-related fatigue, which include (*1*) anemia, (*2*) abnormalities in adenosine triphosphate, (*3*) vagal afferent activation, and (*4*) the interaction of cytokines and serotonin. Cytokine dysregulation, specifically erythropoietin, interleukin, tumor necrosis factor, and interferon, has been implicated in cancer-related fatigue and associated with factors that exacerbate fatigue, including anemia, cachexia, fever, infection, and depression.[18]

Fatigue is often underrecognized and consequently undertreated in clinical settings. Vogelzang et al.[19] surveyed oncology providers and patients and found that 80% of oncology providers believed that fatigue is not adequately assessed or treated. Among cancer patients with fatigue, 50% did not discuss treatment options with their oncologist and only 27% had received any treatment recommendations. Seventy-four percent of cancer patients reported that they believed that fatigue was a symptom they had to endure as a normal consequence of cancer and its treatment. Screening for fatigue in clinical settings using a single item or a brief measure has been demonstrated to be an effective approach for identifying patients who may benefit from clinical attention.[13,20]

Table 11.2. Examples of standardized measures for assessing fatigue

Brief Fatigue Inventory	Mendoza et al.[23]
Fatigue Severity Scale	Krupp et al.[24]
Functional Assessment of Chronic Illness Therapy–Fatigue	Cella,[1] Yellen et al.[8]
Multidimensional Fatigue Inventory	Smets et al.[25]
Multidimensional Fatigue Symptom Inventory	Stein et al.[26]
Piper Fatigue Scale	Piper et al.[27]

Given the diverse etiological factors that contribute to fatigue and its multi-dimensional nature, the comprehensive assessment of patients with fatigue is required for the development of effective treatment interventions.[21] Because fatigue is a subjective sensation, there is no "gold standard" for its measurement.[22] Several self-report measures for the assessment of fatigue have been developed for medical populations and are used for clinical research. A few of these measures are presented in Table 11.2.[1,8,23–27]

Treatment strategies for illness-related fatigue include pharmacological and non-pharmacological interventions, which are summarized in Table 11.3. When factors known to exacerbate illness-related fatigue have been identified, for example, anemia or thyroid dysfunction, they should receive clinical attention prior to implementing interventions aimed at fatigue management. For some patients, treatment of these factors may lead to significant reductions in fatigue. Anemic cancer patients have reported significantly worse fatigue scores than nonanemic cancer patients.[28] Cancer patients with anemia have demonstrated increased energy and improved quality of life following a course of treatment with erythropoietin.[29–33] Patients completing successful treatment for etiological factors with continued fatigue or patients without identified causative factors for their fatigue may benefit from pharmacological and nonpharmacological fatigue management.

Pharmacological treatments for the management of illness-related fatigue include psychostimulants and corticosteroids, although these treatments currently have limited research support.[34] Methylphenidate reduced the sedation associated with opioid administration among cancer patients,[35] improved cognitive functioning and psychomotor slowing among primary brain tumor patients,[36] and has been used to treat fatigue associated with depression in the elderly.[37] Pemoline was effective in a double-blind randomized trial for the treatment of fatigue associated with multiple sclerosis.[38] Modafinil, typically used for the treatment of excessive sleepiness among narcolepsy patients, was superior to placebo at reducing fatigue among 72 patients with multiple sclerosis[39] and is currently being examined for cancer-related fatigue. The use of low-dose corticosteroids, specifically dexamethasone and prednisone, for symptom management among cancer and AIDS patients has been supported by clinical observation and limited data from controlled trials.[40–43] The National Comprehensive

Table 11.3. Treatment strategies to manage fatigue

Cause-specific treatments
  Anemia: erythropoetic therapy, blood transfusion
  Depression: antidepressant medication, psychotherapy
  Thyroid dysfunction: thyroid hormone replacement therapy
  Malnutrition: nutritional assessment and appropriate therapy
  Dehydration: rehydration
  Infection: antibiotic/antiviral therapy

Nonspecific pharmacologic interventions
  Psychostimulants
    Methylphenidate
    Pemoline
    Dextroamphetamine
  Low-dose corticosteroids
    Dexamethasone
    Prednisone
  Selective serotonin-reuptake inhibitors

Nonpharmacological interventions
  Education
  Exercise
  Modify patterns of activity and rest
  Stress management
  Cognitive-behavioral therapy
  Nutritional intervention

Sources: Portenoy and Itri,[34] Atkinson et al.,[44] Cella et al.[54]

Cancer Network practice guidelines for cancer-related fatigue also recommend antidepressants for fatigue management when major depression is present.[44,45] Morrow et al.[45] conducted a randomized, placebo-controlled clinical trial of paroxetine with patients undergoing chemotherapy who reported fatigue following the second chemotherapy cycle. They found that paroxetine reduced symptoms of depression but had no effect on fatigue.

Nonpharmacological interventions include patient education, exercise, modification of activity and rest patterns, stress management and cognitive therapies, and nutritional interventions. Education of cancer patients and their families regarding the anticipated course of illness and treatment side effects has been advocated, particularly for nursing interventions.[34,46] Holley and Borger[47] reported pilot data from a prospective examination of 20 patients who completed an 8-week educational group based on a rehabilitation approach to managing cancer-related fatigue. Statistically significant findings from pre- to postintervention assessments were reported, which included a reduction in fatigue distress and an increase in quality of life.

The use of exercise to ameliorate cancer-related fatigue has been examined among patients receiving high-dose chemotherapy and stem cell support[48] and among breast cancer patients prior to chemotherapy[49] and during the first three cycles of chemotherapy.[14] Patients completing home-based aerobic exercise programs demonstrated reduced intensity of fatigue compared to patients who did not exercise. Graded activity and exercise programs have been demonstrated to improve fatigue among patients with chronic fatigue syndrome.[50]

Psychological interventions, including stress management training and cognitive-behavioral therapy, may offer clinical benefit to patients with fatigue secondary to chronic illness. The effectiveness of psychological interventions for symptom management has been demonstrated in cancer patients[51,52] and individuals with chronic fatigue syndrome.[50]

Short-Term and Long-Term Goals of Clinical Research for the Treatment of Fatigue

Short-term and long-term goals for clinical research in the treatment of fatigue are presented in Table 11.4. Four short-term goals of clinical research are recommended: (1) improved understanding of the etiology of fatigue, (2) a more clear definition of fatigue, (3) improved understanding of the relationships between fatigue and other commonly occurring symptoms, and (4) evaluation of treatment interventions.

Improved understanding of the etiology and the underlying mechanisms of fatigue would assist in (1) identifying patient populations at risk for the development of fatigue, (2) the development of treatment interventions, and (3) the selection of target samples for intervention studies. In discussing the biological basis of fatigue, Gutstein[11] pointed out that very little basic research has been conducted on cancer-related fatigue and suggested new directions for research in this area.

A clearer definition of fatigue and its diagnosis should be developed. Accomplishment of this goal would permit researchers to obtain more accurate estimates of fatigue prevalence. In addition, use of a more clear definition would

Table 11.4. Short-term and long-term goals of clinical research

Short-term goals	Long-term goals
Improved understanding of the etiology of fatigue	Accurate population-based estimates of the prevalence and impact of fatigue
More clear definition of fatigue	Reduce the burden of fatigue
Improved understanding of the relationships between fatigue and co-occurring symptoms	Interdisciplinary research
Evaluation of treatment interventions	Expanded study population to include diverse and underserved populations

lead to the identification of homogenous research samples. This work is in progress by Cella et al.[53,54] and Sadler et al.[55] Together with the Fatigue Coalition, a multidisciplinary group of experts interested in illness-related fatigue, these groups have put forth diagnostic criteria for cancer-related fatigue and have estimated the prevalence of fatigue based on these specific criteria. By standardizing eligibility criteria, this offers methodological benefits for studies examining the mechanisms underlying fatigue and the effectiveness of treatment interventions. Research advances in chronic fatigue syndrome have been impeded by the use of heterogeneous patient samples, which has led to discrepant or contradictory findings from epidemiological, descriptive, and treatment studies and has obscured the identification of laboratory correlates of fatigue.[50] In addition, a clear conceptualization of fatigue would lead to a standard operational definition. The availability of a widely used operational definition for fatigue would allow comparisons across research studies and across disease groups.

The third short-term goal of clinical research in the treatment of fatigue should be to improve our understanding of the relationships between fatigue and other symptoms that often co-occur. Associations between fatigue and depression, cognitive dysfunction, and pain have been well documented in cancer populations.[56] A better grasp of these relationships will lead to an improved understanding of the etiology of fatigue and the development of effective treatment approaches.

As a fourth goal, the empirical evaluation of treatment interventions for fatigue management using sound methodological principles is critical. This will lead to the identification and refinement of effective treatments, reduction in the use of treatments that do not offer symptom relief, and avoidance of treatments that do not have solid empirical support. For example, psychostimulants are often prescribed for cancer-related fatigue based on anecdotal information that they may be helpful. Pemoline and modafinil have been examined in randomized controlled trials for the treatment of fatigue related to multiple sclerosis.[38,39] However, well-controlled clinical trials to evaluate the efficacy of these medications for cancer-related fatigue have not been conducted.[57]

Three long-term goals of clinical research in the treatment of fatigue are suggested: (1) accurate population-based estimates of the prevalence and impact of fatigue, (2) reduced burden associated with fatigue, and (3) increased diversity of clinical research teams and study populations.

Population-based estimates of the prevalence and impact of fatigue are needed. Fatigue is common to many chronic illnesses, as well as in the general population. Data on the prevalence and impact of fatigue among various medical populations would provide direction in how to best utilize resources in terms of clinical research and clinical service delivery. Characteristics of patient subgroups likely to benefit from particular treatments should be identified. In addition, comparisons should be made among disease groups to advance our understanding of this commonly reported symptom.

A second long-term goal should be to reduce the burden associated with fatigue. This goal can be addressed through advances in our knowledge of mechanisms causing fatigue and the relationships between fatigue and symptoms that commonly co-occur as well as adoption of a standard definition and assessment approach, ultimately leading to the development of effective treatments. Because of the subjective nature of fatigue, patients are required to self-report its presence and severity. Developing innovative strategies for the routine screening of patients for fatigue in clinical practice could significantly reduce symptom burden by identifying patients who could benefit from clinical attention and would otherwise go undetected.[19] Well-controlled clinical trials to evaluate treatment interventions could reduce the burden associated with fatigue through the development of fatigue-management strategies.

As a third long-term goal, clinical research in the treatment of fatigue needs to strive for increased diversity in two respects: the use of interdisciplinary clinical research teams for investigation of cancer-related fatigue and increased cultural and ethnic diversity. Fatigue has been examined by a variety of disciplines, such as nursing, medicine, psychology, physical therapy, and occupational therapy. Given the multidimensional nature of fatigue, each discipline makes a unique contribution to its clinical management. The conduct of clinical research on the treatment of fatigue in the context of interdisciplinary teams can prevent the duplication of efforts by promoting communication across disciplines and is likely to enhance the clinical utility of treatment approaches. Clinical practice guidelines for the management of cancer-related fatigue emphasize the importance of interdisciplinary teams in conducting clinical research and in clinical services delivery.[44]

Future clinical research endeavors to advance treatments for fatigue must emphasize the recruitment of diverse samples in terms of culture, ethnicity, and socioeconomic status. This will ensure that patient subgroups that may exist will be adequately represented and that results can be generalized. Rieger[58] suggested enhancing cultural diversity in fatigue studies through conducting studies within cooperative networks or groups, such as the Community Cancer Oncology Program of the National Cancer Institute. For example, the Eastern Cooperative Oncology Group, one of the National Cancer Institute–sponsored national cancer treatment evaluation groups, has recently developed a symptom-management consortium to focus clinical research on symptoms such as fatigue. The inclusion of culturally diverse populations requires that standardized measures for fatigue be developed and made available in multiple languages.

Methodological Issues

Studies conducted to date

Few studies have been conducted to identify the physiological mechanisms underlying fatigue, and most studies conducted to date have been descriptive or correlational in nature. Basic research needs to be conducted on the pathophysiology of fatigue. Advances in the identification of laboratory and neuroimaging correlates of fatigue would likely contribute to the development of treatment interventions.

Research on the prevalence of illness-related fatigue has relied largely on clinic-based samples. Studies using more methodologically rigorous sampling techniques are needed to obtain more accurate estimates of the prevalence of fatigue among various medical populations. Samples used to generate estimates of the prevalence of fatigue have infrequently included ethnic minorities. Future studies should make a concerted effort to increase the ethnic diversity of study populations, to enhance the generalizability of epidemiological findings. Standard approaches to the measurement of fatigue should be used to obtain more accurate estimates of the prevalence and to enhance comparability of research findings across studies, such as the diagnostic criteria developed for cancer-related fatigue.[53,54]

Few randomized controlled trials with fatigue as a primary end point have been conducted to evaluate the range of pharmacological and nonpharmacological interventions suggested for the management of illness-related fatigue. A randomized controlled trial is the gold standard in medical research, and trials of this nature are needed to provide empirical support for commonly used fatigue interventions, such as psychostimulants, corticosteroids, and educational programs. Well-designed phase III studies have been conducted on the effectiveness of epoetin alfa for the treatment of anemia among cancer patients, and some of these trials have included quality of life and fatigue as primary end points.[29–31,33] A prospective evaluation of patients pre- and post-treatment is an alternative to a randomized, controlled trial. Holly and Borger[47] reported pilot data from a study utilizing this design to evaluate an educationally focused rehabilitation program designed to reduce fatigue among cancer patients.

Methodological limitations and approaches for overcoming these limitations

Conducting randomized, placebo-controlled trials can be challenging with clinical populations, particularly in palliative care settings. Ethical issues inherent to palliative care research have been discussed.[59] Threats to the reliability and validity of patient-reported data, the representativeness of study samples, and the interpretability of data obtained from clinical trials will be discussed.

Obtaining data may be difficult from patients who are experiencing severe physical illness, weakness, impaired stamina, or cognitive deterioration. Given the subjective nature of fatigue, its measurement is based on patient self-report. However, the reliability and validity of patient-reported fatigue severity may be compromised in individuals with advanced illness. The use of additional data sources to corroborate patient report, such as family members, friends, caretakers, and treatment staff, may help to address this issue, although proxy sources of data also contain bias.[60]

The representativeness of patient samples recruited for clinical research in fatigue management is limited by attrition, heterogeneity, and selection bias. Attrition due to illness progression or death is inherent to the nature of palliative care research and presents a threat to the validity of research findings from clinical trials conducted in palliative care settings. The absence of patients with more severe illness from post-treatment and follow-up assessments will lead to over-representation of less symptomatic patients, thus biasing treatment studies to evaluate treatment interventions more favorably. Statistical models developed to account for data not missing at random should be utilized. Fairclough[61] reviewed applicable models in discussing the analysis of quality-of-life data from clinical trials.

The heterogeneity of patient samples due to diversity among patients with advanced illness in terms of etiology of fatigue, treatment regimen, co-morbid illnesses, prognosis, and symptoms is an additional threat to the representativeness of research samples.[60] Variations in patient treatment preferences also increase the heterogeneity of clinical research samples, particularly since increased emphasis is placed on patient-centered medical care during the end of life.[62] Patients choosing to receive treatment as part of a clinical trial comprise a biased sample since presumably some patients may decline treatment and it is likely that they differ systematically from the former group. Patients with the capacity to make treatment decisions, including the decision to participate in clinical research, represent a select sample of palliative care patients in that they will have a better health status than patients who are unable to consent to study participation. The use of longitudinal research models with the inclusion of a well-designed pre- and post-treatment fatigue assessment may overcome some of these limitations. Case studies or small samples can be examined using time series analysis, a robust multivariate statistical technique which is well suited for the analysis of repeated symptom assessments.[63,64]

Deterioration as a consequence of disease progression is a threat to the validity of clinical trial data and increases the difficulty in interpreting changes in fatigue over time.[60] For example, fatigue among cancer patients increases over the course of chemotherapy and radiation therapy and as cancer advances.[12–14] Evaluation of a treatment intervention for patients currently receiving treatment for cancer or with advancing disease should take the natural progression of fatigue severity into account. Failure to do so may obscure the detection of treatment benefits. The use of a control group or the availability of normative data with good reliability and validity can address this methodological challenge.

Summary

Fatigue is a symptom commonly associated with medical illness, and its underlying mechanisms are poorly understood. Pharmacological and nonpharmacological treatments currently in use are based on limited research studies. Future research should lead to more accurate estimations of the prevalence and impact of fatigue, reduce the burden of fatigue, and strive for increased diversity. Randomized, placebo-controlled clinical trials are the gold standard in evaluating treatment interventions. However, few trials of this nature have been conducted to examine the effectiveness of medications commonly used for the management of fatigue. Empirical support for exercise in managing fatigue has been reported. Non-pharmacological interventions have not been adequately evaluated. Many challenges to conducting clinical research in the context of palliative care exist, which threaten the reliability, validity, and generalizability of research findings. Use of additional sources of data to corroborate patient reports and of longitudinal research models, including statistical models for managing missing data and time series analysis, may address some of these challenges.

References

1. Cella D. The Functional Assessment of Cancer Therapy–Anemia (FACT-An) scale: a new tool for the assessment of outcomes in cancer anemia and fatigue. Semin Hematol 1997; 34S:13–19.
2. Cella D, Tulsky D, Gray G, et al. The Functional Assessment of Cancer Therapy Scale: development and validation of the general measure. J Clin Oncol, 1993; 11: 570–579.
3. Winningham ML, Nail LM, Burke MB, et al. Fatigue and the cancer experience: the state of the knowledge. Oncol Nurs Forum 1994; 21:23–36.
4. Vogl D, Rosenfeld B, Breitbart W, et al. Symptom prevalence, characteristics, and distress in AIDS outpatients. J Pain Symptom Manage 1999; 18:253–262.
5. Bakshi R, Miletich RS, Henschel K, et al. Fatigue in multiple sclerosis: cross-sectional correlation with brain MRI findings in 71 patients. Neurology 2000; 53:1151–1153.
6. Cella D. Quality of life in cancer patients experiencing fatigue and anemia. Anemia Oncol 1998; March:2–4.
7. Irvine D, Vincent L, Graydon J, et al. The prevalence and correlates of fatigue in patients receiving treatment with chemotherapy and radiation therapy: a comparison with the fatigue experienced by healthy individuals. Cancer Nurs 1994; 17: 367–378.
8. Yellen S, Cella D, Webster K, et al. Measuring fatigue and other anemia-related symptoms with the Functional Assessment of Cancer Therapy (FACT) measurement system. J Pain Symptom Manage 1997; 13:63–74.
9. Breitbart W, McDonald MV, Rosenfeld B, et al. Fatigue in ambulatory AIDS patients. J Pain Symptom Manage 1998; 15:159–167.
10. Yarbro CH. Interventions for fatigue. Eur J Cancer Care 1996; 5:35–38.
11. Gutstein HB. The biologic basis of fatigue. Cancer 2001; 92:1678–1683.
12. Groopman J, Itri L. Chemotherapy-induced anemia in adults: incidence and treatment. J Natl Cancer Inst 1999; 91:1616–1634.
13. Okuyama T, Tanaka K, Akechi T, et al. Fatigue in ambulatory patients with advanced lung cancer: prevalence, correlated factors, and screening. J Pain Symptom Manage 2001; 22:554–564.

14. Schwartz AL, Nail LM, Chen S, et al. Fatigue patterns observed in patients receiving chemotherapy and radiotherapy. Cancer Invest 2000; 18:11–19.
15. Dean GE, Spears L, Ferrell B, et al. Fatigue in patients with cancer receiving interferon alpha. Cancer Pract 1995; 3:164–171.
16. Malik UR, Makower DF, Wadler S. Interferon-mediated fatigue. Cancer 2001; 92: 1664–1668.
17. Morrow GR, Andrews PLR, Hickok J, et al. Fatigue associated with cancer and its treatment. Support Cancer Care 2002 (in press).
18. Kurzrock R. The role of cytokines in cancer-related fatigue. Cancer 2001; 92: 1684–1688.
19. Vogelzang NJ, Breitbart W, Cella D, et al. Patient, caregiver, and oncologist perceptions of cancer-related fatigue: results of a tripart assessment survey. The Fatigue Coalition. Semin Hematol 1997; 34S:4–12.
20. Kirsch KL, Passik S, Holtsclaw E, et al. I get tired for no reason: a single item screening for cancer-related fatigue. J Pain Symptom Manage 2001; 22:931–937.
21. Wagner L, Cella D. Cancer-related fatigue: clinical screening, assessment, and management. In: Marty M, Pecorelli S, eds. ESO Scientific Updates: Fatigue, Asthenia, Exhaustion and Cancer, 5th ed. Oxford: Elsevier Science, 2001:201–214.
22. Neuenschwander H, Bruera E. Asthenia. In: Doyle D, Hanks GWC, MacDonald N, eds. Oxford Textbook of Palliative Medicine, 2nd ed. New York: Oxford University Press, 1998:573–581.
23. Mendoza TR, Wang XS, Cleeland CS, et al. The rapid assessment of fatigue severity in cancer patients: use of the Brief Fatigue Inventory. Cancer 1999; 85:1186–1196.
24. Krupp LB, LaRocca NG, Muir-Nash J, et al. The Fatigue Severity Scale: application to patients with multiple sclerosis and systemic lupus erythematosis. Arch Neurol 1989; 46:1121–1123.
25. Smets EMA, Garssen B, Bonke B, et al. The Multidimensional Fatigue Inventory (MFI): psychometric qualities of an instrument to assess fatigue. J Psychosom Res 1995; 39:315–325.
26. Stein KD, Martin SC, Hann DM, et al. A multidimensional measure of fatigue for use with cancer patients. Cancer Pract 1998; 6:143–152.
27. Piper BF, Dibble SL, Dodd MJ, et al. The revised Piper Fatigue Scale: psychometric evaluation in women with breast cancer. Oncol Nurs Forum 1998; 25:677–684.
28. Cella D, Lai JS, Chang CH, et al. Fatigue in cancer patients compared with fatigue in the general United States population. Cancer 2002; 94:528–538.
29. Demetri GD, Kris M, Wade J, et al. Quality of life benefit in chemotherapy patients treated with epoetin alfa is independent of disease response or tumor type: results from a prospective community oncology study. J Clin Oncol 1998; 16:3412–3425.
30. Dunphy FR, Dunleavy TL, Harrison BR, et al. Erythropoietin reduces anemia and transfusions after chemotherapy with paclitaxel and carboplatin. Cancer 1997; 79:1623–1628.
31. Glaspy J, Bukowski R, Steinberg D, et al. Impact of therapy with epoetin alfa on clinical outcomes of patients with non-myeloid malignancies during cancer chemotherapy in community oncology practice. J Clin Oncol 1997; 15:1218–1234.
32. Littlewood TJ, Bajetta E, Nortier JW, et al. Effects of epoetin alfa on hematologic parameters and quality of life in cancer patients receiving nonplatinum chemotherapy: results of a randomized, double-blind, placebo-controlled trial. J Clin Oncol 2001; 19:2865–2874.

33. Turner R, Anglin P, Burkes R, et al. Epoetin alfa in cancer patients: evidence-based guidelines. J Pain Symptom Manage 2001; 22:954–965.

34. Portenoy RK, Itri LM. Cancer-related fatigue: guidelines for evaluation and management. Oncologist 1999; 4:1–10.

35. Wilwerding MB, Loprinzi CL, Mailliard JA, et al. A randomized, crossover evaluation of methylphenidate in cancer patients receiving strong narcotics. Support Care Cancer 1995; 3:135–138.

36. Meyers CA, Weitzner MA, Valentine AD, et al. Methylphenidate therapy improves cognition, mood, and function of brain tumor patients. J Clin Oncol 1998; 16: 2522–2527.

37. Massand PS, Tesear GE. Use of stimulants in the medically ill. Psychiatr Clin of North Am 1996; 19:515–547.

38. Weinshenker BG, Penman M, Bass B, et al. A double-blind, randomized, crossover trial of pemoline in fatigue associated with multiple sclerosis. Neurology 1992; 42:1468–1471.

39. Rammohan KW, Rosenberg JH, Pollak CP, et al. Provigil (modafinil): efficacy and safety for the treatment of fatigue in patients with multiple sclerosis. Neurology 2000; 54(Suppl 3):A24.

40. Bruera E, Roca E, Cedaro L, et al. Action of oral methylprednisolone in terminal cancer patients: a prospective randomized double-blind study. Cancer Treat Rep 1985; 69:751–754.

41. Bruera E, Macmillan K, Hanson J, et al. A controlled trial of megestrol acetate on appetite, caloric intake, nutritional status, and other symptoms in patients with advanced cancer. Cancer 1995; 66:1279–1282.

42. Tannock I, Gospodarowicz M, Meakin W, et al. Treatment of metastic prostatic cancer with low-dose prednisone: evaluation of pain and quality of life as pragmatic indices of response. J Clin Oncol 1989; 7:590–597.

43. Wagner GJ, Rabkin JG, Rabkin R. Dextroamphetamine as a treatment for depression and low energy in AIDS patients receiving a continuous infusion of narcotics for cancer pain. Pain 1997; 48:163–166.

44. Atkinson A, Barsevick A, Cella D, et al. NCCN practice guidelines for cancer-related fatigue. Oncology 2000; 14:151–161.

45. Morrow GR, Hickok JT, Raubertas RF, et al. Effect of an SSRI antidepressant on fatigue and depression in seven hundred thirty-eight cancer patients treated with chemotherapy: A URCC CCOP study. Proc Am Soc Clin Oncol 2001; 20: 1531.

46. Ream E, Richardson A. From theory to practice: designing interventions to reduce fatigue in patients with cancer. Oncol Nurs Forum 1999; 26:1295–1303.

47. Holley S, Borger D. Energy for living with cancer: preliminary findings of a cancer rehabilitation group intervention study. Oncol Nurs Forum 2001; 28:1393–1396.

48. Dimeo FC, Steiglitz RD, Novelli-Fischer U. Effects of physical activity on the fatigue and psychological status of cancer patients during chemotherapy. Cancer 1999; 85:2273–2277.

49. Schwartz AL. Daily fatigue patterns and effect of exercise in women with breast cancer. Cancer Practice 2000; 8:16–24.

50. Jason LA, Taylor RR. Chronic fatigue syndrome. In: Nezu AM, Nezu CM, Geller PA, eds. Comprehensive Handbook of Psychology, vol 9. Health Psychology, 2002 (in press).

51. Knight SJ. Oncology and hematology. In: Camic P, Knight S, eds. Clinical Handbook of Health Psychology. Seattle: Hofgrefe and Huber, 1998:389–438.
52. Trijsburg RW, van Knippenberg FC, Rijpma SE. Effects of psychological treatment on cancer patients: a critical review. Psychosom Med 1992; 54:489–517.
53. Cella D, Davis K, Breitbart W, et al. Cancer-related fatigue: prevalence of proposed diagnostic criteria in a United States sample of cancer survivors. J Clin Oncol 2001; 19:3385–3391.
54. Cella D, Peterman A, Passik S., et al. Progress toward guidelines for the management of fatigue. Oncology 1998; 12:369–377.
55. Sadler IJ, Jacobsen PB, Booth-Jones M, et al. Preliminary evaluation of a clinical syndrome approach to assessing cancer-related fatigue. J Pain Symptom Manage 2002; 23:406–416.
56. Valentine AD, Meyers CA. Cognitive and mood disturbance as causes and symptoms of fatigue in cancer patients. Cancer 2001; 92:1694–1698.
57. Burks TF. New agents for the treatment of cancer-related fatigue. Cancer 2001; 92: 1714–1718.
58. Rieger PT. Assessment and epidemiologic issues related to fatigue. Cancer 2001; 92: 1733–1736.
59. Casarett DJ, Karlawish JHT. Are special ethical guidelines needed for palliative care research? J Pain Symptom Manage 2000; 20:130–139.
60. Wilkinson EK. Problems of conducting research in palliative care. In: Bosanquet N, Salisbury C, eds. Providing a Palliative Care Service: Towards an Evidence Base. New York: Oxford University Press, 1999:22–29.
61. Fairclough DL. Design and Analysis of Quality of Life Studies in Clinical Trials. Boca Raton, FL: CRC Press, 2002.
62. Teno JM. Palliative care teams: self-reflection—past, present, and future. J Pain Symptom Manage 2002; 23:94–95.
63. Mark MM, Reichardt CS, Sanna LJ. Time-series designs and analyses. In: Tinsley HE, Brown SD, eds. Handbook of Applied Multivariate Statistics and Mathematical Modeling. San Diego: Academic Press, 2000:354–386.
64. Moskowitz DS, Hershberger SL. Modeling Intraindividual Variability with Repeated Measures Data: Methods and Applications. Multivariate Applications Book Series. Mahwah, NJ: Lawrence Erlbaum Associates, 2002.

V

NEUROPSYCHIATRIC AND PSYCHOSOCIAL RESEARCH

12

Depression in the Terminally Ill: Prevalence and Measurement Issues

HARVEY MAX CHOCHINOV

The task of diagnosing clinical depression in the palliative care setting is fraught with a variety of challenges. While sadness and depressed mood may be indicative of an underlying depression, they may also be part of a normal response to the anticipation of one's own death. While periodic sadness is to be expected in these circumstances, such a normal mood state must be distinguished from the entity of clinical or major depression.

The term *depression* can be used in a variety of ways, adding confusion to an already complex issue. In its colloquial form, it is used as a synonym for the affect of sadness. It can also refer to a symptom associated with a wide variety of physical and psychological states. Finally, it also refers to a very specific group of psychiatric syndromes.[1] Given that the latter may represent a highly remediable source of suffering in this patient population,[2] the ability to distinguish these different entities, measure or quantify depression, and make a psychiatric diagnosis when appropriate is critical.

Underdiagnosis of Depression in the Terminally Ill

In spite of the limited number of controlled trials on the treatment of depression in advanced cancer patients,[3–5] all of which have demonstrated therapeutic benefit, clinical depression tends to be largely underdiagnosed among dying patients.[6] Although Derogatis et al.[7] reported that 51% of cancer patients were prescribed psychotropics, antidepressants accounted for only 1% of these medications. In part, this may be due to a sense of therapeutic nihilism, which all too often pervades mood assessments in this particularly vulnerable group of patients; such a stance dismisses even the most severe of mood disturbances as "understandable" when considered in the context of a life-limiting diagnosis.[8]

Another source of therapeutic inaction is the difficulty of making a diagnosis of major depression in this patient population. The diagnostic challenge in patients who are physically ill, particularly terminally ill, is the nonspecificity of somatic symptoms. These symptoms, which include insomnia/hypersomnia, significant weight or appetite change, and fatigue or loss of energy, are diagnostic criteria within the *Diagnostic and Statistical Manual*, fourth edition (DSM-IV), psychiatric classification system, used widely throughout North America.[9] Other symptoms of major depression include depressed mood, markedly diminished interest or pleasure in all or nearly all activities, feelings of worthlessness or excessive or inappropriate guilt, diminished ability to concentrate or indecisiveness, and recurrent thoughts of death or suicide. Whereas somatic symptoms in an otherwise healthy individual might be used to make a diagnosis of major depression, among the terminally ill they may be accounted for by the advancing disease process itself. Thus, measuring depression, in spite of limiting the discussion to one diagnostic system (DSM-IV), remains fraught with controversy.

Measuring Clinical Depression

Four approaches to the evaluation of depressive symptoms in the medically ill have been described: the inclusive, etiological, exclusive, and substitutive.[10] The *inclusive* approach counts all symptoms, be they of physical or psychological origin, toward the diagnosis of depression. This approach is conceptually clear and does not require the clinician to make etiological inferences. It is phenomenological in its approach in that diagnostic decisions are made on the basis of observable phenomena. The inclusive approach tends to maximize inter-rater reliability and to heighten sensitivity at the expense of lowered specificity (that is, false-positives due to incorrectly diagnosing depression in patients who are only physically ill).

The *etiological* approach requires that the clinician include a symptom as part of clinical depression only if it is clearly not a result of a physical illness. This is the approach used in the Structured Clinical Interview for DSM-III-R (SCID).[11] While this approach is theoretically sound, it is difficult in practice to attribute the etiology of symptoms in a reliable way. Although intuitively appropriate, it is difficult to implement in practice.

The *exclusive* approach, which has primarily been used in depression research on cancer patients,[12,13] simply eliminates anorexia and fatigue from the list of nine depressive criteria. Like the inclusive approach, this approach is conceptually straightforward in that it specifies how to apply the criteria. High specificity results from lowering the likelihood of confounding variables contributing to a diagnosis of depression. While this reduces the number of false-positives, it does so at the expense of lowering the sensitivity. In that it is more difficult to reach a critical diagnostic threshold, an excessive number of false-negatives may emerge. This could have the detrimental effect of denying treatment to those who might benefit. While this approach may have applications in the context of research, it may be too restricting for clinical use.

Finally, the *substitutive* approach replaces somatic depressive symptoms with cognitive symptoms, which are less reliant on the underlying physical status. Endicott[14] addressed the lack of specificity of somatic symptoms in cancer patients by proposing nonsomatic alternatives. This approach recommends substituting a change in weight or appetite, sleep disturbance, loss of energy or fatigue, and difficulty in thinking or concentrating with depressed appearance, social withdrawal or decreased talkativeness, brooding, self-pity, pessimism, and lack of reactivity in situations that would normally be pleasurable. While this strategy appears conceptually reasonable, there has been little experience with it to date.

Kathol et al.[15] examined the impact of using various different diagnostic approaches on the reported prevalence rates of depression in a group of 152 cancer patients. When an inclusive approach was used (DSM-III), 38% met the diagnostic criteria for major depression. The etiological approach (as represented by DSM-III-R) yielded a prevalence rate of 29%. A slightly more stringent approach, requiring that patients manifest five (rather than four) of nine symptoms of depression, resulted in an expectedly lower prevalence of 25%. The substitutive approach, using Endicott[14] criteria, yielded a prevalence rate of 36%. These results suggest that the reported rate of clinical depression varies, by as much as 15% in this study, according to the particular manner in which depression is measured. In spite of the longstanding controversy about the nonspecificity of somatic symptoms among the medically ill, this study found little difference in the prevalence of depression comparing the standard versus the substitutive approach.

The diagnostic approach is important not only for measuring the presence of clinical depression but also for the manner in which this system is applied. Zimmerman et al.[16] reported that minor variations across research centers in the specification of operational criteria for individual symptoms of endogenous depression led to large differences in observed prevalence rates and problems in replicating research findings.

Our group studied two of the issues that may influence the measurement and diagnosis of depression in the medically ill, that is, the severity with which symptoms must be expressed before they are considered clinically significant and how to deal with somatic symptoms that may be caused by medical illness.[17] This study used different approaches of case identification to examine prevalence rates for major and minor depression in a group of terminally ill cancer patients. Semistructured diagnostic interviews were conducted with 130 patients receiving palliative care. Diagnoses made according to an inclusive approach were compared with diagnoses made according to Endicott's[14] revised criteria, when either a low-severity or a high-severity threshold for classifying criterion A symptoms (depressed mood or loss of interest) was used. The less stringent low-threshold diagnostic approach greatly increased the overall prevalence of depressive episodes with both the inclusive and the Endicott[14] criteria (26.1%

versus 13%, inclusive approach; 23.1% versus 13%, Endicott[14] approach). With high thresholds, the inclusive and the Endicott[14] criteria were essentially equivalent. It thus appears that small differences between investigators in the application of symptom-severity thresholds can result in large differences in prevalence rates for depression, with somatic symptoms being less of a confounding factor.

Depression Prevalence Studies

The difficulties in measuring depression are further highlighted when one examines the prevalence studies of depression among cancer patients.[12,15,17–25] Rates from as low as 6%[19] to as high has 42%[12] have been reported. Measurement challenges, at least in part accounting for such a wide range of findings, include diagnostic uncertainty, variability in the degree of underlying physical disease burden, and a wide variety of measurement instruments used to quantify the degree of depression. A variety of measurement strategies have been used in these prevalence studies, including self-report instruments [for example, the Beck Depression Inventory (BDI),[24] current and past psychological adjustment scale,[13] Geriatric Mental State Schedule,[20] Present State Examination[21]] and clinician-directed evaluations [for example, clinical interviews using structured questionnaires[13,15] such as the Schedule for Affective Disorders and Schizophrenia (SADS)[17,25]].

In examining the prevalence of clinical depression in the terminally ill[17] and studies of desire for death in this patient population,[25] our group used the SADS interview. This instrument[26] is a semistructured psychiatric diagnostic tool that can be used to make a variety of psychiatric diagnoses. It provides a standardized assessment protocol that can be used across a variety of settings. In general, it has come to be used quite extensively for establishing diagnoses according to explicit criteria. In the hands of a sensitive clinician familiar with discrete psychiatric syndromes, the SADS provides the closest thing to a "gold standard" for psychiatric assessment.

In its complete form, the SADS allows for the diagnosis of 24 discrete syndromes. The full interview can be quite time-consuming, particularly among patients with advanced cancer. For our purposes, we abbreviated the interview by selecting only those sections that were relevant to the diagnosis of depression. In spite of this, among our cohort of patients, the interview took from 30–90 minutes to administer. As such, despite its many advantages pertaining to rigor and standardization, the SADS may be too cumbersome to be used in routine clinical practice among the terminally ill.

Due to the unwieldy nature of the SADS interview and to obtain an independent measure of depression, we also used the BDI.[24] This is a 21-item, self-administered inventory that asks patients to rate the intensity of their attitudes and symptoms of depression over the past week. A 13-item form of the BDI has also been validated.[27] Each item has three options ranked on a scale of 0–3, from lowest to highest intensity, respectively. Items are written at a fifth- to sixth-grade level and take only minutes to complete among otherwise healthy populations. However, in the terminally ill, it often needs to be read to the patient and repeated, with assistance provided in helping to fill in the form. Thus, what under normal circumstances is a brief self-report instrument, among the terminally ill serves as the basis of a 10- to 15-minute circumscribed interview, focused on depressive symptomatology.

Screening Instruments

Screening for clinical depression among the terminally ill is particularly important, considering that this diagnosis is frequency overlooked and represents a source of remediable suffering. The screening literature is plagued by many of the same measurement issues affecting the prevalence studies. A variety of screening instruments have been utilized, including the BDI,[24,27] the General Health Questionnaire-30,[28] the Hospital Anxiety and Depression Scale (HADS),[29] the Carroll Rating Scale (CRS),[30] and mood visual analogue scales (VASs).[31] Lack of screening uniformity along with variable critical threshold "cut-off scores," affecting sensitivity and specificity performance, make for a complex literature.

The HADS was specifically designed for clinically ill populations and has a high proportion of psychological items.[29] Razavi et al.[32] examined the utility of the HADS as a screening tool for major depression in a sample of 210 oncology patients. Their gold standard was a structured diagnostic interview using DSM-III criteria. They reported that 6.8%–25.5% had major depressive disorders. They used receiver operating characteristic (ROC) analysis to generate a curve expressing the relationship between true and false-positives for each score. The ROC curve conveys the ability of the screening instrument to discriminate cases and noncases. A cut-off is then chosen to minimize the sum of false-positives and false-negatives.[33] Razavi et al.[32] reported an optimal cut-off score of 19 for major depression, with a sensitivity of 0.70 and a specificity of 0.75. In spite of a positive predicted value of 0.50, they concluded that the HADS was a simple and sensitive screening test for depression in patients with cancer.

Razavi et al.[34] also studied the HADS in 117 patients with lymphoma. In that instance, the gold standard was adapted from the DSM-III-R. They reported that 6.8% had major depressive or anxiety disorders. Again, they found this to be a useful screening tool for depression in this patient population (ROC cut-off of 10, 84% sensitivity and 64% specificity).

Golden et al.[30] studied the ability of the CRS, a 52-item self-report questionnaire, to screen for depression in 65 gynecological oncology patients. As a "gold standard," they used a semistructured diagnostic interview employing DSM-III criteria. They tested several modifications of the CRS, including a 40-item scale constructed by removing somatic items and an 11-item scale whose components were found to be more frequency-endorsed among depressed patients. Each of these scales was reported to be valid for identifying depression in this patient cohort. The 40-item CRS did not outperform the full scale (87% sensitivity, 62% specificity versus 87% sensitivity, 58% specificity, respectively). While the positive predictive value of all three scales ranged from 38% to 50%, the negative predictive value ranged from 94% to 95%. This implies that this instrument is a good indicator of who is not depressed.

Our group studied brief screening instruments to measure depression in the terminally ill.[31] We compared the performance of four measures for depression in a group of terminally ill patients. The methods compared included (1) a single-item interview assessing depressed mood, (2) a two-item interview assessing depressed mood and loss of interest in activities, (3) a VAS for depressed mood, and (4) the BDI-13 item. Semistructured diagnostic interviews were administered to 197 patients receiving palliative care for advanced cancer. The interview diagnoses served as the standard against which the screening performance of the four methods was assessed. As reported in other depression-screening studies,[30,32,34] the self-report instruments (the BDI and the mood VAS) demonstrated a low positive predictive value (0.27 and 0.17, respectively) and a high negative predictive value (0.96 and 0.92, respectively). Most noteworthy, the single-item interview correctly identified the diagnosis of every patient while not misidentifying any patient, substantially outperforming the questionnaire and VAS measures. Brief screening measures for depression are thus important clinical tools for terminally ill patients. The performance of the single-item interview, which essentially asks patients if they are depressed most of the time, speaks to the importance of mood inquiry in this particularly vulnerable patient population.

Desire for Death

Due to the limited energy level of patients with advanced diseases, expediency must sometimes supersede rigor. Given the lack of an existing measure specifically addressing a desire for death among the terminally ill, we incorporated the following gate question into the SADS[26] interview: "Do you ever wish that your illness would progress more rapidly so that your suffering could be over sooner?" If the patient responded affirmatively to this lead item, a series of follow-up questions was administered to assist the interviewer in clarifying how serious and pervasive was the patient's desire to die. The follow-up included such questions as "Do you pray for an early death," "Do you wish you were already dead," and "Have you discussed with anyone that your desire is to have an early death?" In keeping with the format of other SADS items, the interviewer scored the extent of the desire for death on a six-point rating scale. The reliability of the desire for death rating scale (DDRS) was established by having a second rater attend a random sample of 27 interviews (13.5%, $n = 200$).[26] Perfect concordance was found between raters in scoring the desire for death item. Given the ordinal nature of the DDRS, nonparametric procedures (Spearman's rank order correlation) were required when exploring the relationships between desire for death and depression, pain, and social support.

Occasional wishes that death might come soon were reported by 45% of the study group, indicating that such thoughts do not appear particularly uncommon in this patient population. However, only 17 of 200 patients (8.5%) acknowledged a desire to die that was serious and pervasive. The prevalence of depression among patients endorsing a desire for death was 58.8% compared to 7.7% in patients without such stated desires [$\chi^2(1) = 33.66$, $p < 0.0001$, 95% confidence interval 5.0–60.0]. Seventy-six (76.5) percent of patients with a genuine desire for death reported their pain to be of moderate or greater intensity compared to 46.2% without a desire for death ($\chi^2 = 4.75$, df = 1, $p = 0.03$; odds ratio = 3.8, 95% confidence interval 1.1–14.4). Patients classified as having a serious desire gave significantly lower ratings than other patients on the family support scale but not on the scales pertaining to friends and nursing support. Depression entered first into a logistic regression equation and emerged as the strongest predictor of desire for death (F = 23.33, df = 1, $p < 0.001$). Neither pain nor family support entered into the model, suggesting that they did not make a unique contribution to the regression model once depression had been included. This finding suggests that depression may lie closest to the desire for death in a causal pathway in which pain and family support exert more indirect influences. Prolonged physical pain may increase the risk of depression, while family support may offer protection against it. However, once depression has developed, the emergence of a desire for death may be a more direct step.

Rosenfeld et al.[35] examined the reliability and validity of the Schedule of Attitudes toward Hastened Death (SAHD), a self-report measure of desire for death previously validated in a population of individuals with acquired immunodeficiency syndrome (AIDS), among terminally ill patients with cancer.[35] They interviewed 92 terminally ill cancer patients after admission to a palliative care hospital. The average number of SAHD items endorsed was 4.76 (standard deviation = 4.3); 15 patients (16.3%) endorsed 10 or more items, indicating a high desire for death. Internal consistency was strong (coefficient $\alpha = 0.88$, median item-total correlation = 0.49), as were indices of convergent validity. Total SAHD scores were correlated significantly ($r = 0.67$) with the DDRS and somewhat less so with measures of depression ($r = 0.49$) and hopelessness ($r = 0.55$). Lower correlations were observed between the SAHD and measures of spiritual well-being ($r = -0.42$), quality of life ($r = -0.36$), physical symptoms ($r = 0.38$), and symptom distress ($r = 0.38$). There were no significant correlations between SAHD scores and social support ($r = -0.06$) or pain intensity ($r = 0.16$); however, pain-related functional interference and overall physical functioning were correlated significantly with SAHD scores ($r = 0.31$ and $r = -0.23$, respectively). The SAHD appeared to be a reliable and valid measure of desire for death among terminally ill cancer patients.

While measuring desire for death in the context of a single, cross-sectional study is feasible, doing so on a regular basis, to measure longitudinal trends and shifts in this construct, is unpalatable to most terminally ill patients and their family members. Reframing the question in terms of the "will to live" is a far more positive stance of inquiry, which nevertheless taps into the same essential issues pertaining to the continuing desire (or lack thereof) to live, in spite of the approaching death. Employing a will-to-live VAS, anchored by "no will to live" and "strong will to live," represents a compromise between pursuing measurement rigor (that is, lengthy questionnaires) and clinical expediency. This trend is reflected in other recent developments in palliative care research measurement.

Visual Analogue Scales

A VAS provides a simple mechanism by which subjective experiences can be measured.[36] While they have been used in psychological research for over 70 years,[37] their widespread use was stimulated by the work of Aitken and Zealley[38–40] in their construction of single-item mood scales. These scales were described as "practical," "reliable," and "particularly good for the measurement of change and the observation of its significance."[38] In the palliative care setting, these scales have many obvious advantages. They have been described as quick and simple to construct,[41–43] administer, and score.[43–45] Given our interest in pursuing the temporal stability of will to live and its determinants, the suitability of a will to live VAS for frequent and repeated use is particularly advantageous.[42] Bearing in mind the limited energy of our target population, the ability of VAS instruments to be easily understood[43,45] and to require little motivation for completion by subjects is critical.[43]

The VAS technique was first applied to the assessment of quality of life of cancer patients by Priestman and Baum.[46] They developed a 10-item (and later a 25-item) quality-of-life scale, which they then applied to breast cancer patients receiving chemotherapy.[47] Coates et al.[48] used a subset of this scale to evaluate quality of life in specific forms of cancer. For example, they used a five-item scale to measure general well being, mood, pain, nausea and vomiting, and appetite among patients with melanoma and small cell anaplastic bronchogenic carcinoma. Using an equal weighting of this five-item VAS, they found that it accounted for about one-third of the variance of patients' performance status as measured by a five-point scale developed by the Eastern Cooperative Oncology Group (ECOG). In a similar design, examining a cohort of ovarian cancer patients, the equally weighted averages of VAS scores (general sense of well-being, breathlessness, and physical fatigue) were predictive of the ECOG scores and accounted for over half of the variance. These studies are important for having demonstrated the applicability of VAS techniques in the cancer setting.

While some have argued that VAS instruments measure depression at the expense of the precision and reliability of structured depression scales,[49] many studies have shown high correlations between the VAS-depression and criterion scales, and, thus, very strong support for the validity of VAS instruments when used in both psychiatric and nonpsychiatric populations. High correlations have been demonstrated between VAS-depression and the BDI (0.51–0.76, p < 0.05–0.001),[41,44,50,51] the CRS (–0.68 to –0.71, p < 0.001),[49] the Clinical Global Rating Scale for depression (–0.56 to –0.60, p < 0.001),[49] the Hamilton Depression Scale (–0.63 to –0.88, p < 0.001),[38,48,49] a self-rating depression scale (0.51–0.83, p < 0.001),[52] and the symptom checklist (0.41, p < 0.05).[41]

Establishing the test–retest reliability of the VAS is challenging, particularly in the palliative care setting, where symptoms are highly changeable. In a study using a short time interval (1 hour), Robinson et al.[53] asked subjects to rate their hunger on two occasions during a fasting period in their study of the reliability of VAS-hunger. The correlation between the two rating periods was very high (r = 0.92, p < 0.001). Equivalent test–retest studies with the VAS have not been conducted in palliative care settings. Inter-rater reliability studies have been done, comparing psychiatrist-rated and patient-rated VAS-depression.[44,53] While significant inter-rater reliability was achieved, patient self-ratings were at a significantly higher level than psychiatrist ratings. This speaks to the difficulty of comparing observer and subject ratings. A study that examined the behavior of geriatric patients, using a VAS designed for this purpose, compared the ratings between two-observer measures.[45] They reported high correlations between two nurse observers and between nurse and relative observers (r = 0.89–0.96, p < 0.001).

Visual Analogue Scales and Palliative Care

The brevity and simplicity of VASs are particularly appealing in the palliative care setting. They offer the potential to reliably measure a variety of constructs in a manner suitable to this patient population. Age and the loss of abstract thinking ability,[54] confusion and mental disorganization,[55] and impaired perceptual and memory skills[56] have been cited as possible confounders. In spite of these potential difficulties, Bruera et al.[57] developed a multidimensional instrument, composed of several VASs, to be used in the palliative care setting. They described this approach, known as the Edmonton Symptom Assessment System (ESAS), as a "simple method" for the assessment of symptoms, twice a day, in patients admitted to a palliative care unit. It originally consisted of eight VASs, completed by the patient alone, by the patient with nursing assistance, or by the nurses or relatives at 10:00 AM and 6:00 PM. The ESAS was initially designed to measure levels of pain, activity, nausea, depression, anxiety, drowsiness, appetite, and sense of well-being. This information was then transferred to a graph, which contained assessments of up to 21 days per page. The sum of the scores for all symptoms was defined as the symptom distress score or symptom load. Given the prevalence of dyspnea in terminal cancer, Bruera et al.[57] added a shortness of breath VAS to a revised version of the ESAS. Further revising the ESAS to include a will to live VAS allows this construct to be measured within the context of other frequent sources of symptom distress.[58]

Patients in the palliative care setting are able to complete the ESAS with very little effort within 1–2 minutes. Bruera (personal communication) indicated that ESAS scores independently rated by patients, nurses, and relatives show reasonable concordance. The correlation between observers varied from 0.90 for pain to 0.64 for activity. Bruera (personal communication) also indicated 100% participation in a series of 101 consecutively admitted patients on whom ESAS data were gathered. This speaks both to the simplicity and the acceptability of this particular psychometric instrument for this patient population. Such a recruitment rate is particularly impressive, given that patients in the palliative care setting are frequently too sick or cognitively impaired to meaningfully participate in palliative care research protocols.

Qualitative Methods

The discussion thus far concerning measurement in the terminally ill has focused exclusively on quantitative methods. A consideration of qualitative methods is necessary, given the limitations of quantitative approaches in shedding sufficient understanding on some palliative care issues. There are many issues, including dignity, suffering, meaning, and will to live/desire for death, for which psychometric instruments either do not exist or have limited ability to provide the necessary information required to advance the field of end-of-life care. Qualitative methods reach beyond attempts at numerical quantification and have the methodological capacity to delve into the most complex, and in the palliative care setting critical, of issues.[59]

The quantitative paradigm makes a number of critical assumptions, which include the following: (1) reality is objective and singular, apart from the researcher; (2) the researcher is independent from that which is being researched; (3) the research is value-free and unbiased; (4) the language of research is formal, impersonal, and based on set definitions; and (5) the research process is deductive, static in design, and context-free, thus enabling generalizations, predictions, and understanding which are accurate and reliable through validity and reliability testing.[60] When one is studying fundamentally emotional constructs such as depression and particularly the desire for death among the terminally ill, these quantitative assumptions are deserving of challenge.

A qualitative paradigm provides a context within which the experiences of dying patients can be further explored and understood.[59] This paradigm subsumes a number of critical assumptions, including the following: (1) reality is subjective and multiple as seen by participants in a study, (2) the relationship between researchers and those being researched is interactive, (3) research is value-laden and biased, (4) the language of qualitative research is informal and personal and speaks of evolving decisions, and (5) the research process is inductive and context-bound, thereby seeing the design emerge and categories unfold throughout its course; the accuracy and reliability of the resultant patterns and theories are established through verification.[59]

The qualitative paradigm is associated with a number of specific methodological approaches, including ethnographies, phenomenological studies, and grounded theory, approaches that can, in many instances, overlap. Ethnographies refer to a "systematic process of observing, detailing, describing, documenting, and analyzing the life-ways for particular patterns of a culture (or subculture) in order to grasp the life-ways or patterns of the people in their familiar environment."[61] Ethnographic research always involves face-to-face interviewing, with data collection and analysis taking place in the natural setting. Phenomenological studies are ones in which human experiences are examined by way of detailed descriptions of the people being studied.[59] This approach emphasizes understanding the "lived experience," based on the philosophical works of Husserl, Heidegger, Schuler, Sartre, and Merlau-Ponty.[62] Phenomenological studies involve prolonged, detailed work with a small number of subjects to examine patterns and relationships of meaning.[59]

Grounded theory describes an approach wherein the researcher attempts to derive a theory or understanding using multiple stages of data collection, with the resultant categories of information being continuously refined.[63] This method requires constant comparison of data with emerging categories and theoretical sampling of various different groups to compare, contrast, and maximize the similarities and differences of the information.[59] Given that depression and the desire for death are relatively circumscribed constructs, albeit often vaguely understood, which can emerge in the context of terminal illness, a grounded theory approach may be particularly suitable. Such a qualitative approach allows us to shed the quantitative assumptions that may constrict our understanding of dying patients' adjustment to their approaching death.

Conclusions

Measuring depression in the terminally ill and related constructs, such as desire for death or will to live, is not an easy task. However, our ability to do so is critical if we are to address these issues in patients approaching death. As challenging as physical symptoms are to quantify and research in this patient population, psychological constructs present their own unique set of measurement challenges. Those challenges will likely best be met by employing both qualitative and quantitative modes of clinical investigation.

Several critical areas of research pertaining to these issues require further investigation. Intervention trials that target depression and desire for death as outcome variables are desperately needed. Studies that track desire for death/will to live may provide a better understanding of how these factors shift over the palliative disease trajectory. Finally, quantitative studies that further explicate various components of confronting terminal disease, such as hope, dignity, and suffering, may improve our understanding of the inner life of dying patients.

References

1. McDaniel JS, Brown FW, Cole SA. Assessment of depression and grief reactions in the medically ill. In: Stoudemire A, Fogel BS, eds. Psychiatric Care of the Medical Patient. New York: Oxford University Press, 2000, 149–164.
2. Breitbart W, Levenson JA, Passik SD. Terminally ill cancer patients. In: Breitbart W, Holland JC, eds. Psychiatric Aspects of Symptom Management in Cancer Patients. Washington DC: American Psychiatric Press, 1993, 173–230.
3. Costa D, Mogos I, Toma T. Efficacy and safety of mianserin in the treatment of depression of women with cancer. Acta Psychiatr Scand 1985; 72(Suppl 320):85–92.
4. Evans DL, Nemeroff CB. Use of dexamethasone suppression test using DSM III criteria on an inpatient psychiatric unit. Biol Psychiatry 1983; 18:505–511.
5. Rifkin A, Reardon G, Siris S, et al. Trimipramine in physical illness with depression. J Clin Psychiatry 1985; 46:4–8.
6. Goldberg RJ, Mor V. A survey of psychotropic drug use in terminal cancer patients. Psychosomatics 1985; 26:745–751.
7. Derogatis LR, Abeloff MD, McBeth CD. Cancer patients and their physicians in the perception of psychological symptoms. Psychosomatics 1976; 17:197–201.
8. Breitbart W, Chochinov HM. Psychiatric aspects of palliative care. In: Doyle D, Hanks G, MacDonald N, eds. Oxford Textbook of Palliative Medicine, 2d ed. New York: Oxford University Press, 1998:933–954.
9. American Psychiatric Association. Diagnostic and Statistical Manual of Mental Disorders, 4th ed. Washington DC: American Psychiatric Association, 1994.
10. Cohen-Cole S, Stoudemire A. Major depression and physical illness. Psychiatr Clin North Am 1987; 10:1–17.
11. Spitzer RL, Endicott J, Robins E. Research diagnostic criteria: rationale and reliability. Arch Gen Psychiatry 1978; 35:773–782.
12. Bukberg, JB, Penman D, Holland JC. Depression in hospitalized cancer patients. Psychosom Med 1984; 46:199–212.
13. Plumb M, Holland J. Comparative studies of psychological function in patients with advanced cancer. II. Interviewer-rated current and past psychological symptoms. Psychosom Med 1981; 43:243–276.
14. Endicott J. Measurement of depression in patients with cancer. Cancer 1984; 53:2243–2249.
15. Kathol RG, Mutgi A, Williams J, et al. Diagnosis of major depression in cancer patients according to four sets of criteria. Am J Psychiatry 1990; 147:1021–1024.
16. Zimmerman M, Coryell WH, Black DW. Variability in the application of contemporary diagnostic criteria: endogenous depression as an example. Am J Psychiatry 1990; 147:1173–1179.

17. Chochinov HM, Wilson KG, Enns M, et al. Prevalence of depression in the terminally ill: effects of diagnostic criteria and symptom threshold judgments. Am J Psychiatry 1994; 151:537–540.
18. Bukberg JB, Holland JC. A prevalence study of depression in a cancer hospital population. Proc Am Assoc Cancer 1980; 21:382.
19. Derogatis LR, Morrow GR, et al. The prevalence of psychiatric disorders among cancer patients. JAMA 1983; 249:751–757.
20. Morton RP, Davies ADM, et al. Quality of life in treating head and neck cancer patients: a preliminary report. J Otolaryngol 1984; 9:181–185.
21. Dean C. Psychiatric morbidity following mastectomy: preoperative predictors and types of illness. J Psychosom Res 1987; 31:385–392.
22. Evans DL, McCartney CF, Nemeroff CB, et al. Depression in women treated for gynecological cancer: clinical and neuroendocrine assessment. Am J Psychiatry 1986; 143:447–452.
23. Weddington WW, Segraves KB, Simon MA. Current and time incidence of psychiatric disorders among a group of extremity sarcoma survivors. J Psychosom Res 1986; 30:121–125.
24. Beck AT, Rush AJ, Shaw BF, et al. Cognitive Therapy of Depression. New York: Guilford Press, 1979.
25. Chochinov HM, Wilson KG, Enns M, et al. Desire for death in the terminally ill. Am J Psychiatry 1995; 152:1185–1191.
26. Endicott J, Spitzer RL. A diagnostic interview: the schedule for affective disorders and schizophrenia. Arch Gen Psychiatry 1978; 35:837–844.
27. Beck AT, Steer R, Garbin M. Psychometric properties of the Beck Depression Inventory: twenty-five years of evaluation. Clin Psychol Rev 1988; 8:77–100.
28. Rodin G, Craven J, Littlefield C. Depression in the Medically Ill. New York: Brunner/Mazel, 1991.
29. Zigmond AS, Snaith RP. The hospital anxiety and depression scale. Acta Psychiatr Scand 1983; 67:361.
30. Golden RN, McCartney CF, Haggerty JJ Jr., et al. The detection of depression by patient self-report in women with gynecological cancer. Int J Psychiatry Med 1991; 21:17–27.
31. Chochinov HM, Wilson KG, Enns M, et al. Are you depressed? Screening for depression in the terminally ill. Am J Psychiatry 1997; 154:674–676.
32. Razavi D, Delvaux N, Farvacques C, et al. Screening for adjustment disorders and major depression disorders in cancer inpatients. Br J Psychiatry 1990; 156:79–83.
33. Lynch ME. The assessment and prevalence of affective disorders in advanced cancer. J Palliat Care 1995; 11:10–18.
34. Razavi D, Delvaux N, Farvacques C, et al. Screening for psychiatric disorders in a lymphoma outpatient population. Eur J Cancer 1992; 28A:1869–1872.
35. Rosenfeld B, Breitbart W, Galietta M, et al. The schedule of attitudes toward hastened death: measuring desire for death in terminally ill cancer patients. Cancer 2000; 88:2868–2875.
36. McCormack HM, del Horne DJ, Sheather S. Clinical applications of visual analogue scales: a critical review. Psychol Med 1988; 18:1007–1019.
37. Hayes MH, Patterson DG. Experimental development of the graphic rating method. Psychol Bull 1921; 18:98–99.
38. Aitken RCB. A growing edge of measurement of feelings. Proc R Soc Med 1969; 62:989–996.

39. Zealley AK, Aitken RCB. Measurement of mood. Proc R Soc Med 1969; 62:993–996.
40. Aitken RCB, Zealley AK. Measurement of moods. Br J Hosp Med 1970; iv:215–225.
41. Ahles TA, Ruckdeschel JC, Blanchard EB. Cancer-related pain. II: Assessment with visual analogue scales. J Psychosom Res 1984; 28:121–124.
42. Luria RE. The validity and reliability of the visual analogue mood scale. J Psychiatr Res 1975; 12:51–57.
43. Rampling DJ, Williams RA. Evaluation of group processes using visual analogue scales. Aust N Z J Psychiatry 1977; 11:189–191.
44. Little JC, McPhail NI. Measures of depressive mood at monthly intervals. Br J Psychiatry 1973; 122:447–452.
45. Morrison DP. The Crichton Visual Analogue Scale for the assessment of behaviour in the elderly. Acta Psychiatr Scand 1983; 68:408–413.
46. Priestman TJ, Baum M. Evaluation of quality of life in patients receiving treatment for advanced breast cancer. Lancet 1976; i:899–901.
47. Priestman TJ, Baum M, Jones V, et al. Comparative trial for endocrine versus cytotoxic treatment in advanced breast cancer. BMJ 1977; 1:1248–1250.
48. Coates A, Dillenbeck CF, McNeil DR, et al. On the receiving end. II. Linear analogue self-assessment (LASA) in evaluation of aspects of the quality of life of cancer patients receiving therapy. Eur J Cancer Clin Oncol 1983; 19:1633–1637.
49. Feinberg M, Carroll BJ, Smouse PE, et al. The Carroll rating scale for depression. III. Comparison with other rating instruments. Br J Psychiatry 1981; 138:205–209.
50. Davies B, Burrows G, Poynton C. A comparative study of four depression rating scales. Aust N Z J Psychiatry 1974; 9:21–24.
51. Handley SL, Dunn TL, Waldron G, et al. Tryptophan, cortisol and puerperal mood. Br J Psychiatry 1980; 136:498–508.
52. Malpas A, Legg NJ, Scott DF. Effects of hypnotics on anxious patients. Br J Psychiatry 1974; 124:482–484.
53. Robinson RG, McHugh PR, Folstein MF. Measurement of appetite disturbances in psychiatric disorders. J Psychiatr Res 1975; 12:59–68.
54. Kremer E, Atkinson JH, Ignelzi RJ. Measurement of pain: patient preference does not confound pain measurement. Pain 1981; 10:241–248.
55. Hornblow AR, Kidson MA. The visual analogue scale for anxiety: a validation study. Aust N Z J Psychiatry 1976; 10:339–341.
56. Carlsson AM. Assessment of chronic pain. I. Aspects of the reliability and validity of the visual analogue scale. Pain 1983; 16:87–101.
57. Bruera E, Kuehn N, Miller MJ, et al. The Edmonton Symptom Assessment System (ESAS): a simple method for the assessment of palliative care patients. J Palliat Care 1991; 7:6–9.
58. Chochinov HM, Tataryn D, Clinch JJ, Dudgeon D. Will to live in the terminally ill. Lancet 1999; 354:816–819.
59. Creswell JW. Research Design: Qualitative and Quantitative Approaches. London: Sage Publications, 1994.
60. Glaser BG, Strauss AL. Awareness of Dying. Chicago: Aldine, 1968.
61. Leininger MM. Qualitative Research Methods in Nursing. Orlando, FL: Grune and Stratton, 1985.
62. Nieswiadomy RM. Foundations of Nursing Research, 2d ed. Norwalk, CT: Appleton and Lange, 1993.
63. Strauss A, Corbin J. Basics of Qualitative Research: Grounded Theory Procedures and Techniques. Newbury Park, CA: Sage, 1990.

13

Issues in Measuring Family Care Needs and Satisfaction

LINDA J. KRISTJANSON

Care of dying patients and their families has been described as a unique type of care, requiring special skills and knowledge of health professionals. Hospice care providers consider the patient and family to be the unit of care and endeavor to assess and meet the needs of family members.[1–3] As families witness care provided to an ill family member and receive care themselves in the forms of information, emotional support, and/or respite, they make judgments about the quality of care provided. For health professionals to provide care that addresses the needs of families and promotes their sense of satisfaction with care, it is essential to be able to measure family care needs and family care satisfaction.

There is also evidence that family care variables (such as needs and care satisfaction) may be predictors of family members' health and family functioning during the end stages of the patient's illness and in the early bereavement period.[4,5] Therefore, attention to family care needs and family care satisfaction likely goes far beyond usual assessments of consumer satisfaction, and may be useful in the identification of families who require greater attention and focused interventions.[6] However, such assessment is not simple. Issues associated with the measurement of any family construct challenge healthcare providers and researchers who aim to index the views of this complex aggregate, the family. We explore these issues in the following ways:

1. By discussing specific theoretical and methodological conundrums underpinning measurement problems associated with these two constructs
2. By describing measurement issues common to the assessment of both family care needs and family care satisfaction
3. By suggesting ways in which clinicians might make use of existing tools to assess family care needs and family care satisfaction in a palliative care context

Family Care Needs: Theoretical and Measurement Issues

There is a substantial body of literature that documents the importance of attending to family care needs during a terminal illness.[3,4,7–9] Families have many needs during the cancer illness of a member, and many of these needs may be unmet.[3,10–13] For the most part, families report that their needs are largely met through use of trial-and-error methods.[13,14] There is also a suggestion that family members' whose needs are met are more satisfied with care.[4,15,16] The extent to which a family's needs remain constant over time is less well documented, although there is some evidence that needs are relatively stable during the end stages of the patient's illness.[17,18]

Three theoretical issues that must be addressed when considering the measurement of family care needs include the domain of needs to be assessed, how to assess whether needs have been met, and the most appropriate reliability model that underpins the construct, *need*.

The domain of family care needs

There is a notable lack of consistency in the classification of family care needs. Reported family caregiver needs include patient care needs (comfort needs for the patient, self-care, bathing); practical needs (meal preparation, housework, financial advice, legal advice); and psychological, spiritual, and information needs.[3,9,19,20] A broader need categorization has also been proposed. A review of the literature reveals two inter-related domains: the family's needs in relation to patient care (need to know what treatment the patient is receiving) and the family's own personal needs (need to have their questions answered honestly). These domains have been identified through qualitative methods and further validated in subsequent instrument development and testing studies.[4,10,21,22] Although distinct, assessments of both family care needs and family's needs for patient care are important.

Patient care needs that are important to families include specific physical aspects (a need to have the patient's pain relieved) and psychosocial needs (a need to feel that health professionals care about the patient). The domain of family care needs encompasses physical concerns (someone concerned with family member's health), psychosocial needs (a need to feel there is hope), and practical needs for care assistance (need to have information about what to do for the patient at home). A challenge associated with specifying the domain of family care needs is the temptation to add a lengthy list of possible needs, without attention to producing an abbreviated tool that indexes the most salient needs. A consistent finding, however, is that families are most concerned with patient comfort and pain relief[23–25] and that families who witness a relative's uncontrolled pain experience "vicarious suffering."[26]

A related challenge associated with how to structure the domain of family care needs within an instrument is that family members will rate their own needs for care as less important than the needs of the patient.[27] This should not be interpreted to mean that family members' needs are unimportant or less worthy of measurement. Exclusion of items specific to the family's own care needs would result in a gap in the measurement domain. Rather, relative to the patient's needs, family members rank their own concerns as secondary. Therefore, efforts must be made to allow family members to respond to both subdomains so that health professionals can assess this area completely.

Assessment of needs met

A specific issue facing researchers who measure family care needs is determining the extent to which needs have been met. On the surface, this appears deceptively simple. In reality, it is not so straightforward. Kristjanson and colleagues[10] used a simple dichotomous response option to assess need fulfillment (met, not met) to develop the Family Inventory of Need scale. The rationale for this method was to decrease subject burden on participants who were completing many other questionnaires at the same time. However, this scaling method resulted in less powerful data and incomplete assessment of this question. Since then, the tool has been adapted to allow families to indicate whether the need is met, unmet, or partly met and has resulted in more robust and clinically meaningful data.[4]

A practical necessity for this type of questionnaire is to pair a question about the need with a question about the extent to which the need has been met. Therefore, structuring of the questionnaire to allow family members to read a need statement only once and to reply to two prompts, one about the importance of the need and one about the extent to which it has been met, reduced subject burden. Questions have been raised about whether a need that has been identified as important and has been scored as met is still a need. Family members may also rate some needs as not applicable. Therefore, care must be taken when administering the questionnaire and analyzing data to ensure that appropriate methods are used to handle these complexities.

Choice of reliability model

Internal consistency reliability models are frequently used to assess the reliability of instruments. However, this reliability model assumes that items on a questionnaire are parallel to each other. This model may not be suitable for scales that measure the extent to which needs have been met. For example, an individual may have a high need for information about pain management but rate a need for information about the patient's prognosis as low. Some needs may be met and others not. Having some needs not met may be more serious (need to be informed about changes in the patient's condition) than others (need to feel accepted by health professionals). Therefore, the notion of parallel needs may not fit, and other reliability models might be better considered.

The reliability model most suitable to scales comprised of nonparallel items is an assessment of stability over time using a test–retest procedure,[28] which has been used most often in family needs assessment.[10,29,30] This type of reliability assessment raises questions about the time interval appropriate between testing times and the burden on participants to answer a questionnaire twice. However, given the immaturity of tools used to assess family care needs, further psychometric work is required to determine the extent to which items on the scales are parallel and stable over time.

In summary, these three methodological issues pose particular challenges to clinicians and researchers who measure family care needs: clarify the domain of family care needs, assess the extent to which needs have been met, and choose the most suitable reliability model. Despite these difficulties, some useful advances have been made in recent years, and collaborative work to further refine and test family care needs instruments is essential.

Family Care Satisfaction: Theoretical and Measurement Issues

Family satisfaction with palliative care can be conceptualized as an attitude that lies along a continuum ranging from very satisfied to very dissatisfied.[31] This concept is defined as the evaluation made by a family member about distinct dimensions of care received by both the patient and the family.

A review of the literature related to measurement of satisfaction reveals four issues: multiple- versus single-item tools, direct versus indirect approaches, dimensionality of the concept, and purported acquiescent response sets.[31]

Multiple- versus single-item tools

There is debate regarding the merits of multiple- versus single-item instruments for measuring care satisfaction.[32,33] According to Ware,[32] well-designed multiple-item scales tend to produce greater variability and to be more reliable and valid than single-item measures. In most recent reports of care satisfaction measures, multiple-item scales have been constructed and tested with the aim of accessing various dimensions of care satisfaction and increasing the sensitivity of the measures.[29,31,34]

Direct or indirect measures

Another measurement issue described in the literature is whether to use direct or indirect approaches to measure satisfaction with care. Indirect measures are better suited to macromeasures of medical enterprise and providers at a collective level and direct measures to assess microsatisfaction with services actually received.[35,36] Indirect approaches have been argued to be appropriate for measuring the satisfaction of clients with healthcare based on the belief that direct and indirect approaches result in similar findings. However, research findings indicate that direct and indirect approaches measure two different types of satisfaction.[36] In the context of family satisfaction with palliative care, indirect approaches have been used when researchers measure perceptions of care and report this rating as an indicator of care satisfaction. There is evidence that perceptions of care are distinct from care satisfaction and, although closely related, are not synonymous.[16,30]

Satisfaction assessed by the direct approach requires fewer items than the indirect approach. The direct approach has been used in a number of family satisfaction studies.[4,12,16,34,37] Because family satisfaction with care refers to a specific (micro) type of care actually received, a direct approach for measurement is recommended.

Dimensionality

A third measurement issue to consider is whether care satisfaction is a multidimensional or a unidimensional concept. The patient care satisfaction literature provides inconclusive results regarding the question of whether the concept is multidimensional.[29,32,38–40]

There are a number of different categories or aspects of care: information giving, technical care, symptom management, interpersonal care, inclusion of family in care, pain relief, physical comfort, continuity of care, availability of health professionals, involvement in treatment and care decisions, and quality of life.[31,33,41] For the most part, this literature is limited by inconsistent and poorly specified theoretical definitions of the satisfaction construct and an absence of empirical testing of the factorial composition of satisfaction. Kristjanson[31] examined the structure of the 20-item FAMCARE scale and suggested that family care satisfaction is a unidimensional concept encompassing four subdimensions: information giving, availability of care, psychological care, and physical patient care. These dimensions have been confirmed in subsequent studies.[42] Westra and colleagues[33] refined and tested a tool to measure satisfaction with home care and reported the concept to be unidimensional. Although family care satisfaction may be comprised of some subdimensions, a reliable and valid composite satisfaction score can be attained.

Acquiescent response set

The fourth measurement issue often leveled as a criticism toward satisfaction research is that an acquiescence response set operates, resulting in little variation and a conclusion that most individuals will report that they are satisfied. Indeed, a commonly reported finding is the negatively skewed satisfaction distributions obtained with little variance.[4,29,33,37] This observation raises questions about whether family care satisfaction is a normally distributed construct or a type of "threshold" construct, whereby one would expect that most families are satisfied and only a few are not. This might be a more accurate mirror of clinical care. Westra and colleagues[33] support the view that care satisfaction may be better considered a criterion-related instrument. They suggest that a threshold of 80% or above (or a minimum of 4 on a 5-point scale) might be set as an acceptable response, rather than assuming that an average of 3 on a 5-point scale indicates care satisfaction. The task then becomes how to identify families who are least satisfied with care and determine clinical cut-offs for satisfaction ratings that correlate with other family care constructs. Some preliminary work has been undertaken to examine this point.[4,37]

Early work[15] reported that approximately 20% of family members rate care on the lower end of the distribution. These family members were not unique in terms of sociodemographic variables of disease and treatment variables associated with the patient's care and illness. However, they rated their care needs as less important, and the few needs that they identified were not met. They could be characterized as family members who were passive and uncertain about who to ask for information and about their legitimate role in the care experience.

Subsequent work revealed that family care satisfaction was a predictor of family members' health and family functioning during the palliative care phase of the patient's illness and in the bereavement period 3 months after the patient's death.[4] Most notably, changes in the family members' mental health status were reported. Therefore, further work to identify the extent to which family care satisfaction may help clinicians identify high-need families is justified.

Family care satisfaction may also be unlike other variables in that there is no specific action that can be clearly taken if one is dissatisfied. Family members may feel indebted to health professionals who provide care to the patient and may be reluctant to register a complaint out of fear of retribution to the patient. Family members may be unhappy with care but lack confidence about their abilities to judge. Therefore, there may be a type of cognitive dissonance that limits a family member's willingness to rate the care too low when there is little they are prepared to do or think they can do about a poor evaluation. In these instances, abbreviation of the scale to encourage family members to make use of the entire range of response options would likely not result in an improved distribution. Rather, family members may need this negative skew to allow them a personally/socially tolerable range within which to acceptably express dissatisfaction. Of greater importance may not be the numerical value on the scale but the position of a family member's score relative to the norm.

Notwithstanding these findings, it behooves researchers to make efforts to decrease the possible effects of an acquiescence response set. Some approaches found to be helpful include use of multiple items, ensuring that the person conducting the assessment is not a caregiver, and ensuring that procedures to protect the identity of participants are clearly communicated.

Measurement Issues Common to Assessment of Both Family Care Needs and Satisfaction

A number of measurement issues arise when measuring either family care needs or family care satisfaction. These issues are also commonly confronted when measuring other family care constructs and warrant careful attention.

Definitions of family

Although many authors use the term *family*, assessments are often obtained from individual family members or the family member most involved in the patient's care experience, rather than the family as a whole. In some instances, the family member is a blood or legal relative, and in other situations the family member(s) most affected or involved in the care is not related in these ways. From a clinical perspective, the most important criterion for defining a family or family mem-ber may not be a legal or blood relationship but the functional care-giving relationship that exists. Therefore, a more inclusive definition may be more clinically useful and is often reported in the literature.[37,43,44] Errors occur when one family member's perspective is taken to be the entire family's position and vice versa.

The first step in any family assessment process, therefore, is to be clear about how *family* is defined and to determine the unit of analysis: is it the family as a whole that is to be assessed or individual family members? Although proponents of general systems theory[45] argue that the family is greater than the sum of its parts and that a true family perspective should include some sort of aggregate assessment, for most clinicians, an individual family member's perspective is sought. This approach also allows identification of the degree of congruence among family members. Although some family constructs might require a more holistic/composite family unit measurement approach (assessment of family functioning), care constructs such as family care needs and family care satisfaction appear to be better measured by asking individual family members to respond to questionnaires.

Assessment time frame

A second generic issue involved with measurement of family care constructs in a palliative care context is the time point used as a reference for the respondent. The extent to which family perceptions of palliative care are influenced by prior care experiences in other settings is not documented. As well, it is not known how easily family members can separate in their minds the care provided by different services or teams, especially when the transition between services and care goals is not always explicit or well understood by families. It is also possible that two approaches to care are provided simultaneously (active treatment and palliative support for symptom management), clouding assessments further. Care must be taken when assessing family constructs to help family participants put boundaries around the care experience in a way that matches the aims of the research question or quality-assurance project.[6]

Stability of the construct over time versus stability of the instrument

Given the often rapid changes that occur during the illness trajectory of the patient, assessment of changes in family care constructs over time can become confused with assessment of stability of the tools used to measure the constructs. Generally, the appropriate time frame for test–retest reliability assessments is 2 weeks. This time frame is not feasible for most patients and families in the palliative care phase of illness. Therefore, shorter time intervals are needed between administrations of tools for test–retest evaluations. Most often, a 24-hour time interval or less is required because changes in the patient's condition or in the plan of care can occur that would confound psychometric assessments of the tool. Confusion can also result when researchers are not precise in reporting findings, mixing interpretations about test–retest reliability with comments about the stability of the construct over time.

To date, little work has assessed the stability of family care constructs over time. Further work in this area is needed to determine the time points at which family members might experience the greatest distress, have more critical needs, or be least satisfied with care. Longitudinal designs to address these research questions are indicated.

Burden on family respondents

Clinicians and researchers are faced with challenges of how to assess family care constructs without placing undue burden on individuals who are already experiencing considerable stress. Efforts to develop brief, reliable, and valid instruments are essential. As well, concerns about subject burden limit the number of questionnaires that can be provided to a family member at any one time, resulting in assessments or studies that may be more focused and narrow.

Although palliative care researchers may wish to include a number of questionnaires to assess for confounding variables or possible covariates, they are forced to limit the length of protocols to the fewest questionnaires that are absolutely necessary to reduce participant burden. These abbreviated protocols limit the scope of inquiry. Given this problem, concerted efforts must be made to undertake programmatic research in a sequenced and carefully choreographed manner that builds on prior empirical findings.

Social desirability effect

The social desirability effect is often discussed in relation to assessments of family care constructs. Although concerns about this type of response set are cited in the general psychometric literature, the extent to which it operates within palliative care research is less certain. Ideally, the social desirability effect is best evaluated by administering a parallel tool. However, the subject burden associated with adding this extra tool may seem excessive. Instead, investigators have examined the responses of participants to various questionnaires, to assess the extent to which this type of response set might operate, and have made observations about the candor of participants during the protocol. Some examples of ways in which a social desirability effect would arise include family members wishing to appear as if they are coping well, having few needs, having many needs that are met, and being well satisfied with care.

Family members of advanced cancer populations report a large number of care needs, unmet needs, and a range of perspectives about care and family well-being.[4,5,10,14,31,37,46,47] Observations of data-collection protocols suggest that family members are willing to provide quite candid and honest responses regarding their care experiences.[3,10,31] At a time of such intense distress, family members appear to concentrate on answering questions as accurately and honestly as possible. In contrast to more general surveys with the public about matters that may be less personal, family members of palliative care patients are living through an experience that is central to their life. Their participation in a study about this experience is usually expressed as a desire to share their points of view so that the knowledge generated might help someone else. Therefore, measurement errors associated with a social desirability effect are likely minimal in this population.

Negatively worded items

The general psychometric literature recommends that approximately half the items on questionnaires (such as Likert scales) should be negatively worded. This scale-construction strategy is intended to avoid an automatic response bias whereby participants simply check off answers in an inattentive manner without carefully reading the questions.

Clinical and research experience with family members of advanced cancer patients suggests that this type of response bias is not a problem.[31,33] Further, use of negatively worded items can create confusion for family members, many of whom might be elderly or experiencing difficulties concentrating due to stress and sleep deprivation. Therefore, use of negatively worded items may actually increase response error, rather than avoid a response set. Given the stresses for families associated with the patient's illness, efforts made by clinicians and researchers to simplify questionnaires will result in higher-quality data and more ethically sensitive protocols.

Clinical Assessment of Family Care Needs and Family Care Satisfaction

The transfer of instruments used in research protocols to everyday clinical practice presents a number of issues as well: readiness of the tool for everyday use, guidelines for use of tools within practice, and interface with ongoing research.

Readiness of tools for everyday use

Frequently, a question arises about the readiness of an instrument developed in research for use in everyday clinical practice. Clinicians are often in urgent need of a tool to evaluate and guide practice. Researchers, however, may be cautious about releasing an instrument for use in practice that is still relatively immature. These two realities must be reconciled. Clinicians should expect to use a tool with acceptable reliability to be sure that they are basing practice decisions on stable assessment methods. Therefore, instruments with reliabilities lower than 0.80 should not be incorporated into practice. It is possible, however, for clinicians to work collaboratively with researchers to use instruments in practice while continuing to assess the psychometric properties of the tool. This allows for refinements that are clinically meaningful while ensuring that issues of reliability and validity are addressed on an ongoing basis. This type of collaborative work escalates the pace of instrument development and has potential to result in a more appropriate tool.

Guidelines for use in practice

Guidelines for using instruments may vary in practice from setting to setting. For example, in a medical oncology setting of an inpatient hospital, the frequency of assessment may need to be higher than in a home-based hospice service. Staff may need help to incorporate instruments into practice so that the process fits with usual practice and does not appear to be an artificial or bureaucratic add-on (that is, filling out another form). Although some consistency of use of tools is helpful in detecting patterns across families and care situations, incorporation of the tool into practice must allow for individual tailoring to different patient/family circumstances and should be embedded naturally within the care-giving relationship.

  If the data obtained from use of these tools are not included as part of care planning and health team discussions, the data-collection process involved with instrument competition would be an exercise separate from the care-giving relationship. Therefore, mechanisms must be in place to make the data obtained accessible, visible, and part of team discussions. This can be achieved through use of an accompanying graph or chart that attaches to the patient record (such as the Edmonton Symptom Assessment System).[48] Care settings also need to provide for staff who can collate these data and provide ongoing results to care settings so that care needs and trends can be monitored and addressed.

Interface with ongoing research

The use of assessment tools in clinical practice can be linked to ongoing research programs if collaborative partnerships are fostered and data collection is undertaken in an ethical and systematic manner.

Summary

Measurement of family care needs and family care satisfaction in the context of palliative care is a challenging task. Findings specific to family care needs indicate that families have needs in two domains: concerns about patient care and specific requirements of their own. Family members need to feel confident that the patient's comfort needs are met and that the patient's perceptions of his or her symptoms are attended to carefully. They require liberal amounts of disease and treatment information, provided in doses that they can process and at a pace that is comfortable to them. As well, families benefit from information about the diagnosis, prognosis, treatment options, and expected course of recovery to help lessen their fears and increase their sense of predictability. A consistent theme in the family needs literature is the importance of communication between health professionals and families. Researchers and clinicians who measure these needs must be alert to the comprehensiveness of the domain measured, the clarity with which needs and need fulfillment rankings are made and compared, and unique reliability issues associated with needs assessments.

Family care satisfaction appears to be best measured by a multiple-item tool using a direct, multidimensional approach. Although on the surface family care satisfaction may appear to be a construct that shows little variation, it may be a useful way of identifying family members who are hurting the most and who may not have other ways of expressing their concerns. The finding that approximately 20% of family members may be at the lower end of the satisfaction distribution should be important clinical information to health professionals assigning diminishing health resources to those most in need. Given the fact that this group may be at risk for greater dysfunction and poorer health outcomes themselves, family care satisfaction and the factors that may be associated with this construct, such as family needs, are worthy of further study and clinical investigation.

References

1. Ferrell BR. The family. In: Doyle D, Hanks GWC, MacDonald N, eds. Oxford Textbook of Palliative Medicine. New York: Oxford University Press, 1998: 909–918.

2. Kristjanson LJ, Ashcroft T. The family's cancer journey: a literature review. Cancer Nurs 1994; 17:1–17.
3. Steele RG, Fitch MI. Needs of family caregivers of patients receiving home hospice care for cancer. Oncol Nurs Forum 1996; 23:823–828.
4. Kristjanson LJ, Sloan JA, Dudgeon DJ, et al. Family members' perceptions of palliative cancer care: predictors of family functioning and family members' health. J Palliat Care 1996; 12:10–20.
5. Leonard KM, Enzel S, McTavish J, et al. Prolonged cancer death: a family affair. Cancer Nurs 1995; 18:222–227.
6. Fakhoury WK. Satisfaction with palliative care: what should we be aware of? Int J Nurs Stud 1998; 35:171–176.
7. Grande G, Todd C, Barclay S. Support needs in the last year of life: patient and carer dilemmas. Palliat Med 1997; 11:202–208.
8. Grbich C, Parker D, Maddocks I. Communication and information needs of caregivers of adult family members at diagnosis and during treatment of terminal cancer. Prog Palliat Care 2000; 8:345–350.
9. Osse BHP, Vernooij-Dassen J, de Vree B, et al. Assessment of the need for palliative care as perceived by individual cancer patients and their families. Cancer 2000; 88:900–911.
10. Kristjanson LJ, Atwood JR, Degner LF. Validity and reliability of the Family Inventory of Needs (FIN): measuring the care needs of families of advanced cancer patients. J Nurs Meas 1995; 3:109–126.
11. Longman AJ, Atwood JR, Sherman JB, et al. Care needs of home-based cancer patients and their caregivers. Cancer Nurs 1992; 15:182–190.
12. Meyers JL, Gray LN. The relationships between family primary caregiver characteristics and satisfaction with hospice care, quality of life, and burden. Oncol Nurs Forum 2001; 28:73–82.
13. Rose K. A qualitative analysis of the information needs of informal carers of terminally ill cancer patients. J Clin Nurs 1999; 8:81–88.
14. Scott G. A study of family carers of people with a life-threatening illness 2: the implications of the needs assessment. Int J Palliat Nurs 2001; 7:323–330.
15. Kristjanson LJ, Sloan JA. Determinants of the grief reactions among survivors. J Palliat Care 1991; 7:51–56.
16. Medigovich K, Porock D, Kristjanson LJ, et al. Family members' expectations, perceptions and satisfaction with home hospice care: an Australian replication. J Palliat Care 1999; 15:48–56.
17. Mor V, Masterson-Allen S, Houts P. The changing needs of patients with cancer at home: a longitudinal view. Cancer 1992; 69:829–838.
18. Scott G, Whyler N, Grant G. A study of family carers of people with a life-threatening illness 1: the carers' needs analysis. Int J Palliat Nurs 2001; 7:290–330.
19. Mor V, Masterson-Allen S. The hospice model of care for the terminally ill. Adv Psychosom Med 1988; 18:119–134.
20. Ramirez A, Addington Hall J, Richards M. ABC of palliative care. The carers. BMJ 1998; 316:208–211.
21. Kristjanson LJ. Indicators of quality of palliative care from a family perspective. J Palliat Care 1986; 2:7–19.
22. Kristjanson, LJ. Quality of terminal care: salient indicators identified by families. J Palliat Care 1989; 5:21–30.

23. Bucher JA, Trostle GB, Moore M. Family reports of cancer pain, pain relief, and prescription access. Cancer Pract 1999; 7:71–77.
24. Ferrell BR, Ferrell BA, Rhiner M, et al. Family factors influencing cancer pain management. Postgrad Med J 1991; 67(Suppl. 2):S64–S69.
25. Taylor EJ, Ferrell BR, Grant M, et al. Managing cancer pain at home: the decisions and ethical conflicts of patients, family caregivers, and homecare nurses. Oncol Nurs Forum 1993; 20:919–927.
26. Kristjanson LJ, Avery L. Vicarious pain: the family's perspective. Pain Manage News 1994; 7:1–2.
27. Harrington V, Lackey NR, Gates MF. Needs of caregivers of clinic and hospice cancer patients. Cancer Nurs 1996; 19:118–125.
28. Nunnally JA, Bernstein I. Psychometric Theory, 3rd edition. New York: McGraw Hill, 1994.
29. Geron SM, Smith K, Tennstedt S, et al. The home care satisfaction measure: a client-centered approach to assessing the satisfaction of frail older adults with home care services. J Gerontol B Psychol Sci Soc Sci 2000; 55:S259–S270.
30. Kristjanson LJ. Family Satisfaction with Palliative Care: A Test of Four Alternative Theories. Tucson: University of Arizona, 1991. Dissertation.
31. Kristjanson LJ. Validity and reliability of the FAMCARE scale: measuring family satisfaction with advanced cancer care. Soc Sci Med 1993; 36:693–701.
32. Ware JE Jr. How to survey patient satisfaction. Drug Intell Clin Pharm 1981; 15:892–899.
33. Westra BL, Cullen L, Brody D, et al. Development of the home care client satisfaction instrument. Public Health Nurs 1995; 12:393–399.
34. Tierney RM, Horton SM, Hannan TJ, et al. Relationships between symptom relief, quality of life, and satisfaction with hospice care. Palliat Med 1998; 12:333–344.
35. Pascoe GC. Patient satisfaction in primary health care: a literature review. Eval Program Plann 1984; 6:185–210.
36. Wright JG. Outcomes research: what to measure. World J Surg 1999; 23:1224–1226.
37. Kristjanson LJ, Leis A, Koop P, et al. Family members' care expectations, care perceptions and satisfaction with advanced cancer care: results of a multi-site pilot study. J Palliat Care 1997; 13:4–11.
38. Oberst MR. Patients' perceptions of care: measurement of quality and satisfaction. Cancer 1984; 53:2366–2375.
39. Sherwood G, Adams-McNeill J, Stark PL, et al. Qualitative assessment of hospitalized patients' satisfaction with pain management. Res Nurs Health 2000; 23:486–495.
40. Ware JE Jr, Davies-Avery A, Stewart AL. The measurement and meaning of patient satisfaction: a review of recent literature. Health Med Care Serv Rev 1978; 1:1–15.
41. McCusker J. Development of scales to measure satisfaction and preferences regarding long-term and terminal care. Med Care 1984; 22:476–493.
42. Jarvis H, Burge FI, Scott CA. Evaluating a palliative care program: methodology and limitations. J Palliat Care 1996; 12:23–33.
43. Leis A, Kristjanson LJ, Koop P, et al. Family health and the palliative care trajectory: a research agenda. Can J Clin Oncol 1997; 1:352–360.
44. Kristjanson LJ. The family as the unit of treatment. In: Portenoy R, Bruera E, eds. Topics in Palliative Care, vol 1. New York: Oxford University Press, 1997:245–262.

45. Steinglass P. A systems view of family interaction and psychopathology. In: Jacob I, ed. Family Interaction and Psychopathology. New York: Plenum Press, 1987:21–45.
46. Kissane DW, Bloch S, Dowe DL, et al. The Melbourne Family Grief Study I: perceptions of family functioning in bereavement. Am J Psychol 1996; 153:650–658.
47. Kissane DW, Bloch S, Burns WI, et al. Psychological morbidity in the families of patients with cancer. Psychooncology 1994; 3:47–56.
48. Bruera E, Kuehn N, Miller M, et al. The Edmonton Symptom Assessment system (ESAS): a simple method for the assessment of palliative care patients. J Palliat Care 1991; 7:6–9.

VI

QUALITY-OF-LIFE
RESEARCH

14

Usefulness of Utility in Making Decisions about Palliative Care

THOMAS J. SMITH

Doing a test is like picking one's nose in public: before one does it, one should figure out what one will do with the results if one finds something.

J.N. Bodurtha

Cancer accounts for 23% of all deaths[1] so suffering from this disease will continue. We clearly do not do a satisfactory job of relieving symptoms, with over half of cancer or dying patients having uncontrolled pain.[2-5] Cancer patients and their doctors face an increasing array of choices, which may be mutually exclusive: hospice care, nonhospice palliative care, palliative measures such as erythropoietin and bisphosphonates, palliative chemotherapy, and investigational therapy. At the same time, cancer costs have risen from $35 billion in 1990[6] to an estimated $50 billion in 1996.[7] This increasing demand for services, new technologies, exclusions within types of care, and an aging population have led to an increasing tension about what services to provide, to whom, and on what basis.[8,9]

Cost–effectiveness studies can help lay the framework for the comparison and allocation of resources.[10,11] The standard ways of presenting data are listed in Table 14.1. Cost–effectiveness studies do not generally apply to palliative care, which by definition does not improve "effectiveness" by adding survival. The only way that palliative care can show value for money is by improving the cost–utility ratio, where utility is the value placed on the time spent in a particular state of health. In this chapter, I will define utility, illustrate how utility values are obtained, illustrate some uses of utility in cost–utility studies, and show how utility can be used in patient, payer, and provider decision making. Ultimately, we can ask "Should we do the utility test?"

Table 14.1. Clinical and cost studies and application to palliative care

Type of study	Advantages and disadvantages	Application to palliative care
Clinical outcomes only	Ignores costs. Easy to choose among clearly superior therapies such as cisplatin for testicular cancer; harder among all others that give lesser benefits at high costs.	Very few direct comparisons between interventions.
Cost only (costs of treating pain)	Ignores clinical outcomes. Does not help decision makers choose among clinical strategies.	Does not take into account effectiveness or things that we know work, such as pain medicine, but cannot prove.
Costs and clinical outcomes together		
Cost-minimization	Assumes that two strategies are equal; lowest-cost strategy is preferred.	Very few direct comparisons of any two therapies. (Very few pharmaceutical firms will take the risk of putting their products in competition.[37])
Cost-effectiveness	Compares two strategies; assigns monetary value per additional year of life saved by strategy.	By definition, palliative care does not add years of life, or if so, the effect is minuscule.
Cost-utility	Compares two strategies; assigns monetary value per additional year of life saved by strategy, then estimates the quality of that benefit in dollars/quality-adjusted life year.	There are only two ways to improve ratio: improve utility or decrease costs.
Cost-benefit	Compares two strategies but converts the clinical benefits to money, e.g., a year of life is worth $100,000. Possible but rarely done due to difficulty in assigning monetary value to human life.	Almost certainly unfavorable to palliative care as patients rarely work or generate income.

Methods

I reviewed the medical literature on patient utility, cost–utility, and effectiveness using Medline. I have listed relevant definitions in Table 14.2.

Utilities

Utility is the value given to time in a particular health state. For example, perfect health might be rated as 1.0 on a scale of 0 (dead) to perfect health (1.0); an in-between state of "lung cancer metastatic to bone but generally functional with

Table 14.2. Definitions

Term	Definition	Application in utility
Health state	A type of health, e.g., well, recurrent disease, toxicity from treatment.	May change rapidly, especially as patients "fail" and become rapidly terminal.
Utility	The value placed by a patient on time in a particular state of health, e.g., a day in conference = 0.7 of a normal day.	Requires either a quality-of-life score or a utility score.
Transition probability	The probability of moving from one health state to another, e.g., a woman has a 5% chance in year 1 of going from well to breast cancer recurrence.	Often difficult to find.
Effectiveness	Improvement in relevant outcome, traditionally survival or disease-free survival.	—
Resource utilization	The resources used, e.g., 4 bed days or 35,000 mg morphine.	Accessible.
Cost	What it costs to provide a service, from a societal viewpoint.	Accessible, can be converted from charges using ratio of cost to charges.[38]
Charge	Bills for service, including all costs and profit.	Accessible from hospital, clinic, and provider charges.
Perspective	From whose viewpoint is the analysis done? Could be societal, the norm; health care system; the payer; or the patient.	Should start from a societal viewpoint. Patients may value any health care intervention at any cost, regardless of the consequences on others.

controlled pain" might be rated as 0.63. Utilities are obtained by two general methods: (*1*) the time trade-off and (*2*) the standard gamble. The time trade-off can use a "feelings thermometer" or analogue scale to rate value on a scale of 0 to 1.0. Accompanying questions might ask "How many months of perfect health would you trade for 6 months with lung cancer, bone metastasis, controlled pain?" The standard gamble technique asks patients to choose from two alternatives and attempts to find the time trade-off when the alternatives are judged equal. For instance, patients might be asked " Would you trade 10 months of perfect health for 12 months in your current health state? No? Then how about 9 months?" If 9 "well" months equal 12 "sick" months, then the utility of the sickness state is 0.75.

There are other ways to obtain utilities, including making them up or obtaining them from focus groups of healthcare practitioners[12–15] or patients. For instance, in our work on adjuvant therapy of breast cancer and various forms of

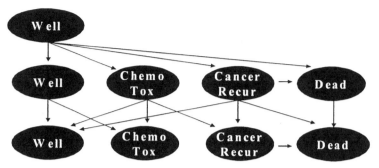

Tally all the value: time x utility value
ex: 3 months x 0.5 = 1.5 months
Compare treatment with no treatment

Figure 14.1. Markov models of transition states.

chemotherapy for non-small cell lung cancer, we did a survey of healthcare professionals, mostly oncology nurses, as "informed consumers." An alternative method has been to estimate baseline values, then to use sensitivity analysis to show that all values favor one type of treatment over another; for example, almost all combinations of utility for recurrence and toxicity from interferon-α favored treatment over placebo.[16] A more usable method has been to transform quality of life (QOL) into utility values. This method requires transforming QOL into a scale of 0–1, then transforming values under 0.85 by multiplying by 1.18 since patients are unwilling to give up time below this value. If the value is >0.85, multiply by 1.0. This simple method uses more readily available QOL data and correlates well with other methods, such as the standard gamble.[17]

Utility (U) values are used to place value on time in a health state. This is shown in Figure 14.1, a typical Markov model,[18] but can be used for spreadsheet analyses or back-of-the-envelope calculations. For breast cancer adjuvant treatment, the baseline survival benefit would be about 19.3 months compared to no treatment. However, since some of that time is spent with toxicity from treatment (U = 0.7), the actual benefit is 19.3 × 0.7 = 14 quality-adjusted months.

Utility values can also be used to estimate cost–effectiveness and cost–utility ratios. The standard cost–effectiveness question is

$$\Delta C/\Delta E \;=\; (C_2 - C_1)/(E_2 - E_1)$$

where C = costs and E = effectiveness of treatment measured in time. When utility, or time multiplied by the utility value, is added, the equation becomes

$$\Delta C/\Delta U$$

where $\Delta U = U_2 - U_1$. For example, a therapy that does not improve survival but increases utility by 10% will increase U by (1 year) × (0.10) = 0.1 year. If this treatment costs an additional \$10,000/year, then the cost–utility ratio is:

$$\Delta C = C_2 - C_1 = \$10,000 = \$100,000/QALY.$$

$$\Delta U = U_2 - U_1 = 0.10$$

where QALY = quality-adjusted life year. Such values can be compared to other medical interventions, as shown in Table 14.3.

Use of utility for patient decision making

Utility values could be used in a real-life situation. For instance, some patients state that "Chemotherapy scares me as much as cancer," so all of their time on chemotherapy would be given a utility of 0. In this case, the benefit falls from 14.0 months to 2.7 quality-adjusted months.[12] At the other end of the spectrum, some women state that "I will do anything to prevent recurrence and do not care how sick you make me." For these women, the time on chemotherapy must have

Table 14.3. Cost–effectiveness and/or cost–utility of some medical interventions

Intervention	Incremental cost-effectiveness (\$US)
Liver transplantation compared to medical management	237,000
Mammography, age <50 years	232,000
Cholestyramine for high cholesterol compared to no treatment	178,000
ABMT compared to standard chemotherapy for limited metastatic breast cancer	116,000
Captopril compared to hydrochlorothiazide for hypertension	82,000
Zidovudine compared to no treatment for HIV	8520–88,500
Dialysis compared to medical management	50,000
Mammography screening for breast cancer age 50–75 years	20,000–50,000
Drug therapy for moderate hypertension	32,600
ABMT compared to salvage chemotherapy for Hodgkin's disease recurrent after MOPP-ABV	21,000
Vinorelbine + cisplatin compared to vindesine + cisplatin	15,500
Chemotherapy for NSCLC compared to best supportive care	−8400–20,000
Adjuvant CMF compared to no treatment for early-stage breast cancer, age 45 years	4900
Adjuvant chemotherapy for stage III colon cancer	2300
Smoking cessation counseling	1300

ABMT, autologous bone marrow transplantation; HIV, human immunodeficiency virus; MOPP-ABV, mechlorethamine, vincristine (Oncovin), procarbazine, prednisone, doxorubicin (Adriamycin), bleomycin, and vincristine; NSCLC, non-small cell lung cancer; CMF, cyclophosphamide, methotrexate, and 5-Fluorouracil.

Source: Smith et al.[10]

Table 14.4. Possible cost–utility ratios for a successful palliative care intervention that increases utility from 0.63 to 0.69

Case Example:

Your clinic has been asked to use a new appetite stimulant, EATMOR. In clinical trials, EATMOR increased weight and quality of life significantly, but it costs $3300 a year. The benefit only comes when the drug is given. The quality-of-life scores can be compressed to a 0–1 score and transformed to utility values. The intervention, which clearly works, does not work at a sufficiently high level or low cost to justify its use compared to other healthcare interventions.[36] Some representative values are listed, with resultant cost–utility ratios.

Incremental effect and cost of intervention ($/utility)	$/QALY	Comment
10,000/0.05	200,000	Too expensive
3300/0.06	55,000	Too expensive, given benchmark of $35,000–50,000[10]
1000/0.05	20,000	Acceptable, requires a 5% change in utility
100/0.05	2000	Acceptable, intervention probably too inexpensive to interest any company

a utility of 1.0, and they would gain 11.2 quality-adjusted months. Because the "scared" person gains a much shorter time but the therapy still costs the same, her cost–utility ratio is $30,000/QALY. The person who does not mind toxicity and wants to avoid recurrence would have a cost–utility ratio better than normal (Table 14.4).

In real life, it is difficult to use these types of patient utility in patient decision making. First, one should ideally use the patient's own utilities. However, there is no easy tool with which to measure utilities and no set of decision analysis models to use the values. If QOL measures are used then transformed to utilities, some method of paying for the measurement of QOL (estimated at $400/patient in most research studies[19]) must be found. Second, there is no simple unchanging number to reflect all of the various and changing health states. Third, to evaluate and rank all health states, the patient should have lived through them all, and this is rarely possible (especially with death). Finally, the impact of sickness and medical interventions on QOL scores is remarkably small; this could reflect that other factors are more important, that the effect is small, or that humans have remarkable adaptive powers. For instance, the change in QOL from complete disappearance of rheumatoid arthritis is only 0.20 and that of becoming 20 years younger, only 0.14.[20]

These values may be useful in other implicit ways, such as illustrating to patients what could happen in the future and quantifying some of the unknown health states, benefits, and toxicities of treatment. There is no reason why costs, charges, or prices should be sacred and unchangeable. We have found that a careful review of the bills and of the services provided can lead to simplification of care and lower costs, thereby changing the cost–effectiveness without changing the effectiveness at all. For example, foregoing "STAT" lab tests gave one-third laboratory savings, and reducing the cost of high-dose chemotherapy for metastatic breast cancer lowered the cost–effectiveness from $116,000/QALY[21] to $70,000/QALY.[22]

Problems with use of patient utilities

There are a limited number of studies on the actual utilities of cancer patients. Jaakimainen et al.[23] described the utilities of seven lung cancer patients obtained using the standard gamble technique (Fig. 14.2). The time these utility values were obtained and whether each of the patients had experienced each health state are not stated. I suspect, if patients in each health state had been asked, that the actual values would be better represented by the line in Figure 14.2; but there are no data.

A different concern is whether we should use patient or societal values since societal resources are being spent. Tsevat and colleagues[24] studied utility values of 80-year-old patients hospitalized but able to cooperate with the SUPPORT study. Of these sick patients, the average U was 0.81. Only 31% of patients rated their current QOL as excellent or very good, but of these, 69% would give up 1 month or less of their current health state (U = 0.92). At the other extreme, 6% were willing to live 2 weeks or less in their current state in exchange for 1 year of wellness (U = 0.04). Surrogates underestimated U values by 25%, for example, 9 instead of 12 months, suggesting that only patients can give reliable answers. These values may force society to ask the question, since it is paying for the care, "If sick 80-year-olds will not trade their health state, then who will?"

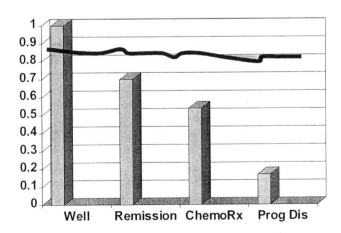

Figure 14.2. Some utility values of lung cancer patients. The line represents what might be found with real patients at every point. Patient values estimated from Goodwin et al.[39]

Also, should we use their values or society's since society is paying for their healthcare? The Institute of Medicine recommendation was to use societal values.[25–27]

Usefulness of provider utilities

The use of provider utilities is attractive since providers are "informed consumers" (in that they know the benefits and toxicities of treatments), and they are available. However, the data suggest that there are major differences in how patients and health-care professionals view treatment choices. Slevin and colleagues[28] showed that patients would be willing to undergo chemotherapy with major toxicity for a 1% chance of long-term survival or a 10% chance of symptom relief. Their providers would require over a 50% chance of benefit to take the same treatment; however, the providers did not have cancer. When the patients were questioned after 3 months of treatment, their choices were the same. Meystre and colleagues[29] showed that hospice patients viewed treatments, such as blood transfusion and radiation, as quite ordinary when hospice nurses rated them as "aggressive." Davies et al.[30,31] showed that glioma patients would still take radiation, even though only about 40% had stabilization and some had intellectual decrements; they pointed out the difficulty of patients making "rational" decisions when faced with a terrifying illness.

Provider utilities may be useful to define the questions to ask and to quantify the benefits from an informed consumer benefit. Again, there is no simple, easy, and inexpensive tool.

Use of payer utilities

The responsibility of payers is different in that they must meet the needs of all patients within a fixed budget. Payers would prefer a single number that represents the composite of all relevant health states, but there is no number that includes all of the complexities of diagnosis, treatment, surveillance, toxicity, recurrence, etc.[32] Any treatments that make such a large change in utilities are likely to be discernible without QOL measures.

Measurement of utilities or QOL may help to reduce biases held by payers. As an example, a common argument by insurers about the cost and effectiveness of high-dose chemotherapy was that QOL was adversely affected. In fact, QOL showed some decrement initially but rapidly returned to premorbid levels.[33]

Potential for bias

There are ways that interested parties can bias a study or comparison to make their product look good. First, ignore global QOL and utility scores since they rarely change. Even clinically successful[34] and cost–effective[35] interventions, like mitoxantrone for metastatic prostate cancer, show no improvement in global

QOL. Second, add as many symptom-specific questions to the utility or QOL instrument as possible. For example, if 10 of 15 questions are about fatigue, then a fatigue intervention is more likely to show an impact. Of course, those interested in studying nausea will want 10 of 15 questions about nausea, pitting symptom relief groups against one another. Third, make an entirely new instrument incorporating the principles above. Fourth, collect only data from the time on treatment, and ignore any potential downstream effects and costs; of course, this could also miss downstream benefits or savings. Finally, set the price of your drug/service at the current one, and do not explore the threshold where the price of the drug would make it cost-saving; that is, keep the price at a level that supports maximum return on investment rather than one that will maximize use, and show only that it falls within accepted guidelines for use.[36]

Conclusion

Utility can be used to rank treatments based on their effect and to calculate cost–utility ratios. Change in utility is difficult to show for palliative care interventions because the effects of the interventions are small, the effects of the disease are large, and current global instruments do not capture the benefit. Perhaps the most practical use is to quantify the benefits and toxicities of various interventions and to illustrate the future health states that the patient is likely to experience. This may be useful in patient decision making but requires an informed, knowledge-seeking patient, who is willing to make choices informed by data. At present, utility and cost–utility are not useful in resource allocation, except as an implicit way to illustrate benefit for comparative cost and clinical decision making.

References

1. Parker SL, Tong T, Bolden S, et al. Cancer statistics. Cancer 1997; 47:5–27.
2. Von Roenn JH, Cleeland CS, Gonin R, et al. Physician attitudes and practice in cancer pain management. A survey from the Eastern Cooperative Oncology Group. Ann Intern Med 1993; 119:121–126.
3. Cleeland CS, Gonin R, Hatfield AK, et al. Pain and its treatment in outpatients with metastatic cancer. N Engl J Med 1994; 330:592–596.
4. Cleeland CS, Gonin R, Baez L, et al. Pain and treatment of pain in minority patients with cancer. Ann Intern Med 1997; 127:813–816.
5. SUPPORT Principal Investigators. A controlled trial to improve care for seriously ill hospitalized patients. The Study to Understand Prognoses and Preferences for Outcomes and Risks of Treatments (SUPPORT). JAMA 1995; 274:1591–1598.
6. Brown ML. The national economic burden of cancer. J Natl Cancer Inst 1990; 82: 1811–1814.
7. Rundle RL. Salick pioneers selling cancer care to HMOs. Wall Street J August 12 1996:B1–B2.

8. Callahan D. Controlling the costs of health care for the elderly—fair means and foul. N Engl J Med 1996; 335:744–746.

9. Levinsky NG. The purpose of advance medical planning—autonomy for patients or limitation of care? N Engl J Med 1996; 335:741–743.

10. Smith TJ, Hillner BE, Desch CE. Efficacy and cost-effectiveness of cancer treatment: rational allocation of resources based on decision analysis. J Natl Cancer Inst 1993; 85:1460–1474.

11. Smith TJ, Desch CE, Hillner BE. Ways to reduce the cost of oncology care without compromising the quality. Cancer Invest 1994; 12:257–265.

12. Hillner BE, Smith TJ. Efficacy and cost-effectiveness of adjuvant chemotherapy in women with node-negative breast cancer. A decision analysis model. N Engl J Med 1991; 324:160–168.

13. Smith TJ, Hillner BE. The efficacy and cost-effectiveness of adjuvant therapy of early breast cancer in premenopausal women. J Clin Oncol 1993; 11:771–776.

14. Smith TJ, Hillner BE, Neighbors DM, et al. An economic evaluation of a randomized clinical trial comparing vinorelbine, vinorelbine plus cisplatin and vindesine plus cisplatin for non-small cell lung cancer. J Clin Oncol 1995; 13:2166–2173.

15. Weeks JC, Tierney MR, Weinstein MC. Cost effectiveness of prophylactic intravenous immune globulin in chronic lymphocytic leukemia. N Engl J Med 1991; 325:81–86.

16. Gelber RD, Goldhirsch A. A new endpoint for the assessment of adjuvant therapy in postmenopausal women with operable breast cancer. J Clin Oncol 1986; 4: 1772–1779.

17. O'Leary JF, Fairclough DL, Jankowski MK, et al. Comparison of time-tradeoff utilities and rating scale values of cancer patients and their relatives: evidence for a possible plateau relationship. Med Decis Making 1995; 15:132–137.

18. Sonnenberg FA, Beck JR. Markov models in medical decision making: a practical guide. Med Decis Making 1993; 13:322–338.

19. Brown M, Glick H, Harrell F, et al. Integrating economic analysis into cancer clinical trials: the NCI-ASCO Economics Workbook. J Natl Cancer Inst 1998; 24:1–28.

20. Testa MA, Simonson DC. Assessment of quality-of-life outcomes. N Engl J Med 1996; 334:835–840.

21. Hillner BE, Smith TJ, Desch CE. Efficacy and cost-effectiveness of autologous bone marrow transplantation in metastatic breast cancer. Estimates using decision-analysis while awaiting clinical trial results. JAMA 1992; 267:2055–2061.

22. Smith TJ, Hillner BE. Decision analysis: a practical example. Oncology 1995; 9(Suppl 11):37–45.

23. Jaakimainen L, Goodwin PJ, Pater J, et al. Counting the costs of chemotherapy in a National Cancer Institute of Canada randomized trial in non-small cell lung cancer. J Clin Oncol 1990; 8:1301–1309.

24. Tsevat J, Dawson N V, Wu AW, et al. Health values of hospitalized patients 80 years or older. JAMA 1998; 279:371–375.

25. Russell LB, Gold MR, Siegel JE, et al. The role of cost-effectiveness analysis in health and medicine. JAMA 1996; 276:1172–1177.

26. Weinstein MC, Siegel JE, Gold MR, et al. Recommendations of the Panel on Cost-Effectiveness in Health and Medicine. JAMA 1996; 276:1253–1258.

27. Siegel JE, Weinstein MC, Russell LB, et al. Recommendations for reporting cost-effectiveness analyses. JAMA 1996; 276:1339–1341.

28. Slevin ML, Stubbs L, Plant HJ, et al. Attitudes to chemotherapy: comparing views of patients with cancer with those of doctors, nurses, and general public. BMJ 1990; 300:1458–1460.
29. Meystre CJN, Burley NMJ, Ahmedzai S. What investigations and procedures do patients in hospices want? Interview based survey of patients and their nurses. BMJ 1997; 315:1202–1203.
30. Davies E, Clarke C, Hopkins A. Malignant cerebral glioma. I: Survival, disability, and morbidity after radiotherapy. BMJ 1996; 313:1507–1512.
31. Davies E, Clarke C, Hopkins A. Malignant cerebral glioma. II: Perspectives of patients and relatives on the value of radiotherapy. BMJ 1996; 313:1512–1516.
32. Brundage MD, Groome PA, Feldman-Stewart D, et al. Decision analysis in locally advanced non-small-cell lung cancer: is it useful? J Clin Oncol 1997; 15:873–883.
33. Zujewski J, Nelson A, Abrams J. Much ado about not … enough data: high-dose chemotherapy with autologous stem cell rescue for breast cancer. J Natl Cancer Inst 1998; 90:200–209.
34. Tannock IF, Osoba D, Stockler M.R, et al. Chemotherapy with mitoxantrone plus prednisone or prednisone alone for symptomatic hormone-resistant prostate cancer: a Canadian randomized trial with palliative end points. J Clin Oncol 1996; 14: 1756–1764.
35. Bloomfield DJ, Krahn MD, Neogi T, et al. Economic evaluation of chemotherapy with mitoxantrone plus prednisone for symptomatic hormone resistant prostate cancer, based on a Canadian randomized trial with palliative endpoints. J Clin Oncol 1997 (in press).
36. Laupacis A, Feeny D, Detsky AS, et al. How attractive does a new technology have to be to warrant adoption and utilization? Tentative guidelines for using clinical and economic evaluation. CMAJ 1992; 146:473–481.
37. Bennett CL, Smith TJ, George SL, et al. Free-riding and the prisoner's dilemma: problems in funding economic analyses of phase III cancer clinical trials. J Clin Oncol 1995; 13:2457–2463.
38. Shwartz M, Young DW, Siegrist R. The ratio of costs to charges: how good a basis for estimating costs? Inquiry 1995; 32:476–481.
39. Goodwin P, et al. Cost effectivness of cancer chemotheray: an economic evaluation of a randomized trial in small-cell lung cancer. J Clin Oncol 1988; 6:1537–1547.

15

Assessing Quality of Life in Palliative Care

S. ROBIN COHEN

Palliative care has been defined as follows[1]:

> the active total care of patients whose disease is not responsive to curative treatment. Control of pain, of other symptoms, and of psychological, social and spiritual problems, is paramount. The goal of palliative care is achievement of the best quality of life for patients and their families.

Therefore, if palliative care providers wish to evaluate the full impact of their care, they must measure changes in quality of life (QOL) as well as improvements in areas specifically targeted by particular interventions (such as pain, depression). Since palliative care considers the family as the unit of care, patient QOL, family member QOL, and the QOL of the family unit are all primary outcomes of palliative care. While problems in specific areas are important to address with specific interventions and specific measures, the best indicator of the quality of whole-person care is the QOL of the care recipient. While family QOL is important, due to the lack of studies in this area, it will not be considered further in this chapter but is briefly covered in Cohen.[2]

The importance of measuring QOL has been widely recognized in the healthcare literature in the last two decades. Unfortunately, this has led to a great pressure to measure QOL at all phases of cancer and human immunodeficiency virus (HIV) disease, even though the measures are not adequately developed to show primary outcomes. We must work to further develop these measures, which can be of great benefit in ensuring patient- and family-centered care and can help us to reach our goal of achieving the best QOL possible for them.

Conceptualizing Quality of Life

The results of large studies of the QOL of Americans[3,4] and more recent qualitative work asking people with cancer or HIV disease to describe what health or

QOL means to them[5–8] suggest that QOL is best defined as subjective well-being. There has been a movement in the healthcare setting to ignore the broader implications of QOL by studying "health-related" QOL. "Health-related QOL refers to the extent to which one's usual or expected physical, emotional, and social well-being are affected by a medical condition or its treatment."[9] However, there is not a direct relationship between a medical condition and its treatment and QOL. Instead, QOL is a measure of the outcome of the *interaction* between the medical condition, and its treatment, and the whole person or family whose QOL is being measured, who form an integral part of the equation that results in QOL. Adding the word *health* before QOL does not allow us to disregard some aspects of the person, such as spiritual well-being, if we consider that people with cancer and HIV disease define *health* as a sense of personal integrity[6] consisting of physical, psychological, and spiritual domains.[5]

Many investigators make the mistake of thinking that contributors to QOL represent QOL. Surely, severe physical symptoms contribute to QOL, but the extent of that contribution will depend on many factors. Therefore, if QOL rather than the symptoms is of interest, it is important to determine how much of an *impact* the symptom has on the respondent, rather than its intensity. If the symptoms themselves are of interest, then a symptom assessment tool rather than a QOL instrument should be used.

Short-Term Goals

The overriding short-term goal in QOL assessment is to develop scientifically sound and practical measures of QOL.

1. Reach a consensus as to what QOL is and what we need to consider when measuring it, to ensure content validity of assessment tools. This must be based on what palliative care patients, their family caregivers, and their families say is important to their respective QOL.
2. Compare results across cultures to determine if there are universal determinants of QOL. If there are, determine whether they are expressed in the same way in different cultures. For example, depression may be a universally important QOL determinant but may be expressed in more somatic terms in some cultures than others.
3. Develop psychometrically sound instruments that are acceptable to the respondents for measuring the QOL of a group of patients, family caregivers, or families. Test properties such as validity, stability (reliability), and responsiveness to change based on hypotheses about QOL. For example, to determine whether the instrument is responsive to change, compare changes in QOL score to the respondent's judgment that QOL has changed, rather than to changes in disease status.
4. Develop QOL instruments that have psychometrically sound subscales, and test to determine whether the judgment of overall QOL is directly re-

lated to a combination of the subscale scores. It is likely that measures that include valid, reliable, and responsive subscales as well as an overall measure of QOL will be most useful in determining the effectiveness of our interventions and services. Overall QOL may remain the same as the patient's physical state deteriorates, but the domains that contribute most to QOL may change.[10–12] There is a greater difference between scores in different domains in those with more advanced disease compared to those at earlier stages of the disease trajectory or who are in remission,[11–13] making it more important to have psychometrically sound subscales in advanced disease.

5. Develop QOL measures that are appropriate for measuring the QOL of individuals so that they can be used as a clinical tool. This measure may be the same as that for measuring the QOL of groups, but it may need to be different.
6. Reach consensus on how to define palliative care patients. To compare results across studies, we need to know whether the patients are the same.

Long-Term Goals

The overriding long-term goal in QOL assessment is to use QOL measures to improve care.

1. Find ways to define and measure the different components of palliative care services so that we can determine those which are most effective at achieving the best QOL for patients and their families.
2. Be able to measure all that may affect QOL in order to be able to control for it in studies that use QOL as an outcome measure.
3. Determine the effects of various types of care on the terminally ill and the overall effect of specific interventions on the patient, family caregiver, or family.
4. Determine which services or interventions are best for different types of patient and family.
5. Use QOL measures designed for the palliative care population to determine effectiveness in studies of the cost–effectiveness of palliative care.
6. Reduce burn-out of the primary family caregivers by monitoring their QOL and acting before a crisis occurs. This has the potential to reduce hospitalization for the patient and to decrease family caregiver problems both while the patient is alive and during the bereavement period.

Studies Defining Palliative Care Patient Quality of Life

We are partway to our goal of defining what is important to the QOL of palliative care patients. There are now several studies wherein people who were terminally ill or had advanced cancer were asked to explain what is most important to their QOL. There is consensus among the results of these studies. The spiritual/existential, social/family relationships, and physical symptoms/functioning domains were listed in all six studies.[8,14–18] The psychological domain was listed as important in all studies except one. Information or communication was listed as important to QOL in two-thirds of the studies. Both Padilla and colleagues[17] and Cohen and colleagues[8] found control, coping, enjoyment of life, and cognitive function to be important to QOL. Cohen and colleagues[8] also included the concept of uncertainty and the domain of environment, while Kaasa and Ahlner-Elmquist[16] mentioned decision making. This list of domains is more comprehensive than that included in most instruments designed to measure "health-related QOL" of people with cancer or acquired immunodeficiency syndrome (AIDS).

Review of Palliative Care Patient Quality of Life Instruments

Without content validity, it is of no use to consider other psychometric properties. If an instrument does not have content validity but its reliability and responsiveness are high, then it is measuring something well but that something is not QOL as the patients define it. The content validity is obvious for instruments that require the respondent to list the areas of his or her life that are most important to QOL, and then to rate his or her current functioning or satisfaction in those areas. This approach is used in the Schedule for the Evaluation of Individual Quality of Life (SEIQoL)[18–20] and the Patient Evaluated Problem Score.[21] While the latter is described as a QOL measure, the respondents are only asked to list their major problems; therefore, it does not really focus on overall QOL, although it is likely to provide other useful information to clinicians. The SEIQoL has been used to measure the QOL of outpatients who were HIV-positive.[19] It requires further testing in the palliative care setting, which has already begun.[18] This measure may be very useful for clinical services trying to ensure that their patients receive individualized care that addresses those areas that are most important to their QOL. Limitations to individualized content instruments are discussed below (see Individualized Versus Standardized Measures).

Standardized instruments that measure QOL with the same set of questions for every respondent do not address the specific concerns of each respondent but can, if they have content validity, inform us about the QOL of groups of people. Unfortunately, no published standardized QOL instruments include all of the domains that are important for palliative care patient QOL as determined in the six studies described in the previous section. Therefore, I will only consider briefly the psychometric properties of those instruments that have the most content validity (they contain items that represent the physical symptoms/functioning, psychological, social/family relationships, and spiritual/existential domains) and are in a format acceptable to palliative care patients (not too long, able to be administered by being read aloud). Several published self-report QOL instruments include items from at least these four domains but have not been developed beyond the initial stage[22,23] or their psychometric properties have not been established in the palliative care setting.[24–26]

The McGill Quality of Life Questionnaire (MQOL) has 16 items that form five submeasures established through factor analysis in three studies: a single item measuring physical well-being and subscales for physical symptoms, psychological well-being, existential well-being, and support.[11–13] The MQOL submeasures appear to have concurrent validity and acceptable test–retest reliability over a period of 2 days. All MQOL scores (Total and submeasures) change significantly when patients say that their QOL has changed, with the exception of the Support subscale, where mean scores indicate a high degree of support at all times.[27] The MQOL Total, Physical Symptoms, Physical Well-being, Psychological Well-being, and Existential Well-being scores were shown to improve significantly during the first week following admission to five Canadian palliative care units.[28] This demonstrates that the effect of palliative care can be demonstrated if appropriate QOL instruments are used.

The McMaster Quality of Life Scale contains 32 items referring to the physical, psychological, cognitive, social, and spiritual/existential domains; but data suggest that the questions can reliably be divided into two subscales: physical and nonphysical QOL.[29] The scale appears to have concurrent validity, to have good test–retest reliability at an interval of 3 hours between tests but less at an interval of 1 week, and to be responsive to changes in QOL.

The original Hospice Quality of Life Index contained 25 items concerning the physical, functional, psychological, social, spiritual, and financial domains as well as an item concerning environment.[30,31] The attempt to weight patient ratings of satisfaction by patient ratings of item importance is laudable, but the method of calculation described would have the counterintuitive result of a higher (better) score for items indicated to be important but about which the patient is dissatisfied than for unimportant items on which satisfaction is rated as low. A more recent version contains 28 items.[32] Factor analysis of data from the Hospice Quality of Life Index showed that not all items load on the factors in a way that allows a clear conceptual distinction between subscales.[30,32] The overall QOL score and the subscale scores were not significantly different at admission to hospice and 3 weeks later.[31]

The revised MQOL (renamed Quality of Life in Life-Threatening Illness—Patient Version, or QOLLTI-P) being developed by the Sociobehavioral Cancer Research Network (SCRN) of the National Cancer Institute of Canada and the palliative care modules developed to add to the Functional Assessment of Cancer Therapy (FACT)[15] may give these instruments complete content validity. However, given that the FACT-General Questionnaire has 27 items, adding items to achieve content validity may render it too lengthy to complete for many palliative care patients. The psychometric properties of these new versions are presently being tested.

Studies Defining Palliative Care Family Member Quality of Life

There are two projects presently under way to develop QOL measures for the family caregivers of cancer patients that are based on the reports of family caregivers themselves as to what is important to them. Both groups are studying the QOL of the primary family caregiver only rather than the QOL of all family members. Weitzner and colleagues[33–35] developed their Caregiver Quality of Life Index—Cancer (CQOLC) questionnaire for family caregivers of patients in the anticancer treatment phase and tested it in a U.S. hospice setting.[36] The content of the CQOLC is based on interviews with 22 patient-caregiver dyads, who were asked to explain how the patient's illness had impacted on the family caregiver's physical, emotional, family, social, and other functioning.[33] One limitation of this approach is that the emphasis is not on overall QOL but rather on changes affecting functioning since the patient was ill. The next two concerns apply only if the tool is to be used with caregivers of palliative care patients but not if the patient is at an earlier phase of the cancer trajectory. First, only family caregiver interviews where the patient also participated were used. Therefore, none of the family caregivers in the study was caring for a patient who was unable to participate due to poor physical or mental condition, which represents a large part of the palliative care population. Second, the family caregiver was excluded "if substances known to affect the central nervous system (i.e., narcotic analgesics, antiemetics, or steroids) were administered to the caregiver or patient 1 week or less before entry into the study." This exclusion criterion is likely to result in few family caregivers of advanced-cancer patients being included.

My SCRN colleagues and I are developing a measure of the QOL of family caregivers of palliative care patients, the Quality of Life in Life-Threatening Illness—Family Caregiver Version (QOLLTI-F) questionnaire to complement our patient QOL instrument (QOLLTI-P). Fifty-nine family caregivers of palliative care patients at home and on palliative care units in three Canadian cities were asked to describe what was important to their QOL at this time and what made a day good or bad. Content analysis revealed many themes, which we grouped into seven domains: state of caregiver, patient well-being, quality of palliative care, outlook, physical environment meets needs, financial, and relationships.[8] The state of the caregiver, patient well-being, quality of palliative care, relationships, and the theme of sense of purpose in life (which falls under the outlook domain) have been shown to be important to family caregivers of advanced-cancer and/or palliative care patients in other studies not focused specifically on QOL.[37]

Review of Palliative Care Family Caregiver Quality of Life Instruments

Some investigators have used modifications of instruments designed for patients to measure family member QOL.[31,38–40] Mohide et al.[41] developed a QOL measure specific to family caregivers that used the time trade-off technique, but this was tested with family caregivers of disabled relatives with chronic degenerative disorders and measured only physical, psychological, and social functioning.

McMillan and Mahon[42,43] developed the four-item Caregiver Quality of Life Index for caregivers of palliative care patients, covering emotional, social, financial, and physical domains, each measured by a single item. Content was based on a literature review and verified by five people who had been the family caregivers of patients who had died 2 years previously. Some important domains are missing, including all that are concerned with patient well-being and care. Furthermore, it remains to be determined whether the single item measuring each domain has sufficient test–retest reliability.

The 35-item CQOLC was tested for validity and test–retest reliability in the anticancer treatment setting, where its psychometric properties appear to be good.[35] There is also evidence for validity and internal consistency reliability in a home hospice setting.[44] In the anticancer treatment setting, factor analysis has revealed five factors: mental/emotional burden, lifestyle disruption, hopefulness, social support, and financial concerns.[34] The CQOLC of Weitzner et al.[35] does not address caregiver physical condition, patient well-being, quality of care, the appropriateness of the environment, or control/helplessness. Since the QOLLTI-F is based on our own qualitative study, we have included all of the relevant domains; but confirmatory evidence of its validity is required, especially in palliative care settings where not all patients have cancer.

Individualized Versus Standardized Measures

The specific contributors to QOL vary tremendously from individual to individual and family to family. In consideration of these individual differences, the argument has been made that it is not useful to measure QOL with standardized instruments and that QOL measures must be individualized, as in SEIQoL, to include the specific contributors that are important to the individual whose QOL is being measured. A similar case has been made that QOL measures must allow the individual to assign weights to each domain indicating its importance.[20,45] This may be the case if one is measuring the QOL of an individual for clinical purposes. Instruments used to inform us about the QOL of individuals must have a higher degree of stability (test–retest reliability) than those required to measure the QOL of groups, where somewhat more measurement error is tolerable because both positive and negative measurement errors will occur and tend to average toward zero. However, for purposes other than clinical care of an individual, such as determining the strengths and weaknesses of a palliative care service, assessing the overall impact of a particular intervention, comparing the effectiveness of palliative care services, and determining what QOL is related to in order to provide better care in the future, it is appropriate to measure the QOL of groups of people. For these purposes, if the questionnaire items have been selected to reflect the areas that palliative care recipients have said are important and are worded in general rather than specific terms so that they are applicable to everyone, then it may not be necessary to have items specific for each person or individual weighting of the domains. If the data are to be grouped, the specifics will be lost in any case and we can measure QOL in more general terms with standardized instruments so that we are comparing groups on the same domains. To date, weighted data have not been used in published studies or have correlated so closely with unweighted data that they did not supply any additional or different information.[31,46] This is the result that would be expected if equal numbers of people weight each of the different domains highly so that the group average weight of each domain is similar. In addition, while some items are inherently important (for example, depression), circumstances that may be important for some people but not others (such as feeling in control) can be phrased to implicitly include a rating of importance by asking "How much of a problem was X for you?" rather than "How much of X is present?" The importance of weighting needs to be directly tested in studies comparing weighted and unweighted scores.

Valid and reliable subscales are particularly important for measuring QOL in the palliative care setting, where QOL related to physical functioning and physical symptoms such as fatigue will inevitably decline but QOL in other domains may improve. Data from studies using the MQOL show that the more advanced the disease, the greater the discrepancy between scores in different domains, for both people with cancer and people with HIV disease.[11-13] The importance of measuring each domain with a separate subscale is therefore greater when the disease is more advanced. With individualized measures, each respondent is evaluating his or her status in areas nominated by himself or herself so that different groups of respondents are not rating their status in the same areas. Therefore, these instruments provide an overall QOL score but do not have subscales.

We can and should directly test whether the total score obtained from individualized QOL measures is more valid than that obtained from standardized measures by comparing them to QOL scores obtained from a valid and reliable questionnaire that directly assesses overall QOL (that is, contains items such as "How has your QOL been?").

Conclusion

Since the goal of palliative care is to achieve the best QOL possible for patients and their families, measures of patient, family member, and overall family QOL are critically important as outcome measures. The availability of valid, acceptable, reliable, and responsive QOL measures will enable studies to ensure that whole-person care is delivered in the palliative setting. Considerable thought, time, and energy have been expended and will continue to be needed to define what is important to the QOL of palliative care patients, their family members, and their families as a whole, to create measures that have content validity. We are well on the way to having the patient QOL measures we need. The process has begun for the QOL of family members. We are still waiting for someone to take up the formidable challenge of measuring overall family QOL.

Acknowledgments

The author gratefully acknowledges salary support for herself from the Canadian Institutes of Health Research and National Cancer Institute of Canada through the Dorothy J. Lamont Award.

References

1. WHO Expert Committee. Cancer Pain Relief and Palliative Care. WHO Technical Report Series 804. Geneva: World Health Organization, 1990.
2. Cohen SR. Defining and measuring quality of life in palliative care. In: Bruera E, Portenoy RK, eds. Topics in Palliative Care, vol 5. New York: Oxford University Press, 2001:137–156.
3. Cantril H. The Pattern of Human Concerns. Piscataway, NJ: Rutgers University Press, 1965.
4. Campbell A, Converse PE, Rodgers WL. The Quality of American Life. New York: Russell Sage Foundation, 1976.
5. Fryback PB. Health for people with a terminal diagnosis. Nurs Sci Q 1993; 6: 147–159.
6. Kagawa-Singer M. Redefining health: living with cancer. Soc Sci Med 1993; 37: 295–304.
7. Cohen SR, Bunston T, Leis A. Domains relevant to the quality of life of the family caregivers of palliative care patients with cancer. J Palliat Care 1998; 14:104.
8. Cohen SR, Leis A. What determines the quality of life of terminally ill cancer patients from their own perspective? J Palliat Care 2002; 18:48–58.
9. Cella DF. Measuring quality of life in palliative care. Semin Oncol 1995; 22:73–81.
10. Krietler S, Chaitchick S, Rapoport Y, et al. Life satisfaction and health in cancer patients, orthopedic patients and healthy individuals. Soc Sci Med 1993; 36:547–556.
11. Cohen SR, Hassan SA, Lapointe BJ, et al. Quality of life in HIV disease as measured by the McGill Quality of Life Questionnaire. AIDS 1996; 10:1421–1427.
12. Cohen SR, Mount BM, Tomas J, et al. Existential well-being is an important determinant of quality of life: evidence from the McGill Quality of Life Questionnaire. Cancer 1996; 77:576–586.
13. Cohen SR, Mount BM, Bruera E, et al. Validity of the McGill Quality of Life Questionnaire in the palliative care setting: a multi-centre Canadian study demonstrating the importance of the existential domain. Palliat Med 1997; 11:3–20.
14. Chaturvedi SK. What's important for quality of life to Indians—in relation to cancer. Soc Sci Med 1991; 33:91–94.
15. Greisinger AJ, Lorimor RJ, Aday LA, et al. Terminally ill cancer patients. Their most important concerns. Cancer Pract 1997; 5:147–154.

16. Kaasa S, Ahlner-Elmquist M. European Organization for Research and Treatment of Cancer (EORTC)—Social support and spiritual well-being domains. J Palliat Care 1998; 14:111–112.

17. Padilla GV, Ferrell B, Grant MM, et al. Defining the content domain of quality of life for cancer patients with pain. Cancer Nurs 1990; 13:108–115.

18. Waldron D, O'Boyle CA, Kearney M, et al. Quality of life measurement in advanced cancer: assessing the individual. J Clin Oncol 1999; 17:3603–3611.

19. Hickey AM, Bury G, O'Boyle CA, et al. A new short form individual quality of life measure (SEIQoL-DW): application in a cohort of individuals with HIV/AIDS. BMJ 1996; 313:29–33.

20. McGee HM, O'Boyle CA, Hickey A, et al. Assessing the quality of life of the individual: the SEIQoL with a healthy and gastroenterology unit population. Psychol Med 1991; 21:749–759.

21. Rathbone GV, Horsley S, Goacher J. A self-evaluated assessment suitable for seriously ill hospice patients. Palliat Med 1994; 8:29–34.

22. Kaasa S, Maastekaasa A, Stokke I, et al. Validation of a quality of life questionnaire for use in clinical trials for treatment of patients with inoperable lung cancer. Eur J Cancer Clin Oncol 1988; 24:691–701.

23. MacAdam DB, Smith M. An initial assessment of suffering in terminal illness. Palliat Med 1987; 1:37–47.

24. Ferrans CE. Development of a quality of life index for patients with cancer. Oncol Nurs Forum 1990; 17:15–21.

25. Ferrell B, Grant M, Padilla G, et al. The experience of pain and perceptions of quality of life: validation of a conceptual model. Hospice J 1991; 7:9–24.

26. Skevington SM, MacArthur P, Somerset M. Developing items for the WHOQOL: an investigation of contemporary beliefs about quality of life related to health in Britain. Br J Health Psychol 1997; 2:55–72.

27. Cohen SR, Mount BM. Living with cancer: "good" days and "bad" days—what produces them? Can the McGill Quality of Life Questionnaire distinguish between them? Cancer 2000; 89:1854–1865.

28. Cohen SR, Boston P, Mount BM, et al. Changes in quality of life following admission to palliative care units. Palliat Med 2001; 15:363–371.

29. Sterkenburg CA. A reliability and validity study of the McMaster Quality of Life Scale (MQLS) for a palliative population. J Palliat Care 1996; 12:18–25.

30. McMillan SC. The quality of life of patients with cancer receiving hospice care. Oncol Nurs Forum 1996; 23:1221–1228.

31. McMillan SC, Mahon M. Measuring quality of life in hospice patients using a newly developed Hospice Quality of Life Index. Qual Life Res 1994; 3:437–447.

32. McMillan SC, Weitzner M. Quality of life in cancer patients. Use of a revised hospice index. Cancer Pract 1998; 6:282–288.

33. Weitzner MA, Meyers CA, Steinbruecker S, et al. Developing a care giver quality-of-life instrument—preliminary steps. Cancer Pract 1997; 5:25–31.

34. Weitzner M, Stein K, Jacobsen P, et al. Development of a family caregiver quality of life instrument: psychometric properties and preliminary factorial structure. Qual Life Res 1998; 7:673–674.

35. Weitzner MA, Jacobsen PB, Wagner H Jr, et al. The Caregiver Quality of Life Index–Cancer (CQOLC) scale: development and validation of an instrument to measure quality of life of the family caregiver of patients with cancer. Qual Life Res 1999; 8:55–63.

36. Weitzner MA, McMillan SC, Jacobsen PB. Family caregiver quality of life: differences between curative and palliative cancer treatment settings. J Pain Symptom Manage 1999; 17:418–428.

37. Leis AM, Kristjanson L, Koop PM, et al. Family health and the palliative care trajectory: a cancer research agenda. Cancer Prev Control 1997; 1:352–360.

38. Kornblith AB, Herr HW, Ofman US, et al. Quality of life of patients with prostate cancer and their spouses. Cancer 1994; 73:2791–2802.

39. Reele BL. Effect of counseling on quality of life for individuals with cancer and their families. Cancer Nurs 1994; 17:101–112.

40. Zacharias DR, Gilg CA, Foxall MJ. Quality of life and coping in patients with gynecologic cancer and their spouses. Oncol Nurs Forum 1994; 21:1699–1706.

41. Mohide EA, Torrance GW, Streiner DL, et al. Measuring the wellbeing of family caregivers using the time trade-off technique. J Clin Epidemiol 1988; 41:475–482.

42. McMillan SC, Mahon M. The impact of hospice services on the quality of life of primary caregivers. Oncol Nurs Forum 1994; 21:1189–1195.

43. McMillan SC. Quality of life of primary caregivers of hospice patients with cancer. Cancer Pract 1996; 4:191–198.

44. Weitzner MA, McMillan SC. The Caregiver Quality of Life Index–Cancer (CQOLC) scale: revalidation in a home hospice setting. J Palliat Care 1999; 15:13–20.

45. Joyce CRB, O'Boyle CA, McGee H. Individual Quality of Life. Approaches to Conceptualisation and Assessment. Amsterdam: Harwood, 1999.

46. Cella D. The Functional Assessment of Cancer Therapy–Anemia (FACT-An) scale: a new tool for the assessment of outcomes in cancer anemia and fatigue. Semin Hematol 1997; 34(Suppl 2):13–19.

16

Assessing Decision-Making Capacity in the Setting of Palliative Care Research

DAVID J. CASARETT

Investigators face numerous methodological challenges in designing palliative care research, but as other chapters in this volume demonstrate, these challenges are surmountable if care is taken from the design stage forward. For instance, there is enough experience in the design of these sorts of studies to make evidence-based recommendations regarding eligibility criteria, subject selection, and measurement. These methodological challenges have received considerable attention, and the field is making steady progress in overcoming them. However, less attention has been devoted to obtaining informed consent in this patient population.

It is useful to consider informed consent as one aspect of a study's methods because, like procedures for random assignment or measurement, informed consent must be considered at the earliest stages of design. First, this is because decisions that investigators make about informed consent will affect other aspects of a protocol, including eligibility criteria and planned recruitment strategies.[1] The reverse is true as well because when studies enroll patients who are likely to lack decision-making capacity (such as those with delirium or dementia), investigators must consider how procedures for recruitment will affect the process of informed consent and the involvement of a surrogate. Therefore, informed consent should be considered a methodological issue, like sample size, eligibility, and measurement.

Of course, informed consent is not the only ethical challenge that palliative care investigators will face in designing a study. Indeed, investigators are likely to face a variety of difficult questions. However, many of these other questions have received considerable attention elsewhere[2–9] and are the subject of guidelines and position statements.[5,6] In contrast, there is very little practical advice for palliative care researchers regarding the methodological challenges of informed consent. This is unfortunate because institutional review boards typically scrutinize the informed consent process very closely, particularly when a study involves patients near the end of life. Therefore, this chapter focuses on the challenges of obtaining adequate informed consent from patients who are involved in palliative medicine research.

In considering the methodological challenges posed by informed consent in palliative medicine research, it is useful to examine three inter-related but distinct problems that investigators must solve in a study's design. First, to obtain adequate informed consent, investigators must assess a patient's decision-making capacity, either formally or informally. That is, investigators must ensure that patients are able to understand information about a study, appreciate how that information applies to them, and reason through that information to arrive at a choice that is consistent with their preferences. Second, investigators must consider alternative procedures for informed consent (such as advance consent or surrogate consent) that can be employed in the event that a patient lacks decision-making capacity. Third, in designing any study, investigators must tailor these two procedures, assessing capacity and developing alternative procedures for consent, to the study's risks and potential benefits as well as to the characteristics of the population of patients that will be recruited.[5,6] That is, procedures to ensure adequate informed consent should be employed in a way that is rational and evidence-based.

This chapter begins with a discussion of why concerns about informed consent are warranted in palliative medicine research and why, therefore, procedures for informed consent should be considered a key methodological challenge. Next, procedures for assessing decision-making capacity are discussed, followed by an outline of provisions that can be made for patients who lack capacity. The chapter concludes with recommendations to guide the judicious use of these procedures in the design of palliative care studies.

Informed Consent for Palliative Care Research in Perspective

There are at least two reasons why informed consent deserves careful consideration in the design of palliative care studies. First, patients who enroll in palliative care studies are often seriously ill, with one or more life-threatening medical conditions.[10-16] Available data from a variety of other seriously ill patient populations suggest that they often lack sufficient understanding to participate in research.[17-21] Limited additional data suggest that other domains of decision-making capacity (appreciation, reasoning, and the ability to express a consistent choice) may be impaired as well in seriously ill patients.[22,23] Second, patients involved in these studies are drawn from a population with a high prevalence of characteristics that may make informed consent difficult. For instance, patients near the end of life are generally older, and age is a strong predictor of impaired understanding in a variety of settings and for many kinds of research.[21] In addition, cognitive impairment is common in patients with serious illness, particularly patients near the end of life.[24-28] These factors may make it more difficult for these patients to give adequate informed consent.

This does not mean that palliative care research presents informed consent challenges that are significantly different from, or greater than, the challenges posed by research that involves other patient populations. In fact, informed consent also poses substantial methodological challenges in studies that involve patients with dementia,[29,30] patients with psychiatric illness,[31,32] and patients in the intensive care setting,[33] among others. Therefore, the challenges of informed consent are not necessarily greater in palliative medicine studies than in other kinds of research[5,6]; nevertheless, they deserve careful consideration.

Assessing Decision-Making Capacity for Clinical Research

The process of informed consent, which is required for virtually all research, is intended to ensure that a patient's decision to enroll is consistent with his or her autonomous preferences.[34,35] That is, informed consent is the process by which a patient's autonomy is respected. Broadly, informed consent is based on three conditions:[35] (*1*) all relevant information must be disclosed, (*2*) the patient should be free from coercion or undue inducement, and (*3*) the patient must have adequate decision-making capacity.

It is this last element, decision-making capacity, that is the foundation of the informed consent process. The term *decision-making capacity* refers to a patient's ability to make decisions that are consistent with his or her autonomous preferences. Decision-making capacity is further specified as patients' ability to understand information about a study, to appreciate how that information applies to them, to reason through that information to arrive at a choice that is consistent with their preferences, and to express a consistent choice.

The Structured Capacity-Assessment Interview

An investigator can assess these domains using either an unstructured interview or a series of scripted interview instruments. Although a variety of such instruments have been proposed, only one, the MacArthur Competency Assessment Tool (MacCAT), has been studied in a range of clinical settings.[36] It is also the only instrument that has been modified for clinical research (the MacCAT-CR).[37,38] Therefore, the MacCAT-CR offers the best available guide for the assessment of decision-making capacity in clinical research.

Capacity assessments need not use the MacCAT-CR or any interview instrument. Indeed, when psychiatrists are asked to assess capacity in the mental health setting, they typically use unstructured interviewing techniques, and investigators in other fields can do the same. Nevertheless, the MacCAT-CR offers a guide that many investigators and clinicians may find helpful in guiding their own interviews. Therefore, the MacCAT-CR will be used as a guide for the discussion of capacity assessment below, with the proviso that it can also be used more informally, as the template for an interview.

The MacCAT-CR consists of a set of scripted interview questions, divided into four sections that relate to each of the four domains of decision-making capacity. Because studies vary, the basic MacCAT-CR interview questions must be adapted to fit a particular study design. Once the questions have been modified, however, the MacCAT-CR structure can be used in a standardized way to assess each of the four domains of capacity for all patients who enroll.

To illustrate the MacCAT-CR structure and scoring process, a typical MacCAT-CR interview is described below. This interview is designed for a randomized controlled trial of a case-management intervention. Patients who enroll in this trial would be randomly assigned to receive either their usual care or their usual care plus the services of an interdisciplinary case-management team. Patients who enroll could expect closer follow-up and more individualized care if they are assigned to the intervention. All subjects would be required to make additional study visits and to complete telephone health-status surveys.

The MacCAT-CR structure and scoring for this study are summarized in Table 16.1. The questions are scored on a scale of 0–2. Incorrect and correct responses are scored as 0 and 2, respectively. Responses that are difficult to interpret, even after attempts to clarify them, are scored as 1.

When palliative care investigators assess a patient's decision-making capacity, the most fundamental domain is the ability to express a choice. This domain is also the easiest for patients to achieve and the easiest to measure. A patient who is able to express a choice can reach a decision and maintain that decision over a reasonable amount of time. What constitutes a reasonable amount of time is not clear. However, a useful heuristic for research is that a patient should be able to make and maintain a choice throughout the informed consent process. This ensures that a patient retains the right to withdraw from a study at any time, without raising doubts about his or her decision-making capacity.

The second domain is the patient's ability to understand relevant information. At a minimum, patients must be able to understand the study's key risks and potential benefits. They must also understand the alternatives to participating (such as continuing with their usual care) and the key risks and benefits of those alternatives. Patients' understanding might be assessed for a variety of other kinds of information as well, including additional procedures required by the study and random assignment of treatment (Table 16.1). In the MacCAT-CR interview, understanding is assessed for 11 areas, two of which (study procedures and risks or burdens) are assessed with two questions each.

One useful guide to the kinds of information that should be understood is the Common Rule, which is the federal statute that governs most research conducted in the United States.[39] Although the Common Rule does not specify the kinds of information that must be understood, it does describe the kinds of information that must be disclosed. These categories of information are summarized in Table

Table 16.1. Questions to assess decision-making capacity for the study described in the text (possible score for each item)

Understanding (total possible score = 26)
    The subject understands:
        the purpose of the study is to test the effectiveness of a case-management intervention (2)
        the study lasts 1 year (2)
        the study requires two additional procedures (two questions) (4)
        the effectiveness of the intervention is unknown (2)
        not all subjects will receive the intervention (2)
        subjects who do not receive the intervention must complete surveys and undergo health
            evaluations (2)
        the intervention will be assigned at random (2)
        how the study results will benefit future patients (2)
        how subjects in the study may benefit (2)
        the study imposes two additional burdens (two questions) (4)
        subjects can refuse to participate or can withdraw from the study without penalty (2)
Appreciation (total possible score = 6)
    The subject appreciates that he or she:
        would not be asked to be in the study solely for his or her personal benefit (2)
        would not be assigned to receive the intervention or not based on his or her needs (2)
        can refuse to participate or can withdraw from the study without penalty (2)
Reasoning (total possible score = 8)
    The subject is able to:
        describe two reasonable consequences of participating in the study (2)
        compare the merits of participating versus not participating (2)
        give two examples of the impact of participating on his or her everyday life (2)
        express a choice that is consistent with the consequences that he or she has described (2)
Choice (total possible score = 2)
    The subject is able to express a choice about whether or not to enroll (2)

16.2, and investigators who assess a patient's understanding may wish to use this list as a guide.

Third, patients must be able to appreciate how relevant information applies to their own situation. The three questions that are used to assess appreciation are essentially modifications of three understanding questions: those related to the study's purpose, procedures for random assignment, and ability to refuse or withdraw. Thus, a patient must understand not only that a study's purpose is to produce generalizable knowledge but also appreciate that this means he or she is not being asked to participate in the study for his or her own benefit. Similarly, understanding the concept of random assignment must be accompanied by an appreciation that the treatment will be randomly assigned. Finally, even if the patient understands that patients in general are free to refuse to participate, he or she must appreciate that he or she is free to participate as well. Although not part of the MacCAT-CR interview, appreciation of other facts may be important as well. For instance, a patient may understand that a surgical procedure, such as a

Table 16.2. Kinds of information for which understanding might be assessed

---

A. Core elements for disclosure

1. A statement that the study involves research, an explanation of the purposes of the research, the expected duration of the subject's participation, a description of the procedures to be followed, and identification of any procedures which are experimental
2. A description of any reasonably foreseeable risks or discomforts to the subject
3. A description of any benefits to the subject or to others that may reasonably be expected
4. A disclosure of appropriate alternative procedures or courses of treatment, if any, that might be advantageous to the subject
5. A statement describing the extent, if any, to which confidentiality of records identifying the subject will be maintained
6. An explanation as to whether any compensation or medical treatments are available if injury occurs
7. An explanation of whom to contact for answers to pertinent questions about the research and research subjects' rights or in the event of a research-related injury to the subject
8. A statement that participation is voluntary and that the subject may refuse or withdraw without penalty or loss of benefits to which the subject is otherwise entitled

B. Additional elements for disclosure, depending on study design

1. A statement that the particular treatment or procedure may involve risks to the subject (or to the embryo or fetus if the subject is or may become pregnant), which are currently unforeseeable
2. Anticipated circumstances under which the subject's participation may be terminated by the investigator without regard to the subject's consent
3. Any additional costs to the subject that may result from participation in the research
4. The consequences of a subject's decision to withdraw from the research and procedures for orderly termination of participation by the subject
5. A statement that significant new findings developed during the course of the research, which may relate to the subject's willingness to continue participation, will be provided to the subject
6. The approximate number of subjects involved in the study

Source: Department of Health and Human Services.[39]

nerve block, entails risks. The patient may be convinced, though, that those risks do not apply. For instance, the patient may place such trust in the surgeon that he or she feels immune to harm. Therefore, in studies that entail significant risks, it is important to confirm that understanding is accompanied by adequate appreciation.

The domain of capacity that is most difficult for patients to achieve is that of reasoning. It is also the most difficult to assess, but there are two aspects of reasoning that offer useful guides for palliative care investigators. First, patients should be able to anticipate how being in a study will affect their daily lives. For instance, patients who enroll in the trial described above should be able to anticipate how the additional clinic visits, the telephone contacts, and the personalized attention would affect daily life. Second, patients should be able to justify their decision. For instance, a patient who decides to enroll in a study should be able to explain how being in the study is better than not being in the study. This question actually has two components: (*1*) patients must be able to remember and summarize study features that are important to them (that is, they must be able to recall that patients who enroll in the trial may have access to more personalized care from the interdisciplinary team) and (*2*) patients must be able to compare this service with their usual care. For instance, because a patient is enrolled in hospice, she may already receive care from an interdisciplinary team and, therefore, see no advantage in enrolling in the study. Finally, these preferences must be consistent with the choice made. For instance, patients who enroll in a trial should be able to demonstrate in these reasoning questions that, overall, they believe the advantages of enrolling outweigh any disadvantages.

Making Summary Judgments about Capacity

The questions described above and in Table 16.1 provide evidence of each of the four domains of capacity. However, assessments of these four domains by themselves are of limited usefulness for clinicians and investigators. This is because investigators must ultimately decide whether a patient is able to give consent to participate in a study, and this decision is dichotomous. Therefore, investigators must translate assessments about the four domains of capacity into an overall summary judgment that a patient has capacity or not. This is difficult for two reasons.

First, these domains cannot be combined into a summary score. In part, this is because there is no consensus about how each of these domains should be weighted in an overall assessment of capacity. A formula for a summary score has also been elusive because there is no clear hierarchy of abilities. As a result, one patient who is able to understand may show limited ability to reason, while another will demonstrate the opposite pattern. Therefore, the results of a capacity interview can be discussed only in terms of four distinct assessments.

Second, investigators will find it difficult to make an overall judgment of a patient's capacity because there are no generally agreed-upon thresholds for each of the four domains. As a result, investigators will find it difficult to determine whether a patient who answers only some of the understanding questions correctly has adequate understanding to give informed consent for a study. These judgments are easier at the extremes, when a patient answers almost all questions either correctly or incorrectly; but examinations of decision-making capacity in a variety of settings have found that most patients fall somewhere in between on at least one domain of capacity.[40–43] Thus, a patient might understand the risks and potential benefits of participating in a study but may fail to understand the random assignment it entails and that he or she can withdraw at any time. This patient has partial understanding, and an overall determination of capacity should consider this as well as the ability to appreciate, reason, and express a choice.

Therefore, the results of a capacity assessment provide only the raw material for an assessment of capacity. An investigator's final determination requires a careful but subjective synthesis within and across the four domains described above. Before making that determination, though, investigators should consider two questions.

First, investigators should consider the relative importance of the elements of decision-making capacity that were assessed. In practical terms, this means that they should identify key elements of understanding, appreciation, and reasoning that are essential for a particular study. For instance, the investigators for a trial of a pharmacological treatment for dyspnea might conclude that any subject who enrolls must demonstrate both understanding and appreciation of the procedures of random assignment and blinding that will be used and the use of a placebo control. They might conclude that these elements, together with a few others, are essential. By making these sorts of decisions a priori, investigators can streamline the process of assessing decision-making capacity and facilitate summary judgments.

Second, investigators can take steps to enhance decision-making capacity during the informed consent process. A good capacity assessment points out a patient's strengths and weaknesses. That is, it identifies areas that deserve additional attention. In a sense, the informed consent process can be viewed as a teaching exercise in which information is disclosed and used by patients. Viewed in this light, a capacity assessment provides a measure of the effectiveness of the investigator's teaching efforts. For instance, for the patient above, the investigator could make an extra effort to clarify the process of random assignment that would be used in a trial. The investigator can also help the patient to anticipate the consequences of enrolling. With additional teaching, capacity can be improved to levels that can be agreed upon as acceptable.

When Prospective Subjects Lack Decision-Making Capacity

In some cases, prospective subjects will lack adequate decision-making capacity, even after extensive teaching. For instance, when studies recruit patients with certain conditions, such as delirium or dementia, investigators face challenges of informed consent that are likely to be insurmountable. Under these circumstances, it is important to consider alternatives to the usual process of informed consent. In general, the two alternative strategies are surrogate consent and advance consent.

The most widely used procedure for respecting the autonomous preferences of patients who cannot give informed consent themselves is to rely on surrogate consent. Surrogate consent is justified by appeals to the surrogate's substituted judgment about what the patient would have decided if he or she had been able to participate in the informed consent process. The ethical robustness of this approach is only as sound as the surrogate's knowledge of the patient's preferences. Unfortunately, available data cast doubt on the accuracy of these judgments.[44] The utility of surrogate consent is also limited by variation among states regarding its acceptability for research. For these reasons, it offers only a partial solution for investigators.

For certain studies, advance consent offers another way to respect the autonomy of patients who are unable to give informed consent at the time of enrollment. The term *advance consent* refers to consent that is obtained for a particular study before the patient is actually enrolled. For instance, a patient might give consent at the time of hospital admission for enrollment in a randomized controlled trial of treatments for delirium. Eligible patients who were at risk of developing delirium consented in advance to a specific study in which they were enrolled if they developed delirium during their index hospitalization. Advance consent should be distinguished from research advance directives, which provide more general guidance about a patient's preferences regarding research participation in general. Because research advance directives are so broad, they are unlikely to provide information about preferences that will help investigators and family members to discern a patient's preferences about a particular study. In addition, because they may be completed months or years before the opportunity to enroll in a study, research advance directives, like other advance directives, admit the possibility that the patient's preferences and goals have changed.

Because advance consent is obtained for a specific study a short period of time before enrollment, this procedure should be the preferred mechanism for obtaining consent from patients who will lack decision-making capacity. Indeed, advance consent offer substantial promise in facilitating research on syndromes like delirium, the death rattle, or other symptoms at the very end of life, when consent is often impossible to obtain. Nevertheless, when advance consent is used, investigators may wish to supplement it with additional evidence of patient preferences. For instance, even if a patient has already given consent to participate in a study, investigators can still obtain *assent*, which refers to knowledge of the study and absence of visible signs of disagreement. Investigators may also wish to obtain the consent of the surrogate, using the procedures described above.

Determining When Formal Capacity Assessments Are Necessary

The assessment of decision-making capacity described above is not lengthy or difficult to administer. Nevertheless, it does require a series of standard questions or that investigators adapt the MacCAT-CR for their own study. Moreover, it requires time spent completing and scoring the interview. For these reasons, it is not practical to require that all patients who enroll in palliative care research should undergo a capacity assessment. Instead, the need for a formal capacity assessment should be based on two essential features: the prevalence of impaired decision-making capacity in the population that will be recruited and the balance of risks and potential benefits that a study offers.[5]

Guide 1: characteristics associated with decision-making capacity

In determining the need for a formal assessment of decision-making capacity, investigators may find it useful to first consider the characteristics of the patient who would be recruited. Broadly, these can be divided into premorbid characteristics and those related to the patient's current health status. Of all the characteristics that describe a patient's premorbid condition, the two most clearly associated with the four domains of decision-making capacity are age and education.[21,45-49] Specifically, increasing age and limited formal education appear to be the strongest predictors of poor understanding and inadequate decision-making capacity. Therefore, as in other research settings, investigators whose studies recruit from older populations and from those who lack advanced formal education, formal assessments of capacity are more useful.

Understanding and other domains of decision-making capacity also appear to be influenced by a patient's current health state. Of these, the single most important characteristic appears to be cognitive function. Numerous studies have found that cognitive function is related to understanding,[46,49] and equally strong relationships have been found with other domains of decision-making capacity.

These relationships are of particular concern for palliative care investigators because cognitive impairment occurs in 10%–40% of patients in the final months and in up to 85% of patients in the last days of life.[24,26] Cognitive impairment may be difficult to identify in palliative care research because mental status may vary over time.[50] Indeed, a waxing and waning course is a defining feature of delirium, which is common near the end of life. Investigators who conduct trials of delirium medications will encounter these challenges even more frequently if trials are designed to evaluate treatments for which some degree of impairment is an inclusion criterion.[51,52]

These challenges may be compounded in prospective studies that require participation over days or weeks. In these studies, even if patients have the capacity to consent at the time of enrollment, they may not retain that capacity throughout the study. This is particularly true if the pharmacological agents that are being evaluated, such as opioids, benzodiazepines, or corticosteroids, cause cognitive impairment.[53,54] Thus, days or weeks after patients give consent to participate, they may be unable to understand changes in their condition clearly enough to withdraw. The result can be a "Ulysses contract" of sorts, in which research subjects find it easier to enroll than they do to withdraw.[55]

Guide 2: risks and potential benefits of a study

In determining whether an assessment of understanding or decision-making capacity is necessary, investigators and institutional review boards can also consider the balance of the risks and potential benefits that the study offers. In general, an individual should have greater capacity as risks increase in proportion to potential benefits.[56,57] Phrased somewhat differently, clinicians should require greater evidence of decision-making capacity.[58] This is often referred to as the "sliding scale" rule of informed consent and offers a useful guide for the design of informed consent procedures for palliative care research.

This rule is typically operationalized by describing a study's balance of risks and potential benefits as belonging to one of three categories. First, some studies pose only minimal risks.[39] Risks are minimal if they are no greater than those that a patient would face in his or her daily life and routine medical care. Examples of minimal-risk studies include those that consist of surveys or interviews and those that involve educational or similar interventions. These sorts of study require few, if any, additional safeguards of the informed consent process,[5,6] and assessments of understanding or decision-making capacity should not be required.

Other studies pose greater than minimal risks, and these are held to a higher standard of informed consent. These studies are described as either having potential benefits or not. Examples of studies that pose greater than minimal risks but also offer potential benefits include most drug trials and trials of other therapeutic interventions. Studies that pose greater than minimal risks and that do not offer potential benefits are relatively uncommon in palliative care research, but examples include pharmacokinetic studies[59] and descriptive studies that may be very burdensome to subjects.[60] In general, studies that pose greater than minimal risks are held to higher standards of consent if they do not offer subjects any potential benefits.

Combining guides 1 and 2

The American Academy of Hospice and Palliative Medicine position statement on the ethics of palliative care research provides recommendations for consent procedures that are designed to be useful for investigators and institutional review boards.[5] These recommendations incorporate both guides described above in proposing three levels of informed consent safeguards.

First, for studies that pose minimal risks, no additional safeguards are needed. Thus, for most survey studies, the usual processes of informed consent should be adequate, with an informal assessment of understanding.

Second, for studies that pose greater than minimal risks and that offer potential benefits, procedures of informed consent should be determined by the characteristics of the patient population. For example, a study that recruits younger, ambulatory patients from an outpatient oncology clinic in an affluent neighborhood could employ minimal additional consent safeguards. For that study, a simple 5- to 10-item multiple-choice "consent quiz" to assess understanding should be sufficient. However, for a study that recruits patients in an inpatient hospice who are near the end of life, additional safeguards would be appropriate. Depending on the population, these safeguards might include scripted questions to assess understanding or a more formal assessment of capacity.

Third, for studies that pose greater than minimal risks without potential benefits, a formal capacity assessment is indicated. This capacity assessment could be performed by the investigator or a designee. It could include a formal assessment (using the MacCAT-CR) or an informal assessment, using a semistructured interview.

Conclusion

The goals of good end-of-life care are to relieve suffering and to improve quality of life. However, access to palliative care is poor, and standards to guide palliative care have not been clearly established. At least in part, these deficiencies exist because of a lack of solid evidence on which to base clinical decisions.[7,61] Therefore, there is an urgent need for a standard of care and increased access to quality care.

However, as the other chapters in this volume demonstrate, investigators face a variety of methodological challenges in the design of this research. These challenges are significant, but they are also surmountable with careful planning and design. The methodological challenges of the informed consent process, and specifically assessments of decision-making capacity, are no different. That is, they are also surmountable if attention is paid to them in the design of palliative care studies.

For these challenges to be addressed in an organized and productive way, though, it will be important to frame the issues involved appropriately. First, it will be important to consider informed consent and decision-making capacity as elements of a study's methods and design. By integrating ethical considerations into a study's design, investigators will have more opportunities to develop new and innovative ways of overcoming challenges of informed consent than they do if consent requirements are only imposed reactively by institutional review boards. Second, it will be important to avoid the widespread assumption that there are unique ethical challenges of informed consent in palliative care research.[2,8] Although some have objected to this extreme position,[3,4,7] many providers, institutional review boards, and investigators remain uncertain about the ethics of research that involves dying patients. As long as the ethical challenges of palliative care research are viewed as unique and as uniquely intractable, investigators will find it very difficult to develop innovative approaches for use in this patient population. Indeed, the view that palliative care research poses uniquely difficult ethical challenges is also likely to impede progress in palliative care research and to delay the development of a coherent foundation of data on which to base clinical decisions.

Acknowledgments

Dr. Casarett is supported by a Health Services Research Career Development Award from the Department of Veterans Affairs, by a John Hartford Foundation Scholarship, by a Paul Beeson Physician Scholars Award; and by grants from the Department of Veterans Affairs, The National Institutes of Health, the Greenwall Foundation, and the Commonwealth Fund.

References

1. Casarett DJ, Karlawish J. Beyond informed consent: the ethical design of pain research. Pain Med 2001; 2:138–146.
2. Annas GJ. Some Choice: Law, Medicine, and the Market. New York: Oxford University Press, 1998.
3. Casarett D. Beyond vulnerability: the ethics of end of life research. J Pain Symptom Manage 1999; 18:143–145.
4. Casarett D, Karlawish J. Are special ethical guidelines needed for palliative care research? J Pain Symptom Manage 2000; 20:130–139.
5. Casarett D. Position statement of the American Academy of Hospice and Palliative Medicine: the ethics of palliative care research under review.
6. Casarett D, Kirschling J, Levetown M, et al. NHPCO Task Force Statement on Hospice Participation in Research. J Palliat Med 2001; 4:441–449.
7. Mount B, Cohen R, MacDonald N, et al. Ethical issues in palliative care research revisited. Palliat Med 1995; 9:165–170.
8. de Raeve L. Ethical issues in palliative care research. Palliat Med 1994; 8:298–305.
9. Casarett DJ, Karlawish J, Sankar P, et al. Should open label extension studies be required in the design of clinical drug trials? 2001; 23:1–5.
10. Ashby M, Fleming B, Wood M, et al. Plasma morphine and glucuronide (M3G and M6G) concentrations in hospice inpatients. J Pain Symptom Manage 1997; 14: 157–167.
11. Kravitz RL, Delafield JP, Hays RD, et al. Bedside charting of pain levels in hospitalized patients with cancer: a randomized controlled trial. J Pain Symptom Manage 1996; 11:81–87.
12. Lipton A, Theriault RL, Hortobagyi GN, et al. Pamidronate prevents skeletal complications and is effective palliative treatment in women with breast carcinoma and osteolytic bone metastases: long term follow-up of two randomized, placebo-controlled trials. Cancer 2000; 88:1082–1090.
13. Maddocks I, Somogyi A, Abbott F, et al. Attenuation of morphine-induced delirium in palliative care by substitution with infusion of oxycodone. J Pain Symptom Manage 1996; 12:182–189.
14. Payne R, Mathias SD, Pasta DJ, et al. Quality of life and cancer pain: satisfaction and side effects with transdermal fentanyl versus oral morphine. J Clin Oncol 1998; 16: 1588–1593.

15. Raftery JP, Addington-Hall JM, MacDonald LD, et al. A randomized controlled trial of the cost–effectiveness of a district co-ordinating service for terminally ill cancer patients. Palliat Med 1996; 10:151–161.

16. Twycross R, Harcourt J, Bergl S. A survey of pain in patients with advanced cancer. J Pain Symptom Manage 1996; 12:273–282.

17. Aaronson NK, Visser-Pol E, Leenhouts GH, et al. Telephone-based nursing intervention improves the effectiveness of the informed consent process in cancer clinical trials. J Clin Oncol 1996; 14:984–996.

18. Cassileth BR, Zupkis RV, Sutton-Smith K, et al. Informed consent—why are its goals imperfectly realized? N Engl J Med 1980; 302:896–900.

19. Ockene IS, Miner J, Shannon T, et al. The consent process in the Thrombolysis in Myocardial Infarction (TIMI phase I) trial. Clin Res 1991; 39:13–17.

20. Schaeffer MH, Krantz DS, Wichman A, et al. The impact of disease severity on the informed consent process in clinical research. Am J Med 1996; 100:261–268.

21. Sugarman J, McCrory DC, Hubal RC. Getting meaningful informed consent from older adults: a structured literature review of empirical research. J Am Geriatr Soc 1998; 46:517–524.

22. Fitten LJ, Lusky R, Hamann C. Assessing treatment decision-making capacity in elderly nursing home residents. J Am Geriatr Soc 1990; 38:1097–1104.

23. Grisso T, Appelbaum PS. The MacArthur Treatment Competence Study III. Law Hum Behav 1995; 19:149–174.

24. Breitbart W, Bruera E, Chochinov H, et al. Neuropsychiatric syndromes and psychological symptoms in patients with advanced cancer. J Pain Symptom Manage 1995; 10:131–141.

25. Massie MJ, Holland J, Glass E. Delirium in terminally ill cancer patients. Am J Psychiatry 1983; 140:1048–1050.

26. Pereira J, Hanson J, Bruera E. The frequency and clinical course of cognitive impairment in patients with terminal cancer. Cancer 1997; 79:835–842.

27. Weinrich S, Sarna L. Delirium in the older patient with cancer. Cancer 1994; 74: 2079–2091.

28. Casarett D, Inouye S. Diagnosis and management of delirium near the end of life. Ann Intern Med 2001; 135:32–40.

29. Marson DC, Schmitt FA, Ingram KK, et al. Determining the competency of Alzheimer patients to consent to treatment and research. Alzheimer Dis Assoc Disord 1994; 8:5–18.

30. High DM, Whitehouse PJ, Post SG, et al. Guidelines for addressing ethical and legal issues in Alzheimer disease research: a position paper. Alzheimer Dis Assoc Disord 1994; 8:66–74.

31. Benson P, Roth L, Winslade W. Informed consent in psychiatric research: preliminary findings from an ongoing investigation. Soc Sci Med 1985; 20:1331–1341.

32. Elliott C. Caring about risks: are severely depressed patients competent to consent to research? Arch Gen Psychiatry 1997; 54:113–116.

33. Lemaire F, Blanch L, Cohen SL, et al. Informed consent for research purposes in intensive care patients in Europe—part II. An official statement of the European Society of Intensive Care Medicine Working Group on Ethics. Intensive Care Med 1997; 23:435–439.

34. National Commission for the Protection of Human Subjects of Biomedical and Behavioral Research. Belmont Report. Ethical Principles and Guidelines for the Protection of Human Subjects of Research. Washington DC: Government Printing Office, 1979.
35. Faden RR, Beauchamp TL. A History and Theory of Informed Consent. New York: Oxford University Press, 1986.
36. Grisso T, Appelbaum PS, Hill-Fotouhi C. The MacCAT-T: a clinical tool to assess patients' capacities to make treatment decisions. Psychiatric Serv 1997; 48: 1415–1419.
37. Carpenter W, Gold J, Lahti A, et al. Decisional capacity for informed consent in schizophrenia research. Arch Gen Psychiatry 2000; 57:533–538.
38. Kim S, Caine E, Currier G, et al. Assessing the competence of persons with Alzheimer's disease in providing informed consent for participation in research. Am J Psychiatry 2001; 158:712–717.
39. Department of Health and Human Services. The Common Rule. Protection of Human Subjects, title 45, part 46. Revised, Code of Federal Regulation. Washington DC: Government Printing Office, 1991.
40. Appelbaum PS, Grisso T, Frank E, et al. Competence of depressed patients for consent to research. Am J Psychiatry 1999; 156:1380–1384.
41. Frank L, Smyer M, Grisso T, et al. Measurement of advance directive and medical treatment decision-making capacity of older adults. J Ment Health Aging 1999; 5:257–274.
42. Grisso T, Appelbaum PS. Assessing Competence to Consent to Treatment. New York: Oxford University Press, 1998.
43. Grisso T, Appelbaum PS. Comparison of standards for assessing patients' capacities to make treament decisions. Am J Psychiatry 1995; 152:1033–1037.
44. Warren JW, Sobal J, Tenney JH, et al. Informed consent by proxy. An issue in research with elderly patients. N Engl J Med 1986; 315:1124–1128.
45. Davis TC, Holcombe RF, Berkel HJ, et al. Informed consent for clinical trials: a comparative study of standard versus simplified forms. J Natl Cancer Inst 1998; 90: 668–674.
46. Krynski M, Tymchuk A, Ouslander J. How informed can consent be? New light on comprehension among elderly people making decisions about enteral tube feeding. Gerontologist 1994; 34:36–43.
47. Miller CK, O'Donnell DC, Searight HR, et al. The Deaconess Informed Consent Comprehension Test: an assessment tool for clinical research subjects. Pharmacotherapy 1996; 16:872–878.
48. Miller CK, Grable D, Schwartz R, et al. Comprehension and recall of the informational content of the informed consent document: an evaluation of 168 patients in a controlled clinical trial. J Clin Res Drug Dev 1994; 8:237–248.
49. Taub HA, Baker MT. Effect of repeated testing upon comprehension of informed consent materials by elderly volunteers. Exp Aging Res 1983; 9:135–138.
50. Bruera E, Franco JJ, Maltoni M, et al. Changing pattern of agitated impaired mental status in patients with advanced cancer: association with cognitive monitoring, hydration, and opioid rotation. J Pain Symptom Manage 1995; 10:287–291.

51. Breitbart W, Marotta R, Platt MM, et al. A double-blind trial of haloperidol, chlor-
    promazine, and lorazepam in the treatment of delirium in hospitalized AIDS pa-
    tients. Am J Psychiatry 1996; 153:231–237.
52. Chong SF, Bretscher ME, Mailliard JA, et al. Pilot study evaluating local anesthetics
    administered systemically for treatment of pain in patients with advanced cancer.
    J Pain Symptom Manage 1997; 13:112–117.
53. Bruera E, MacMillan K, Kuchn N, et al. The cognitive effects of the administration
    of narcotics. Pain 1989; 39:13–16.
54. Stiefel FC, Breitbart W, Holland, JC. Corticosteroids in cancer: neuropsychiatric
    complications. Cancer Invest 1989; 7:479–491.
55. Dresser R. Bound to treatment: the Ulysses contract. Hastings Cent Rep 1984; 14:
    13–16.
56. Buchanan AE, Brock DW. Deciding for Others. The Ethics of Surrogate Decision
    Making. Cambridge: Cambridge University Press, 1989.
57. Gaylin W. The competence of children: no longer all or none. Hastings Cent Rep
    1982; 12:33–38.
58. Beauchamp TL, Childress JF. Principles of Biomedical Ethics. Oxford: Oxford Uni-
    versity Press, 1994.
59. Hoffman M, Xu JC, Smith C, et al. A pharmacodynamic study of morphine and its
    glucuronide metabolites after single morphine dosing in cancer patients with pain.
    Cancer Invest 1997; 15:542–547.
60. Wood M, Ashby M, Somogyi A, et al. Neuropsychological and pharmacokinetic as-
    sessment of hospice inpatients receiving morphine. J Pain Symptom Manage 1998;
    16:112–120.
61. Field MJ, Cassell CK. Approaching Death. Improving Care at the End of Life.
    Washington DC: National Academy Press, 1997.

VII

RESEARCH ISSUES IN END-OF-LIFE CARE AND ETHICAL DECISION MAKING

17

Research in Advance Care Planning

LINDA L. EMANUEL

Planning for illness involving decisional incapacity has been widely endorsed, at least in principle. How best to accomplish it has been less clear, however. To remedy this lack of practical guidance, considerable research has been devoted to the field. This chapter addresses seven areas of research in advance care planning, each of which has enjoyed progress but needs further research: (1) theoretical development of the rationale for advance care planning, (2) considerations regarding the conditions under which advance directives can be authentic, (3) epidemiological tracking of indicators and outcome measures, (4) issues concerning ethnicity and culture, (5) guidance for clinical practices, (6) outcome measures, and (7) policy development. Inquiry within the different areas entails the use of different methodologies. Within each area, a summary perspective on research methods and development is offered, as well as some directions for future research.

Theoretical Development

Surviving interests

Early controversy in the field of advance directives centered on the questions of how a person could know their wishes for future possible states of decisional incapacity and how durable such wishes would have to be over time and in the face of new illness. Studies repeatedly showed that durability of decisions was imperfect, especially when individuals were asked to consider illness scenarios other than their current health. Proportions of decisions that remained stable over 2-month to 2-year intervals fell below 80%. Kappa analyses resulted in values mostly in the 0.2 range, indicating that for many decision pairs over time there was more than chance correlation but less durability than is usually expected of, for instance, clinical tests that are repeated or re-read.

The solution to this problem was less procedural than theoretical. An understanding clarified the problem, namely, that advance directives draw their justification from the notion of surviving interests in the same way that estate wills are justified. Advance directives are not supposed to be about knowing the wishes of individuals who either are without wishes or who have wishes but no sufficient decisional capacity. Advance directives are supposed to be about the wishes that a person has in real time for their future possible states, just as estate wills are about wishes formulated in real time for a future demise. In this understanding it is clear that, contrary to early thoughts, advance directives do not assist very much in cases where patients have wishes, whether they have decisional competence or not. In such cases, advance directives are not more than one set of indicators among others for decision making by substituted judgment or best-interest standards. Instead, advance directives have authenticity if they were arrived at properly in real time and if the principal (now the patient) has lost capacity to have any wishes. Thus, advance directives have full, authentic applicability only if the patient is unconscious or so profoundly demented that there is no reasonable possibility that he or she has wishes.

Advisory and statutory documents

With respect to authenticity, a separate confusion arose early in the development of the field. As the notion of a living will spread, it was backed by state statutes across the country. Many people came to understand that documents that were drawn up to meet the specifics of state statutes were the only documents that were legally binding. In fact, under constitutional law, any authentic statement of the person's wishes is binding. The helpful theoretical construct that moved the issue forward was the distinction between an advisory document and a statutory document. An *advisory document* aims to record, as accurately as possible, the wishes of the person and is honored under constitutional law, while a *statutory document* usually aims to protect the physician from legal liability if he or she follows the patient's wishes even if those wishes depart from the norms of intervention. These two purposes so differ that the corresponding documents are quite different. However, the purposes are complementary, and it is generally a good idea to combine the two, either by binding documents together or by creating a composite form.

Instructions and proxy designations

Another conceptual controversy in the field centered on the question of whether the principal (patient) can best secure other surviving interests by proxy designation or by instructions for the future. A series of studies, using survey methodology and hypothetical scenarios, indicated that proxies very often do not know the wishes of the patient.[1-4] Surveys further indicated that proxies face considerable burdens, which might include decision regret, emotional attachment, or conflicts of interest, that can prevent implementation of patient wishes. However, great difficulties in knowing one's own preferences, articulating and recording them, and getting them understood and implemented undermine the possibilities for the alternative instructional approach. The conceptual issue that arose in the context of this debate was whether or not designation of a person to make decisions on the principal's behalf is any different from the traditional physician/family decision making on behalf of the patient. Further, is proxy designation the extension of autonomy that is intended by advance directives?

Expositional scholarship settled this controversy reasonably well. Proxy designation is a form of autonomy that is entirely consistent with the living will movement and suitable when the principal either cannot use the instructional process will or prefers to give a full range of decision-making powers to a chosen trusted person. At the same time, the proxy role is much easier if there are some guiding instructions. Conversely, use of the guiding instructions is more likely if there is a proxy to negotiate the desired use.[5] Further, there are individuals who may not have a trusted person they wish to choose. In short, the need to choose between the approaches is mostly unnecessary, and individuals are likely to do best with a combination approach. The focus of choice can instead be on where the balance between the approaches should be. For instance, a proxy may be asked to use extensive judgment or to be greatly guided by detailed instructions.[6]

Advance care planning as an intervention

Advance care planning was seen as an intervention to secure autonomous decision making beyond the onset of incapacity. As it began to be used, some additional purposes for the process became apparent. Anecdotal evidence indicates that an advance care planning discussion can be helpful for bringing coherence to a distressed person's chaotic thinking and peace to anxious states of mind. Indeed, patients who have asked for physician-assisted suicide but who really wanted some form of control or reassurance or a strategy to avoid burdensomeness and indignity have found alternative plans in this process and have dropped what turned out to be a mistakenly motivated interest. Further research should assess how advance care planning can be used as a clinical intervention and to assist a patient who is seeking medical decisions that foster quality of life in a larger sphere of personal meaning.[7]

Advanced care planning as a process more than an event

Advanced care planning began as a movement to make advance directives. The emphasis was heavily on documents, and the assumption was that an event was needed, namely, to make out and file the documents. Gradually, it became clear that advance care planning needs to be a process of communication, the goal of which is to have a core team of people working toward a common goal of patient-centered care.[8–14] Whether that common goal is documented or not is less important than whether it exists and works.

Advance care planning as part of a larger framework

As progress has been made in end-of-life care, advance care planning has fallen into place within a larger framework. Several studies have asked patients, family caregivers, and healthcare professionals about the domains of experience that are important to them.[15–17] One of these provided a framework of domains as they perceived the world of illness and care. This was based on the results of focus group discussions and then modified by questionnaire data from patients and family caregivers. Advance care planning was just one part among others within the domain of medical provider interventions. Thus, like all clinical interventions, advance care planning must be understood in context. Once portrayed as a potential solution to a panorama of problems, advanced care planning is now understood to have a much smaller but nonetheless real place among other clinical interventions.

Another feature that these findings have in common will need to be taken into account in future research on advance care planning. Each study confirmed that patients consider as important not only the physical aspects of their illness and care but also their mental, social, and existential aspects and the nature of the therapeutic relationship. Advance care planning discussions, worksheets, and documents should accommodate not only physical interventions but relational issues. For instance, research has not evaluated how helpful it would be for patients to express advance care planning preferences in terms of their ability to relate or the burden of care on their family. Some research has suggested advantages to family-based advance care planning.[18]

Authenticity of Prior Wishes

Based on the clarification that prior wishes carry authority if they are a valid rendition of real-time wishes for the future, the question as to how to judge the authenticity of prior wishes became much simpler. Early concerns about the fact that people change and/or simply change their minds fell into place as concerns about methodology rather than about authenticity.

Validity

Real-time wishes, whether for the present or the future, are valid if they represent the balanced outcomes of a person's inner disposition. The best methods for arriving at objective experiences of subjective phenomena have been well worked out in the field of psychometrics and can be readily applied to advance care planning. By providing worksheets that have been subjected to testing for

Table 17.1. Evaluation for validity

Instrument	Advance directive
Face	User understanding
Content	Focus groups, experts, scenarios
Construct	Decision-making modes: goals, treatments, values, etc.
Predictive/criterion-related	Factor analysis, extrapolation
Test–retest	Durability

validation, patients can be guided toward understanding and expressing their wishes accurately and usefully.[19–21]

Instruments that record subjective phenomena have to be able to cover the intended area (content validity), pose questions that represent what they seem to in the subject's eyes (face validity), use wording (framing) that is unbiased, and use questions that relate sensibly to each other (construct, criterion-related or predictive validity). In addition, they must produce equivalent findings from one test to another, absent other change (test–retest reliability). These methods are readily adapted to advance care planning worksheets (Table 17.1). Worksheets can be tested for content, face validity, and unbiased framing in the usual way. The necessity of this is underscored by studies showing that many patients did not understand their advance directives[22,23] and, more recently, indicating the need to include information about prognosis and disability outcomes when planning for illness or care scenarios.[24] Construct and criterion-related validity can be assessed by factor analysis, asking how sensible are the clinical decisions elicited from patients and how accurately one decision can predict another.[25–27] The latter is particularly important in advance care planning since the clinical circumstances eventually may not be covered in a document. Studies of the durability of wishes over time provide a rigorous version of test–retest reliability.[28,29]

Types of documents

There are a few of advance care planning documents that have been subjected to validity evaluations. Each can be used both as worksheets/workbooks and as formal documentation if the patient so wishes. Some of these worksheets are generic and aim to cover all major types of scenario under which prior wishes acquire authority.[30–33] Others are tailored for specific illness categories, in particular renal failure, chronic obstructive pulmonary disease, cancer, and human immunodeficiency virus disease.[34–37] Different documents, and indeed processes, are needed for children.[38] All validated documents use fairly detailed scenario-based formats; general statements are not predictive of specific wishes.[39,40]

Another approach to validated planning might involve the use of protocols, which could be quite similar to clinical protocols. This approach bears future research inquiry.

Epidemiology

Advance care planning studies have relied heavily on epidemiological approaches. Evidence concerning the documentation of wishes, proxy designation, conversations, and honored wishes has occupied much of the literature.

Documentation

Both before and soon after the federal government passed the Patient Self-Determination Act of 1990, in which patients were to be routinely asked if they had advance care planning documents, the prevalence of documentation was low. It grew from about one in five to one in four patients in a range of studies.[41,42] This was true both for treatment preferences and for proxy designation. Strategies for increased use have been tried.[43-48] The prevalence appears to be growing, or at least is significantly higher, for terminal patients.

Conversations

Conversations have been rare, too, especially those between patients and physicians but also those between patients and family members. Conversations with lawyers may be more common since most advance care planning documentation is drawn up by lawyers, along with estate planning papers.

Treatment choices

Epidemiological studies can also examine the decisions people make, whether in surveys about hypothetical circumstances or in reality. Actual decisions can be studied by record review or by post-fact reporting. Prospective or cohort studies can compare prior wishes with decisions made. Cohort studies are difficult due to the need for controls, but they can be done if it is clear which controls are selected, whether illness category/severity, physician, prior wish, or other feature.

Ethnographic Studies

Non-Western cultures

The celebration of autonomy that undergirds advance care planning is characteristic of Western cultures. Social scientists and others were correctly concerned to point out that advance care planning may not be well suited to specific ethnic groups and, in general, to many non-Western cultures.

Social science methodology

Ethnographic methodology entered the field of advance care planning using in-depth interviews and observational, descriptive, and narrative approaches. Traditional survey and record review methodologies were also turned to this area.

Some findings and their limits

The first prominent ethnologic finding in advance care planning was the difference between life-sustaining treatments desired by African Americans and by white Americans.[49,50] That African Americans wanted more interventions and were less inclined toward advance care planning was confirmed in several studies.[51,52] The difference was partly ascribable to a mistrust of the healthcare system by minority groups. However, there has been difficulty finding tangible evidence of mistrust in a subsequent end-of-life study, in which African-American subjects reported their trust to be higher than white Americans. Further inquiry with in-depth interviews and narrative approaches may reveal more profound relationships to culture and history than has yet been discovered.

A second wave of studies examined the role of extended family or family leaders in advance care planning. They generally confirmed that cultures with a prominent place for family and a lesser place for autonomy than in Western culture needed different approaches to advance care planning.[53] Future studies may provide a range of culture-specific approaches and worksheets to accommodate inter- and intracultural differences. Some ethnographic studies in the area have been conducted among the Navajo. The Navajo culture tends to avoid discussing future poor outcomes, to avoid inducing them.[54] Storytelling approaches using the third person to accomplish aspects of advance care planning may be productive and might warrant a well-designed study.

What works

Some studies have examined how well different approaches work in raising the topic of advance care planning, including by whom, with whom, and in what setting and illness state. These have tended to be survey-based studies or record reviews, relying on a combination of reported comfort with the process and documented advance care plans. Others have compared what expert and nonexpert clinicians do when they conduct advance care planning. Others have used educational interventions.[55]

Recommendations

Integrated scholarship, drawing on knowledge of the clinical process in general and on studies using all of the above methodologies, has begun to define the processes of advance care planning. Recommendations for how to do advance care planning have become quite specific. One group of researchers have recommended a five-step process: (1) raising the topic; (2) conducting a core discussion between patient, proxy, and physicians; (3) following through with review and documentation after reflection on the patient's own time; (4) review at intervals or when major life changes have occurred; and (5) implementation.[56]

Communication

Poor communication is documented in advance care planning. Structured deliberation has been described and recommended, analogizing the clinical methods of advance care planning to the clinical methods involved in taking a medical history. Some of the shifts involved in communicating bad news to patients may be helpful. Research in this area has come largely from anthropology and psychology, using traditional social science methods.

Outcomes

Process versus event outcomes

As advance care planning became understood as a process not an event, the inadequacy of the usual outcome measures, such as documents in the medical record, became more apparent. Far from being a document, the desired outcomes became much softer and harder to study. The goals of advance care planning include not just a strict match between prior wish and eventual decision but a more intangible state of settledness by the patient, readiness for the role by the proxy, and team functioning by the physician. A desired outcome of advance care plans might be that a person's legacy is not interrupted or that the "total pain" of physical, psychological, and social suffering be minimized. Indeed, since advance care planning is a process, a fair outcome measure might be how well the process was followed.

Autonomous wishes

Most studies assumed that a mismatch between prior wishes and eventual decisions constituted a failure of advance care planning, but this may be a mistake. If the patient and family were settled, ready, and content with the process and outcome, a mismatch may be not too important. Many studies based on a kappa analysis of unmatched wishes may need to be redone with more sensitive and appropriate measures.

A scale

There is some progress toward defining scales for the experience of dying.[57,58] From the earlier mentioned study of dying patients, it appears that several dimensions have measurable scales that can be developed: social connection, provider communication, psychological distress, the patient–physician relationship, sense of purpose, spirituality, and interpersonal resolve. An ultimate test of advance care planning would be to see an impact on this total dying experience scale or an equivalent of it.

Policy

Examining and guiding policy

A number of studies have used epidemiological and survey research to examine policy. Studies of the Patient Self-Determination Act and systems for raising the topic of advance care planning fall into this category. Such studies and comparisons with other types of planning, such as estate planning, have spawned predictions on which approaches to policy have been based. These policy studies have, in turn, been based on research methodologies more suited to economics and political theory. These methods, however, also draw largely on epidemiological and survey data.

Community directives

The speculation that the prevalence of advance care planning would have a ceiling about where the prevalence of estate planning among patients has prompted a proposal for a community-based approach. In this approach, patients' prior wishes would define a default approach for patients who had no personal planning prior to becoming unconscious or wishless. Calculations of prior and posterior probabilities using methods developed for ascertaining test specificity and sensitivity showed that this approach had a good chance of honoring the wishes of patients who had never specifically expressed them.

Cost

Popular assumption that patients generally want less intervention than was standard and that use of life-sustaining intervention is more expensive than comfort care supported a belief that advance care planning might cut the cost of care at the end of life. The data did not clearly support this assumption.[59] An analysis based on patients' actual wishes, received intervention, and cost at the end of life from government (Medicare) statistics provided an economic study. The estimate indicated that cost savings would be minimal. Noting that 1.49 million patients over 65 years of age die each year and that these individuals have an average healthcare cost of $29,300 and estimating generously a maximum savings of 27%, which would amount to $11.8 billion. This represents, of the $546 billion total U.S. health spending, a maximum savings of approximately 2%. Another study indicated that although individual patient preferences for treatment may diverge from their received treatment, patients studied as a group have little divergence between preferences and received treatment.[60] Advance care planning continues to be promoted but not so much as a cost-saving strategy.

Education and implementation

One very large study, the Study to Understand Prognosis and Preferences for Outcomes and Risks of Treatment (SUPPORT), has documented poor practices and outcomes for advance care planning. With studies available to serve as a base, it should be possible to advance a campaign of education and implementation of advance care planning and measure outcomes to monitor progress.[61] A number of such programs are now under way, affirming the role of the empirical studies which have guided the field to this point.[62]

Summary

In sum, research in advance care planning has covered a range of methodologies, from applied philosophy to epidemiology and survey methodology, from ethnology to economics and policy analysis. This research has allowed clarification of the theoretical basis for advance care planning, has constrained its appropriate scope and cautioned its harmony across ethnicities, and has defined a paradigm for a good clinical process and demanded better outcomes for future study. Last but not least, it has effectively guided policy and clinical direction.

References

1. Ouslander JG, Tymchuk AJ, Rahbar B. Health care decisions among elderly long-term care residents and their potential proxies. Arch Intern Med 1989; 149: 1367–1372.
2. Emanuel EJ, Emanuel LL. Proxy decision making for incompetent patients: an ethical and empirical analysis. JAMA 1992; 267:2067–2071.
3. Uhlmann RF, Pearlman RA, Cain KC. Physicians' and spouses' predictions of elderly patients' resuscitation preferences. J Gerontol 1988; 5:1115–1221.
4. Moss AH, Oppenhiemer EA, Casey P, et al. Patients with amyotrophic lateral sclerosis receiving long-term mechanical ventilation. Chest 1996; 110:249–255.
5. Teno JM, Stevens M, Spernak S, et al. Role of written advance directives in decision making. J Gen Intern Med 1998; 13:439–446.
6. Sehgal A, Galbraith A, Chesney M, et al. How strictly do dialysis patients want their advance directives followed? JAMA 1992; 267:59–63.
7. Moss AH, Oppenheimer EA, Casey P, et al. Patients with amyotrophic lateral sclerosis receiving long-term mechanical ventilation. Chest 1996; 110:249–255.
8. Emanuel LL. Structured deliberation to improve decision-making for the seriously ill. Hastings Cent Rep 1995; 25(Suppl):S14–S18.
9. Virmani J, Schneiderman LJ, Kaplan RM. Relationship of advance directives to physician–patient communication. Arch Intern Med 1994; 154:909–913.

10. Ewer M, Taubert K. Advance directives in the intensive care unit of a tertiary cancer center. Cancer 1995; 76:1268–1274.

11. Hoffman JC, Wenger HS, Davis RB, et al. Patient preferences for communication with physicians about end of life decisions. Ann Intern Med 1997; 127:1–12.

12. Singer RA, Martin DK, Lavery J, et al. Reconceptualizing advance care planning from the patient's perspective. Arch Intern Med 1998; 158:879–884.

13. Tulsky JA, Fischer GS, Rose MR, et al. Opening the black box: how do physicians communicate about advance directives. Ann Intern Med 1998; 129:441–449.

14. Teno JM, Stevens M, Spernak S, et al. Role of written advance directives in decision making. J Gen Intern Med 1998; 13:439–446.

15. Emanuel EJ, Emanuel LL. The promise of a good death. Lancet 1998; 351(Suppl II):21–29.

16. Steinhauser KC, Clipp EC, McNeilly M, et al. In search of a good death: observations of patients, families, and providers. Ann Intern Med 2000; 132:825–832.

17. Singer PA, Martin DK, Velner MJ. Quality end of life care: patients' perspective. JAMA 1999; 281:163–168.

18. Hines SC, Glover JJ, Holley JL, et al. Dialysis patients' preferences for family-based advance care planning. Ann Intern Med 1999; 130:825–828.

19. Emanuel LL. Advance directives: evaluating their moral and empirical validity. Hastings Cent Rep 1994; 24:S27–S29.

20. Alpert H, Hoijtink H, Fischer G, et al. Psychometric analysis of an advance directive. Med Care 1996; 34:1057–1065.

21. Patrick DL, Pearlman RA, Starks HE, et al. Validation of preferences for life-sustaining treatment: implications for advance care planning. Ann Intern Med 1997; 127:509–517.

22. Ott BB, Hardie TL. Readability of advance directive documents. J Nurs Schol 1997; 29:53.

23. Jacobson JA, White BE, Battin MP, et al. Patients' understanding and use of advance directives. West J Med 1994; 160:232–236.

24. Fried TR, Bradley EH, Towle VR, et al. Understanding the treatment preferences of seriously ill patients. N Engl J Med 2002; 346:1061–1066.

25. Alpert HR, Hoijtink H, Fischer GS, et al. Psychometric analysis of an advance directives. Med Care 1996; 34:1057–1065.

26. Fischer GS, Alpert HR, Stoeckle JD, et al. Can goals of care be used to predict interventions preferences in an advance directive? Arch Intern Med 1997; 157: 801–807.

27. Patrick DL, Perlman RA, Starks HE, et al. Validation of preferences for life-sustaining treatment: implications for advanced care planning. Ann Intern Med 1997; 127:509–517.

28. Emanuel LL, Emanuel EJ, Stoeckle JD, et al. Advance directives: stability of patients' treatment choices. Arch Intern Med 1994; 154:209–217.

29. Everhart MA, Pearlman RA. Stability of patient preferences regarding life-sustaining treatments. Chest 1990; 97:159–164.

30. Emanuel LL, Emanuel EJ. The medical directive: a new comprehensive advance care document. JAMA 1989; 261:3288–3293.

31. Pearlman R, Starks H, Cain K, et al. Your Life, Your Choices-Planning for Future Medical Decisions. Patient Decision Support. www.patientdecision.com, 1999.

32. Molloy DW, Mepham V. Let Me Decide. Toronto: Penguin, 1992.
33. Singer PA. The Joint Centre for Bioethics Living Will Form. www.utoronto.ca/jcb/
    _lwdisclaimer/canchap5.htm.
34. Berry SR, Singer PA. The cancer-specific advance directive. Cancer 1998; 82:
    1570–1577.
35. Holley JL, Stackiewicz L, Dacko C, et al. Factors influencing dialysis patients' com-
    pletion of advance directives. Am J Kidney Dis 1997; 30:356–360.
36. Singer PA, Thiel EC, Salit I, et al. The HIV-specific advance directive. J Gen Intern
    Med 1997; 12:729–735.
37. Singer PA. Disease-specific advance directives. Lancet 1994; 344:594–596.
38. Wharton RH, Levine KR, Buka S, et al. Advance care planning for children with spe-
    cial health care needs: a survey of parental attitudes. Pediatrics 1996; 97:682–687.
39. Schneiderman LJ, Pearlman RA, Kaplan RM, et al. Relationship of general advance
    directive instructions to specific life-sustaining treatment preferences in patients
    with serious illness. Arch Intern Med 1992; 152:2114–2122.
40. Martin DK, Emanuel LL, Singer PA. Planning for the end of life. Lancet 2000;
    356:1672–1676.
41. Emanuel EJ, Weinberg DS, Gonin R, et al. How well is the Patient Self-
    Determination Act working? An early assessment. Am J Med 1993; 95:619–628.
42. Teno JM, Branco KJ, More V, et al. Changes in advance care planning in nursing
    homes before and after the Patient Self-Determination Act: report of a 10 state
    survey. J Am Geriatr Soc 1997; 45:939–944.
43. Sulmasy DP, Song KY, Marx ES, et al. Strategies to promote the use of advance di-
    rectives in a residency outpatient practice. J Gen Intern Med 1996; 11:657–663.
44. Duffield P, Podzamsky JE. The completion of advance directives in primary care.
    J Fam Pract 1996; 42:378–384.
45. Heffner JE, Fahy B, Hilling L, et al. Outcomes of advance directive education of pul-
    monary rehabilitation patients. Am J Respir Crit Care Med 1997; 155:1055–1059.
46. Heffner JE, Fahy B, Barbieri C. Advance directives education during pulmonary re-
    habilitation. Chest 1996; 109:373–379.
47. Hare J, Nelson C. Will outpatients complete a living will. A comparison of two inter-
    ventions. J Gen Intern Med 1991; 6:41–46.
48. Dexter PR, Wolinsky FD, Gramelspacher FP, et al. Effectiveness of computer-
    generated reminders for increasing about advance directives and completion of
    advance directive forms. Ann Intern Med 1998; 128:102–110.
49. Garrett J, Harris R, Norburn J, et al. Life sustaining treatments during terminal ill-
    ness: who wants what? J Gen Intern Med 1993; 8:361–368.
50. Eleazer GP, Hornung CA, Egbert CB, et al. The relationship between ethnicity and
    advance directives in a frail older population. J Am Geriatr Soc 1996; 44:938–943.
51. Hanson LC. The use of living wills at the end-of-life: a national study. Arch Intern
    Med 1996; 156:1018–1022.
52. McKinley ED, Garrett JM, Evans AT, et al. Differences in end-of-life decision mak-
    ing among black and white ambulatory cancer patients. J Gen Intern Med 1996;
    11:651–656.
53. Blackhall LJ, Murphy ST, Frank G, et al. Ethnicity and attitude toward patient au-
    tonomy. JAMA 1995; 274:820–825.
54. Carresse JA, Rhodes LA. Western bioethics on the Navajo reservation: benefit or
    harm? JAMA 1995; 274:826–829.

55. Landry FJ, Kroenke K, Lucas C, et al. Increasing the use of advance directives in medical outpatients. J Gen Intern Med 1997; 12:412–415.

56. Emanuel LL, Danis M, Pearlman RA, et al. Advance care planning as a process: structuring the discussion in practice. J Am Geriatr Soc 1995; 43:440–446.

57. Teno J, Landrum K. Toolkit of instruments to measure care toward the end-of-life. Center to Improve Care of the Dying, 1996.

58. Byock I. Missoula-Vitas Quality Index. Version 255 of Life at the End of Life Instrument. Vitas Healthcare Corporation, Missoula, MT, 1995.

59. Danis M, Patrick DL, Southerland LI, et al. Patients' and families preferences for medical intensive care. JAMA 1988; 260:797–802.

60. Alpert HR, Emanuel L. Comparing utilization of life-sustaining treatments with patient and public preferences. J Gen Intern Med 1998; 13:175–181.

61. Baldwin DC. The role of the physician in end-of-life care: what more can we do? J Health Care Law and Policy 1999; 2:258–267.

18

Research to Improve End-of-Life Care in the United States: Toward a More Behavioral and Ecological Paradigm

MILDRED Z. SOLOMON

This chapter begins with a brief historical overview of the way in which end-of-life care has been conceptualized by policy makers, bioethicists, and researchers in the United States. It then takes up the question of how best to design and evaluate intervention studies aimed at improving end-of-life care. The chapter makes two related arguments:

1. The bioethical focus on case-based clinical ethics coupled with emphasis in the United States on patient self-determination created a bias toward research focused predominantly on decision making about the use or withdrawal of life-sustaining treatments, rather than on the organizational and broader, systemic factors that are more likely to determine good end-of-life care services.
2. Reliance on a strictly biomedical model of research has constrained improvement efforts and should be expanded to include methods drawn from the social sciences and from the specialized fields of physician behavior change, organizational development, and continuous quality improvement.

The chapter concludes with a call for a more behavioral and ecological model of research rather than a strictly biomedical model. The proposed paradigm offers an eclectic range of strategies for designing and testing end-of-life care improvement efforts, focused not only on improving clinical decision making but also on delivering high-quality services to dying patients and families.

Historical Context: Early Reliance on Case-Based Ethical Analysis

In the United States, the Karen Ann Quinlan case of 1976[1] was the first to bring end-of-life care to national attention. Since then, there have been more than 200 so-called right-to-die cases that have made their way through the U.S. courts. With some important exceptions, nearly all of these cases have shared a similar profile: families urging healthcare providers to forego or withdraw life-prolonging medical interventions that they believed were not in the best interest of their loved one. With near consistency, landmark court decisions, including the U.S. Supreme Court decision in the case of Nancy Beth Cruzan,[2] have up-held patients' and families' rights to forgo medical treatments of all kinds, ranging from ventilatory support to artificial nutrition and hydration.

In addition to the growing legal framework, the 1980s was a time of intense policy formation, including the publication in 1983 of a report by a special presidential commission which set forth guidelines for making decisions about the use of life-sustaining treatments.[3] Ethics centers produced important national policy documents,[4] as did many leading healthcare institutions,[5-7] specially formed state task forces,[8] and professional associations.[9-15] Through these activities and publications, there developed a broad societal consensus in the United States that decisions to use or forgo life-sustaining treatments should be based on individual assessments of the patient's prognosis, patients' and families' values, clinicians' judgments, and mutually agreed-upon goals of care and that patients should receive a wide range of palliative services to ease the dying process.

This ideal was widely espoused for many years, but not until the late 1980s and early 90s did empirical studies begin to examine how end-of-life decisions are actually made in everyday clinical practice or to what extent patients receive good palliative care. In fact, until the late 1980s, these questions were not even conceived as empirical ones but, rather, as normative questions about what principles should be used to guide clinical practice decisions.

The major clinical ethics text of the 1980s[16] identified four bioethical principles (autonomy, beneficence, non-maleficence, and justice) to guide physicians and other healthcare professionals as they help patients and families confront end-of-life dilemmas. Dilemmas were defined as situations in which equally compelling but inherently conflicting values were at stake, such as the classic confrontation between a patient wishing to forgo treatment and a physician or family member who believes that the patient's desires are not in his or her best interest. Resolution of such cases centered on the question of how best to reconcile two apparently contradictory values, in this case the clash between a desire to uphold the patient's right to self-determination and concern about his or her long-term best interest. The method for resolving such dilemmas was to develop a solution that best accommodated both values or to come up with a reasoned argument for privileging one value over the other in the particular context of that case.

In other words, in the 15 years after the Quinlan case, end-of-life care in the United States was conceived, primarily, as a process of ethical analysis and personal decision making. Policy makers, bioethicists, and many researchers framed the challenge of improving end-of-life care as one of getting better at making ethical decisions about the use of life-sustaining treatments and ascertaining with as much precision as possible what patients themselves would want. This conceptual starting point was very different from how end-of-life care has been conceived in many other countries, such as the United Kingdom and Canada, where the emphasis has been on preparing healthcare professionals with the necessary knowledge and skills and holding healthcare organizations accountable for delivering palliative care services.

This emphasis on decision making and personal autonomy grows directly out of the political and cultural context in the United States, with its strong emphasis on individualism. The focus on personal decision making soon translated into a strong interest in advance directives: asking patients to create living wills (treatment-preference documents) and to designate someone to speak for them when they are no longer able to speak for themselves (durable powers of attorney for healthcare). These two main forms of advance directive were seen as the means for enhancing decision making and assuring that patients would receive the kind and level of care that they wanted. Research interest in advance directives was greatly stimulated by the passage of a federal law, the Patient Self-Determination Act of 1991, which required that all healthcare institutions receiving Medicare or Medicaid reimbursements must inform patients, upon admission, of their rights under state law to execute advance directives.[17]

Given this historical context, it is not surprising that most of the intervention studies designed in the early 1990s to improve end-of-life care in the United States focused almost exclusively on advance care planning; sharing information among physicians, patients, and nurses; and personal decision making on the part of families about the use of life-sustaining treatments. The largest and best-known of these was the Study to Understand Prognoses and Preferences in Outcomes and Risks of Treatment (SUPPORT).[18] Analysis of both SUPPORT's conceptual premises and its research methods provides important insights into some of the challenges of conducting end-of-life research and suggests important directions for future research initiatives.

Intervention Research: Trying to Improve End-of-Life Care

The SUPPORT study was distinguished by the size of its sample (9000 patients in the intensive care units of five academic health centers), the rigor of its data-collection methods, and its volume of both resource utilization and patient-level outcome data. During phase I, baseline data on a broad range of interesting variables established that hospital care of seriously ill patients was far from satisfactory. For example, half of all phase I patients who could communicate experienced moderate or severe pain at least half of the time during their last 3 days of life. Although 31% of phase I patients expressed a preference not to be resuscitated, slightly fewer than half of their physicians knew that their patients had this preference. Do-not-resuscitate (DNR) orders were written very late, in 46% of cases only 2 days before death, providing no time for hospice services or a return home before death.

Based on these findings, the SUPPORT investigators designed an intervention to improve outcomes for seriously ill patients with at least a 50% chance of dying within 6 months. The intervention had three components: (*1*) nurse facilitators were trained to hold advance care planning conversations about the use of life-prolonging interventions and encouraged to improve pain management, but as of this writing, the particular methods that the nurses were supposed to use to ensure that pain would be well managed have not been described in SUPPORT's published papers; (*2*) doctors were provided with short written reports, which summarized their own patients' treatment preferences and desires for information; (*3*) a computer-generated report was provided to physicians, which described their specific patients' probability of surviving up to 6 months, likelihood of being severely functionally impaired at 2 months, and probability of surviving cardiopulmonary resuscitation (CPR).

Designed as a randomized controlled trial (RCT), patients and their physicians were randomized by physician specialty group to receive either the intervention or usual medical care. Statistical analyses allowed the researchers to control for a variety of factors related to the randomization scheme, including imbalances between groups at baseline. Startlingly, the phase II results showed no impact of the intervention in the experimental sites on any of the designated outcome measures, which were timing of DNR orders, physician–patient agreement on DNR orders, number of undesirable days in the intensive care unit, prevalence or severity of pain, and amount of healthcare resources consumed.

How can these results be explained?

There are two ways to answer this question, each equally important. One is to consider the basic premises about the nature of the end-of-life care problem, prevalent at the time the SUPPORT team began its research. This analysis will lead to a conceptual critique of the prevailing philosophical assumptions that shaped the investigators' decisions about the purpose, content, and structural components of the intervention. The second important way to answer the question is to take a detailed look at SUPPORT's research design, which greatly influenced how the intervention was implemented and evaluated. In the final section of the chapter, I demonstrate how conceptual premises and research methods are related concerns. Considering them in relation to one another points the way to a new, more eclectic research paradigm that extends beyond the predominant biomedical model upon which most research in palliative care is currently based.

A conceptual critique: limitations of the bioethical premise

A number of descriptive research studies taking place roughly at the same time that SUPPORT was conducting its intervention now provide additional important data. First, there is evidence that, historically, end-of-life researchers (and policy makers) placed too much hope in advance directives as a means for improving end-of-life care. Despite their widespread promotion, depending on the particular study, only somewhere between 15% and 25% of people report having executed a formal advance directive,[19–22] though this can rise to as high as 40% among hospitalized patients.[23,24] (One particularly impressive project in LaCrosse, Wisconsin, succeeded in ensuring that 81% of decedents had some form of advance directive in the medical record, usually a proxy document indicating that durable power of attorney for healthcare had been established for a surrogate decision maker.[25])

Second, Blackhall et al.[26] as well as Koenig and Gates-William[27] revealed that the emphasis on individualism and personalized decision making that underpins the advance directive movement is simply not of paramount importance in many cultures and, in fact, may run counter to deeply held notions of family and community and of the respect, loyalty, and protection children owe their parents. This research suggests that the relevant ethical focus may not be on truth telling or ascertaining with certainty what the individual would want but, rather, on love, support, and care. For many families, the key questions are "Have I supported my mother or father?" and "Have I been a good daughter or son?" Many dying patients may not want to know the details of their prognosis or to make their own autonomous decisions about treatment options. For them, family needs, obligations, and responsibilities may be of greater importance.[28,29]

Third, there are certain overly habituated treatment patterns, that is, medical interventions that are routinely nearly unconsciously offered without regard to the patient's long-term best interests or an open appraisal of what would constitute reasonable goals of care. For example, in the nursing home setting studied by Aronheim and colleagues,[30] artificial nutrition and hydration was nearly universally offered to patients with dementia who lost the ability to swallow or who experienced aspiration pneumonia, despite data showing that enteral tube feedings did not decrease the rate of aspiration pneumonia.

Other invasive treatments routinely provided to patients in the final days and hours of life, without adequate discussion, include widespread use of systemic antibiotics,[31] seemingly disproportionate rates of CPR,[18] and excessively lengthy periods of ventilatory support.[32–34] Many reasons have been provided for this, including the speculation, backed by some interesting data, that the number of hospital beds in a region is the main predictor of whether dying patients will be transferred to the hospital, where they nearly inevitably receive these kinds of life-prolonging intervention.[35]

A focus on decision making and information transfer, without new procedures and protocols to interrupt these "default" patterns, is likely to be ineffective. This problem seems evident in the SUPPORT study, where, despite the talking the nurses did with patients and families about pain and the reports on patient treatment preferences they put into the physician notes, no changes in practice patterns were detected. New procedures, such as routine pain assessments, use of a 10-point pain rating scale, and patient follow-up to see if offered treatments were effective, might have had a greater impact. However, these steps were not built into the intervention, perhaps because the underlying philosophical assumptions of the study were directed, consciously or unconsciously, on decision making rather than on restructuring the system of care.

A methodological critique: limitations of the prevailing biomedical model

Methodologically, the SUPPORT investigators were operating from within a strictly biomedical model of inquiry, akin to drug trials. However, behavior-change interventions are not the same as drug trials. Studies that aim to change individual and organizational behavior are fundamentally social science experiments, involving complex human interactions. Therefore, incorporation of key principles and research methods drawn from the social sciences is likely to enhance their chances for success. The following five points illustrate some of the problems researchers can experience from over-reliance on a strict biomedical model of research and some of the assistance to be gained from drawing upon a broader range of methods to design and test palliative care improvement efforts.

Process data are critical for interpreting results
Randomized controlled trials (RCTs) create the experimental conditions necessary for drawing valid inferences about whether an intervention succeeded or failed in meeting its objectives. However, RCTs cannot say why or how such an effect has occurred. They speak to whether something can be causally linked, but they do not provide the data necessary for understanding the mechanisms responsible for that causal linkage.[36–39] To understand the reasons for the success or failure of an intervention, it is necessary to move beyond examination of the results to a detailed analysis of the content and implementation strategies employed by the intervention.

Unfortunately, there are not enough published data about the SUPPORT strategies or implementation processes to determine why the intervention did not change behavior. For example, it is unclear how the nurses were supposed to improve pain management. As noted above, it does not appear that any mechanisms, other than talking with patients or families and developing a written report for the physicians, were employed. Furthermore, the majority of physicians never read either the treatment preference or the prognostic reports. It could well be that with a change in the way the written reports were delivered to the physicians, a shift in the communication patterns between physicians and nurses, a revision in the nursing protocol, or a different orientation in the patient interviews, wholly different results would have followed.[40]

Triangulation of data sources is important

All interventions require that formative research be conducted to determine how best to design the intervention so that it can address identified problems, harness available resources, and benefit from available leverage points. The SUPPORT investigators interviewed physicians to learn what they perceived to be their needs, and the physicians advised them that if doctors had prognostic data and information about patient preferences, decision making and care near the end of life would be improved. The investigators took the physicians at their word and made prognostic data and information about patient preferences the central features of the intervention.

While physicians are certainly a key group to interview in the formative stages of intervention design, their views are not all that should be considered. Physicians are part of a larger system, involving many other disciplines and subject to many influences, some explicit and others functioning only implicitly in ways that physicians or other healthcare professionals may not consciously recognize. It is important to *triangulate* data sources, which means that investigators purposefully sample the opinions of different organizational players and examine their views in relationship to one another. A combination of interviews with healthcare professionals from different disciplines plus direct observation is often the best approach to detect actual practices as well as beliefs.

Pilot phases are important, and when necessary, intervention redesign is permissible

Unlike drug trials, in intervention research of many types, it is recognized as appropriate for researchers to observe the implementation of the intervention carefully, both in pilot phases beforehand and during the study period itself. This allows for redesign along the way if necessary.[41] For example, when it was discovered that physicians were not reviewing the prognostic and preference data, there might have been ways to modify the implementation plan to address this problem. For evaluation purposes, time-series data collected throughout the study period could provide insight into whether there were any intervention effects associated with changes the researchers made mid-course in the implementation process.

Group randomization is a valid and powerful design

In SUPPORT, randomization occurred by physician specialty group, which meant that within the same institution some physicians and physician groups received the intervention and some did not. Under these circumstances, investigators are likely to be very concerned about contamination between the treatment and control groups and, therefore, to hold back from some of the more public and vigorous steps they might have taken to ensure that the intervention was adopted and fully implemented. Randomizing the intervention to treatment and control institutions, rather than to units within the same institution, would have allowed the researchers to design and implement a far more robust intervention.

Group randomization is particularly important because change is hard to achieve and usually requires substantial buy-in from highly visible organizational leaders. When an intervention is introduced to only a part of an institution, the implementers' hands are tied. It becomes more difficult to recruit the necessary leaders within the organization as champions for the cause and to build the social momentum that is so important in organizational improvement efforts. Unfortunately, group randomization studies are often inappropriately dismissed by medical researchers as "quasi-experimental," even though they employ randomization and despite the fact that the validity of quasi-experiments has long been established.[42]

Theories of physician behavior change and principles of organizational development should inform intervention design

An excellent summary of 44 systematic reviews of the behavior-change literature demonstrates that a small number of fairly robust inferences can be drawn about what does and does not work.[43] A key finding, affirmed in theories of adult learning,[44,45] physician behavior change,[46] and organizational development, is that nearly all successful improvement efforts are locally invented (or adapted) by the participants, who must feel that they are the ones creating the change. If participants see themselves as the agents of change, the changes they institute are far more likely to become adopted and maintained.

In addition to the importance of self-agency, a second principle is clear: effective change efforts are most often highly particularized, depending on sophisticated consideration of the lines of authority, influence, and status with the organization and on other sociological, political, cultural, financial, and administrative factors. Recognizing the importance of fitting the intervention to the particular circumstances of a given institution, National Health Services researchers in the United Kingdom have advocated that all behavior-change interventions begin with what they call a "diagnostic analysis," to identify factors likely to influence the proposed change.[43] Other researchers have also pointed out that the gap between evidence-based guidelines and actual practice will be difficult to surmount, unless would-be change agents develop highly particularized opportunities for local "actors" to engage with new knowledge in contexts that are meaningful to them.[47] They underscore that successful interventions often require time-intensive, politically sensitive approaches to build buy-in: there is no "one size fits all" model that can be imposed from the outside.

Though they differ in their details, successful interventions have many underlying features in common, including visible endorsement by the institution's leadership, a group clearly designated to be accountable for the institution's success or failure in meeting its own goals; strong interdisciplinary collaboration; and specific cues to action that trigger new routines and protocols, which become integrated into everyday habits. Successful routines become a part of "how we provide care here" and do not depend on the initiative of single champions, who can too easily burn out or move away.

Furthermore, a single change is rarely enough. Multiple reinforcing strategies, usually applied in combination, are often required. Involving the target audience in collecting and interpreting data about their own practices[46] as well as establishing accountability and responsibility for meeting performance goals are also important.

As the discussion so far indicates, the conditions for promoting change most robustly are not always conducive to the conditions necessary for randomized evaluation designs. Given the complexity of research that must take human motivation into account, drug trials are not a good analogue. A strictly biomedical model for future research will not suffice.

Toward a More Behavioral and Ecological Research Paradigm

For nearly 20 years, from the Karen Ann Quinlan case in the middle 1970s until the middle 1990s (with the publication of the SUPPORT results), most policy makers and advocates for better end-of-life care in the United States conceptualized the problem of improving end-of-life care as one of clinical decision making. The goal was to enable patients and the families of incapacitated patients to make their own choices based on the principles of autonomy and substituted judgment. These principles were central in SUPPORT, which placed so high a premium on eliciting patient preferences.

The growing empirical research base suggests that this framework was built on an overly rationalistic, overly individualistic concept of healthcare, one that is not shared by all segments of our pluralistic society. Furthermore, there is now evidence that the major problem may not be inadequate preparation for decision making but inadequate services. What we have seen as a problem of choice may in fact be a problem of poor healthcare options and inadequate preparation of healthcare professionals in the skills needed to deliver those services.

It is, of course, important to enhance healthcare providers', patients', and families' ability to think about the choices they inevitably face near the end of life with greater ethical, legal, and interpersonal sophistication. However, the focus needs to extend from making hard choices about what treatments will be withdrawn to structuring what the healthcare system will provide. There need to be assurances that good pain and symptom management is in place, that patients' depression and emotional suffering will be noticed, and that bereavement support will be available. We need to ensure that there will be adequate continuity of care for patients and families when they change care settings and that a healthcare system's incentives, both financial and otherwise, are aligned with the provision of quality care.

Given this more complex view of the problem, it is time to modify the autonomy/clinical ethics paradigm and to shift to what I have called elsewhere a "behavioral and ecological" paradigm.[40] By "behavioral" I mean to signal the centrality of understanding the psychology of human motivation, team building, and the role that incentives of various types play in shaping action, the behaviors of both healthcare providers and patients/families. Behavioral is also meant to contrast with the overly rational view of illness experiences that bioethics and clinical medicine have often assumed. This prevailing view tends to overestimate the role that information, and even consciously espoused values, play in how people actually experience illness. It often assumes that people make decisions in instances where they themselves feel they are a part of something that cannot be controlled. For people in such circumstances, the concept of decision making poorly captures their own existential reality. By "ecological" I mean to underscore the importance of taking a holistic, systemic perspective that recognizes the dynamic interplay of the multiple factors that shape the behavior of individuals and institutions. An ecological paradigm recognizes the critical importance of talking with patients and families about their individual preferences, but it would also place an equally strong focus on redesigning the healthcare environment, both within institutions and in the broader environment affecting organizational and practitioner behavior.

How might such redesign proceed? In this final section, I suggest several possible directions.

Continuous quality improvement

The RCT design should not necessarily be seen as the gold standard in end-of-life care research. First, RCTs do not yield information until the trial is complete, when it is often too late or very expensive to learn from mistakes. In contrast, continuously collected data can provide "quick and dirty," but often accurate, information about how change efforts are doing.[48]

More importantly, as noted above, collecting data about one's own practices and then making changes on the basis of that information is an empowering experience, which treats participants as agents of their own change, not as subjects in a research study. Certainly, the physician behavior-change literature has demonstrated that physicians are most responsive when they are in charge of their own improvement efforts. Since self-initiation, reflection, and accountability are central in continuous quality improvement (CQI), this is an approach that should be highly motivating for physicians but only if it is applied not just to administrative matters (such as shorter wait times) but also to clinical issues of concern to physicians themselves.

Recognizing the potential application of CQI to end-of-life care, the SUPPORT researchers have taken a leadership role in moving the field in this direction. Working with nearly 50 healthcare organizations, through a yearlong collaboration cosponsored by the Institute for Healthcare Improvement and the Rand Center to Improve the Care of the Dying, Lynn et al.[49] have stimulated a wide variety of systematic improvements on behalf of better palliative care.

Through this collaboration and the efforts of others over the last few years, many CQI efforts have been initiated. For example, the United Hospital Fund of New York has worked intensively with five New York City hospitals, experimenting with new procedures and protocols, many embedded within a CQI context.[50]

In addition, over the last several years, the Decisions Near the End of Life National Coordinating Center (http://www.edc.org/cae) has provided assistance and educational resources to more than 200 hospitals and nursing homes. For example, as part of their involvement in the Decisions initiative, Dowdy et al.[32] achieved impressive improvement in advance care planning, the quality of end-of-life decision making, and lower resource utilization when they established an institutional routine requiring a mandatory conversation about goals of care. The purpose of their intervention was to ensure that the attending physician would speak with the family (or patient if he or she were able) about their understanding of the patient's prognosis and would seek consensus with the family on appropriate goals for care. The important factor in this intervention's success was that the conversation was not left to occur by happenstance, dependent on the interest, skill, or time of individual physicians, who vary greatly in their willingness and comfort levels with conversations of this sort. Instead, objective criteria (96 hours of continuous mechanical ventilation) were used to trigger an institutional mechanism: an interdisciplinary ethics consult team comprised of healthcare professionals who are comfortable holding end-of-life discussions was established.

Another example comes from a Harvard teaching hospital, which served as one of the original Decisions Near the End of Life field-test sites. Holloran et al.[34] demonstrated that routine, retrospective case discussions by residents in the surgical intensive care unit significantly improved the quality of the decision-making process, as evidenced by enhanced information in the medical chart and a reduced length of stay due to family decisions to terminate life-prolonging interventions and/or to transfer patients home. Although cost savings were not part of the original goal of this intervention, $1.74 million was saved over a 2-year period.[51]

Special palliative care options, developed for long-term care patients with advanced dementia, have demonstrated higher quality of life and lower resource utilization.[52,53] Hammes et al.[54] achieved impressive increases in advance care planning through a set of communitywide initiatives, which included CQI strategies, and many nurses have played a leadership role in applying CQI to pain and symptom management.[55–57] Given the emerging interest in CQI and the growing recognition that processes of care are a critical focus, there is now a peer-reviewed online journal (*Innovations in End-of-Life Care*, http://www.edc.org/lastacts) that regularly critiques worldwide efforts, focusing on institutional processes as well as outcomes.[58]

The CQI strategies are being adopted in part because there is growing recognition that they may prove more effective than more distant, hands-off research studies, which do not allow for self-agency and local customization. However, as CQI efforts with respect to end-of-life care grow, we will need to grapple with how best to evaluate their effectiveness.

New criteria for evaluating CQI interventions

One of the most difficult future challenges researchers will have to solve is how best to evaluate the effectiveness of CQI efforts without benefit of randomized designs and often with very small sample sizes. In the absence of a controlled design, what inferences can reasonably be drawn about reliability, validity, and generalizability? Even if small-scale CQI or CQI-type interventions cannot produce generalizable results, to what other criteria should they be held accountable? What standards should there be for publishing outcome data drawn from CQI studies? In short, what constitutes rigor? Answering these kinds of methodological questions is well beyond the scope of this chapter. It is important, however, to note the problem as it will require creative thinking over the coming years.

Valid quality indicators and outcome measures

Some quality indicators are obvious and moderately easy to collect: chart review to detect whether pain is being assessed routinely is a straightforward measure. Unit or population-based audits are also a simple, direct way to determine prevalence and severity of pain and to ascertain whether treatments are effective.

However, many possible measures in the end-of-life care arena are not so straightforward. For example, some quality-of-life tools have tended to overemphasize the medical and functional aspects of quality of life, failed to take into account the differential weighting that patients give to different quality-of-life domains, or failed to recognize that patients' assessments of quality of life may change over time as disease progresses. Furthermore, even carefully constructed quality-of-life tools have the potential for misuse. For example, there may be attempts to use them to impose treatment decisions on a particular patient, rather than as a way of learning how patients see themselves or as a way of assessing how well the healthcare organization is providing care.

There are other examples of how important it is to scrutinize the validity of proposed measures. For example, some investigators might assume that an overall increase in DNR orders or the writing of DNR orders earlier would be a sign of an improved process of decision making. However, the opposite could be true. More DNR orders, particularly in the context of capitated care, could arise equally as a consequence of a poorer decision-making process.

As researchers in this field, it will be important to continually work to determine whether the use of a measure has any misleading or harmful effects that could arise either from misinterpreting the meaning of the measure or from using the data for an inappropriate purpose. Outcome measures should be assessed in terms of their psychometric qualities but also in terms of their overall face validity and ethical impact. To help interpret patient-level and resource utilization-level outcome data, related structure and process data should also be collected, to the extent possible. Particularly when indirect measures, such as timing of DNR orders, are used to assess quality of care, they should be examined in combination with information about what patients and families said they wanted and in light of morbidity and mortality data, to detect any inappropriate effects on patient survival.

Impact of the external environment on the behavior of clinicians and organizations

This chapter has focused on intervention research aimed at improving end-of-life care within healthcare institutions. However, an ecological approach also points out the need to examine external factors that may, consciously or unconsciously, influence clinician and organizational behavior. The chilling effect of hypervigilant regulation of narcotic prescription writing on physicians' willingness to use opioids is well known. In addition, there is a need to better understand and differentiate among the various financial incentives that managed-care organizations use to shape physician behavior. Some may appropriately encourage the adoption of practices that could benefit patients and families near the end of life (such as reimbursements for holding an advance care planning conversation during an office visit), while others may inappropriately restrict clinical judgment and the patient's best interest. In other words, to what extent do financial incentives, currently in use, support or impede quality of care?

Moreover, how do various types of payment methods encourage or discourage access to needed services, both for people already enrolled in managed-care organizations as well as for those who may not be actively recruited because of concerns about the expected high cost of their care? Future research should focus on developing and testing risk-adjustment mechanisms and other sorts of payment method, to ensure that access to care is available for those most in need of it.[59,60]

In addition to payment structures and their impact on care delivery, many other questions relate to patterns of resource utilization and referral. We know very little, for example, about what predicts site of death (home, hospital, hospice, or nursing home) or referral to hospice.

As these examples demonstrate, the range of questions that could be helpful is long and varied. The point is that, in addition to suggesting new research methods, a more behavioral and ecological paradigm helps to focus attention on what constitutes significant research questions. Ideally, it would be helpful for investigators with diverse disciplinary training but a common interest in end-of-life care to work together to define a comprehensive research agenda that could be undertaken in a coordinated fashion. Such an agenda would help to create priorities for funding, minimize duplication, and create the means for learning more quickly from the proliferation of what may otherwise remain largely isolated efforts.

Conclusion

The biomedical model of inquiry requires a distant, hands-off approach to behavior change, which can easily impede the design and implementation of interventions robust enough to make an impact. Recognizing the psychological, social, cultural, and political complexity of improvement efforts in end-of-life care, medicine should reach beyond itself to embrace methods developed by other disciplines. We need a more behavioral and ecological paradigm, one that acknowledges and consciously plans for the multifaceted systemic and organizational factors that must be coordinated to sustain meaningful improvements. Fortunately, there is a rich literature in adult learning, theories of physician practice change, organizational development, and CQI that can, and should, guide future research efforts. Now, we must develop interdisciplinary research teams of social scientists and clinicians to define and undertake this agenda.

References

1. In re Quinlan, 70 NJ 10, 355 A2nd 647, cert denied sub nom, Garzer v. New Jersey, 429 US 922, 1976.
2. Cruzan v. Director Missouri Department of Health, 497 US 111, 110 Sup Ct 2841, 1990.
3. President's Commission for the Study of Ethical Problems in Medicine and Biomedical and Behavioral Research. Deciding to Forego Life-Sustaining Treatment: Ethical, Medical and Legal Issues in Treatment Decisions. Washington DC: US Government Printing Office, 1983.
4. The Hastings Center. Guidelines on the Termination of Life-Sustaining Treatment and the Care of the Dying. Bloomington: Indiana University Press, 1987.
5. Ruark J, Raffin T, Stanford University Medical Center Committee on Ethics. Initiating and withdrawing life support: principles and practice in adult medicine. N Engl J Med 1988; 318:25–30.
6. Uhlmann R, Cassel C, McDonald W. Some treatment withholding implications of no-code orders in an academic hospital. Crit Care Med 1984; 12:879–881.
7. Wanzer S, Adelstein S, Cranford R. The physician's responsibility toward hopelessly ill patients. N Engl J Med 1984; 310:955–959.
8. New York State Task Force on Life and Law. Life-Sustaining Treatment: Making Decisions and Appointing a Health Care Agent. New York: July, 1987.
9. American Medical Association. Current Opinions of the Council on Ethical and Judicial Affairs of the American Medical Association: Withholding or Withdrawing Life Prolonging Treatment. Chicago: American Medical Association, 1992.
10. American Nurses' Association. American Nurses' Association Task Force on the Nurse's Role in End of Life Decisions. Position Statement on Foregoing Artificial Nutrition and Hydration. Washington DC: American Nurses' Association, 1992.
11. American Thoracic Society Bioethics Task Force. Withholding and withdrawing life-sustaining therapy. Am Rev Respir Dis 1991; 144:726–731.

12. American College of Chest Physicians/Society of Critical Care Medicine Consensus Panel. Ethical and moral guidelines for the initiation, continuation, and withdrawal of intensive care. Chest 1990; 97:946–958.
13. American College of Physicians Ethics Committee. American College of Physicians Ethics manual—part 2. The physician and society. Ann Intern Med 1989; 3: 327–335.
14. American Dietetic Association. Issues in feeding the terminally ill adult. J Am Diet Assoc 1987; 87:78–85.
15. California Nurses' Association Ethics Committee. Statement on the Nurse's Role in Withholding and Withdrawing Life-Sustaining Treatment and Care of the Dying. Bloomington: Indiana University Press, 1987.
16. Beauchamp T, Childress J. Principles of Biomedical Ethics. New York: Oxford University Press, 1983.
17. McCloskey EL. The patient self-determination act. Kennedy Inst Ethics J 1991; 1: 163–169.
18. SUPPORT Principal Investigators. A controlled trial to improve care for seriously ill hospitalized patients: the Study to Understand Prognosis and Preferences for Outcomes and Risks of Treatments (SUPPORT). JAMA 1995; 274:591–598.
19. Emanuel L, Barry M, Stoeckle J, et al. Advance directives for medical care: a case for greater use. N Engl J Med 1991; 324:889–895.
20. Stelter KL, Elliott BA, Bruno CA. Living will completion in older adults. Arch Intern Med 1992; 152:954–959.
21. Gordon G, Dunn P. Advance directives and the patient self-determination act. Hosp Pract (Off Ed) 1992 Apr 30; 27(4A):39–42.
22. Miles SM, Koepp R, Weber EP. Advance end-of-life treatment planning: a research review. Arch Intern Med 1996; 156:1062–1069.
23. Emanuel E, Weinberg D, Gonin R, et al. How well is the patient self-determination act working? An early assessment. Am J Med 1993 Dec; 95:619–628.
24. Cohen-Mansfield J, Droge J, Billing N. The utilization of the durable power of attorney for health care among hospitalized elderly patients. J Am Geriatr Soc 1991; 39:1174–1178.
25. Hammes BJ, Rooney BL. Death and end-of-life planning in one midwestern community. Arch Intern Med 1998; 158:383–390.
26. Blackhall L, Murphy S, Frank G, et al. Ethnicity and attitudes toward patient autonomy. JAMA 1995; 274:820–825.
27. Koenig B, Gates-Williams J. Understanding cultural differences in caring for the dying. West J Med 1995; 63:244–249.
28. Solomon MZ. From what's neutral to what's meaningful: reflections on a study of medical interpreters. J Clin Ethics 1997; 8:88–93.
29. Solomon MZ. Why are advance directives a non-issue outside the United States? In: Solomon MZ, Romer AL, Heller KS, eds. Innovations in End-of-Life Care, Vol. 1. New York: Mary Ann Liebert Publishing Company, 2000; 3(1):111–114. Also available at www.edc.org/lastacts.
30. Ahronheim J, Morris J, Baskin S, et al. Lung infection in patients with advanced dementia: relation to feeding tubes and severity of dementia. Gerontologist 1996; 36, Special Issue II:208.
31. Ahronheim J, Morrison S, Basking J, et al. Treatment of the dying in the acute care hospital. Arch Intern Med 1996; 156:2094–2100.

32. Dowdy MD, Robertson C, Bander JA. A study of proactive ethics consultation for critically and terminally ill patients with extended lengths of stay. Crit Care Med 1998; 26:252–259.

33. Solomon MZ, O'Donnell L, Jennings B, et al. Decisions near the end of life: professional views on life-sustaining treatments. Am J Public Health 1993; 83:14–23.

34. Holloran SD, Starkey GW, Burke PA, et al. An educational intervention in the surgical intensive care unit to improve ethical decisions. Surgery 1995; 118:294–299.

35. Pritchard RS, Fisher ES, Teno JM, et al. Influence of patient preferences and local health system characteristics on the place of death: Study to Understand Prognoses and Preferences for Outcomes and Risks of Treatment. J Am Geriatr Soc 1998; 46:1242–1250.

36. Maxwell J. Qualitative Research Design: An Interactive Approach. London: Sage, 1996.

37. Cook T. Postpositivist critical multiplism. In: Shotland RL, Marks MM, eds. Social Science and Social Policy. Thousand Oaks, CA: Sage, 1985:21–62.

38. Huberman AM, Miles MB. Assessing local causality in qualitative research. In: Berg DN, Smith KK, eds. The Self in Social Inquiry: Researching Methods. Thousand Oaks, CA: Sage, 1985:351–381.

39. Shadish WR. Source of evaluation practice: needs, purposes, questions and technology. In: Bickman L, Weatherford DL, eds. Evaluating Early Intervention Programs for Severely Handicapped Children and Their Families. Austin, TX: Pro-Ed, 1986:149–183.

40. Solomon MZ. The enormity of the task: support and changing practice. Hastings Cent Rep 1995; 25:S28–S32.

41. Office of Cancer Communications, National Cancer Institute. Making Health Communications Programs Work: A Planner's Guide. Washington DC: US Department of Health and Human Services, 1989.

42. Cook T, Cambell D. Quasi-experimentation: Design and Analysis Issues for Field Settings. Skokie, IL: Rand McNally, 1979.

43. University of York National Health Service Centre for Reviews and Dissemination. Effective Health Care: Getting Evidence into Practice, vol 5. Plymouth: Royal Society of Medicine Press, 1999, www.york.ac.uk/inst/crd

44. Crass K. Adults as learners: Increasing Participation and Facilitating Learning. San Francisco: Jossey-Bass, 1981.

45. Morris Baskett H, Marsick V. New Directions for Adult and Continuing Education. Professionals' Ways of Knowing: New Findings on How to Improve Professional Education, vol 55. San Francisco: Jossey-Bass, 1992.

46. Eisenberg J. Doctors' Decisions and the Cost of Medical Care: The Reasons for Doctors' Practice Patterns and Ways to Change them. Ann Arbor, MI: Health Administration Press, 1986.

47. Wood M, Ferlie E, Fitzgerald L. Achieving clinical behavior change: a case of becoming indeterminate. Soc Sci Med 1998; 47:1729–1738.

48. Kritchevsky S, Simmons B. Continuous quality improvement: concepts and applications for physician care. JAMA 1991; 266:1817–1823.

49. Lynn J, Schuster JL, Kabcenell A. Improving Care for the End of Life: A Sourcebook for Health Care Managers and Clinics. New York: Oxford University Press, 2000.

50. Zuckerman C, MacKinnon A. Challenge of Caring for Patients Near the End of Life: Findings from the Hospital Palliative Care Initiative. New York: United Hospital Fund of New York, 1998.

51. Holloran S. Reply to Dr. Gordon. BIOMED-L Digest Jan-Feb 1997:www.BIOMED-L@listserv.nodak.edu.

52. Volicer L, Collard A, Hurley A, et al. Impact of special care unit for patients with advanced Alzheimer's disease on patients' discomfort and costs. J Am Geriatr Soc 1994; 42:597–603.

53. Hurley A, Volicer L, Romer AL. Caring for patients with advanced dementia: implications of innovative research for practice—an interview with Ann Hurley, RN, DNSc, and Ladislav Volicer, MD, PhD. Innovations in End-of-Life Care 1999; 1(1): www.edc.org/lastacts.

54. Hammes B, Romer AL. The lessons from Respecting Your Choices: An interview with Bernard "Bud" Hammes, PhD, from La Crosse, Wisconsin. Innovations in End-of-Life Care, 1999; 1(1):www.edc.org/lastacts.

55. Bookbinder M, Romer AL. Raising the standard of care for imminently dying patients using quality improvement: Aa interview with Marilyn Bookbinder. Innovations in End-of-Life Care, 2001; 3:www.edc.org/lastacts.

56. Bookbinder M, Coyle N, Kiss M, et al. Implementing national standards for cancer pain management: program model and evaluation. J Pain Symptom Manage 1996; 12:334–347.

57. Dufault MA, Willey-Lessne C. Using a collaborative research utilization model to develop and test the effects of clinical pathways for pain management. J Nurs Care Qual 1999; 13:19–33.

58. Solomon MZ. Innovations in end-of-life care: improving quality by focusing on the process of change. J Palliat Med 2000; 3:111–114.

59. Solomon MZ, Romer AL, Sellers D, et al. Meeting the Challenge: Twelve Recommendations for Improving End-of-Life Care in Managed Care. Newton, MA: EDC, 1999. Available at http://www.edc.org/CAE/meetingchallenge

60. Solomon MZ. Leading the way: managed care for patients near the end of life. Am J Managed Care 2001; 7:1162–1164.

19

Studying Desire for Death: Methodological Issues in End-Of-Life Research

BARRY ROSENFELD

With the growing public, political, and medical interest in physician-assisted suicide, euthanasia, and other end-of-life issues, the importance of empirical research related to end-of-life care has become increasingly apparent. The need, even demand, for such research has resulted in a rapidly growing empirical literature addressing many end-of-life issues. Unfortunately, this literature has been plagued by methodological problems which have limited its usefulness and accuracy.[1] This chapter reviews a number of the primary methodological issues that accompany such complex areas as physician-assisted suicide and the desire for death. The primary issues covered here involve difficulties selecting and operationalizing dependent variables (what to study), sampling issues (who to study and when to conduct the research), and confounding influences on the measurement of relevant variables (how to measure relevant variables). In addition, statistical/data analytic issues, which are not necessarily unique to desire for death/assisted suicide research, are no less problematic in this literature and are briefly reviewed. Two caveats warrant note: first, the order in which these issues are presented is not intended to reflect their relative importance but, rather, to provide a coherent framework for organizing the methodological issues and concerns discussed and, second, this review is not intended as a criticism of existing studies (although some criticism is inherent in any review) but, rather, to facilitate the development of future research studies.

What to Study (Operationalizing Dependent Variables)

Research addressing end-of-life issues, in general, and the desire for death among terminally ill individuals, in particular, has become increasingly sophisticated over the past decade. This growing sophistication is perhaps best exemplified in the gradual evolution of dependent variables used in assisted suicide research. Early research on assisted suicide and euthanasia typically involved hypothetical questions and vignettes, such as asking whether an individual would consider suicide or assisted suicide at some future, often undeclared point.[2,3] Other variants of the hypothetical vignette methodology have provided subjects with a series of vignettes, each of which differs in nature, and analyzed differences in the response rates to each.[4,5] Although hypothetical vignette methodologies are useful for quantifying the proportion of respondents who might approve of euthanasia under certain conditions, most studies have delved further, analyzing demographic and clinical characteristics of subjects who approve of assisted suicide or anticipate possible future interest. However, the significance of analyzing whether variables such as current pain and depression predict hypothetical future interest in assisted suicide is far from clear.

Moreover, interest in (or approval of) assisted suicide or euthanasia under a set of hypothetical conditions does not necessarily correspond to an actual interest in hastened death. In several studies, dramatic differences have emerged between the frequency with which patients indicate a willingness to consider assisted suicide in hypothetical vignettes and their current interest in hastened death.[6,7] For example, in their study of 100 patients with amyotrophic lateral sclerosis (ALS), Ganzini and colleagues[7] found that 55% would "consider" assisted suicide, yet only one individual (1%) was actually interested in hastening death at the time of study participation. A related issue in hypothetical decisions concerns the validity of these hypothetical preferences: does a patient's speculation as to how he or she might behave in the future actually correspond to later behavior? Not surprisingly, medically ill individuals often change their minds about what interventions they do and do not want when they are actually forced to confront the situation.[8] While the potential for changing preferences does not invalidate advance directives (such as living wills, do-not-resuscitate [DNR] orders, etc.), the potential for systematic biases in end-of-life research based on hypothetical vignettes or decision making clearly exists.

In response to these concerns, a growing number of researchers have begun studying actual requests for assisted suicide and current desire for hastened death as an alternative to hypothetical vignette methodologies. Not surprisingly, these two methodologies (requests for assisted suicide and desire for hastened death) have produced somewhat different but largely complementary results.

Studying requests for (or completed) assisted suicide

Studies of actual requests for assisted suicide first arose in the Netherlands, although these studies were largely descriptive, documenting the frequency of assisted suicide and euthanasia as well as the primary reasons behind patient requests.[9] With the 1997 enactment of the Oregon Death with Dignity Act (ODDA), a handful of studies have described the characteristics and outcomes of cases in which assisted suicide has been requested in the United States.[10,11]

For example, Ganzini and colleagues[12] described the results of a survey of Oregon physicians, in which respondents were asked to recount cases where their patients had requested assisted suicide. Responding physicians were asked to recall the reasons behind their patients' requests as well as what, if any, interventions took place in response. Of course, the limitations of physician recollection are no doubt apparent. Not only are physicians likely to report only the most salient or "legitimate" reasons but they may be genuinely unaware of other, unreported factors (such as depression, concerns about becoming a burden to family).

A potentially more useful methodology might involve interviewing the patients themselves who request assisted suicide rather than relying on physician recall. Of course, the ability to systematically study individuals who request assisted suicide is clearly limited by ethical and practical constraints. For example, Lee and Werth[13] analyzed data from Oregon residents who sought guidance from a nonprofit agency (Compassion in Dying) in accessing the ODDA. Although their study was limited in terms of the nature of the data available, they had considerably more information than was described in the "official" report issued by the Oregon Health Division.[10] For example, they compared individuals who contacted the agency and ultimately ended their life using the ODDA versus those who sought information from the agency but died of other causes. Nevertheless, the limitations in this study in terms of sample representativeness (only a subset of Oregonians who utilized the ODDA were included) clearly highlight the difficulties in conducting systematic research with this population.

A central question that faces potential researchers is whether asking physicians to refer their terminally ill and likely quite distressed (physically or psychologically) patients to a research study is either ethical or practical. Only one such study, as yet unpublished,[14] has been reported, and this study suffers from some of the same sample limitations that plagued Lee and Werth.[13] Back and Gordon[14] interviewed patients and/or family members before and after the patient ingested a fatal medication. While this innovative methodology has produced very interesting, though preliminary, findings, the generalizability of the results is certainly questionable. First, in many cases, only family members were available for interview, resulting in data with many of the same limitations noted in studies of physicians described above. In addition, the majority of patients studied were solicited from outside of Oregon and, therefore, ending their lives (with a physician's assistance) despite the illegal status of assisted suicide. There may be important differences between individuals who seek assisted suicide in jurisdictions where such actions are legal and those who do so despite the illegality. Finally, because of potential ethical and legal concerns, no interviews with physicians were included in this study, leaving open to question the accuracy of the medical information reported (such as life expectancy, existing treatment options). Despite these potential limitations, this methodology is likely to be used increasingly, particularly in settings where assisted suicide has been legalized.

Desire for hastened death

An alternative methodology, increasingly used in settings where assisted suicide is illegal, involves studying desire for hastened death. The construct of desire for hastened death was first operationalized by Chochinov and colleagues[15] in their seminal study of terminally ill cancer patients and further refined by Rosenfeld and colleagues.[16,17] Desire for hastened death is thought to underlie not only requests for assisted suicide but suicidal ideation that does not involve a physician and hopes or efforts to speed one's death that may be characterized as "passive" (such as refusal of treatment other than palliative care, DNR orders, termination of artificial nutrition and hydration). By studying desire for hastened death, researchers can identify individuals who might consider assisted suicide as well as those who might wish for a more rapid death but have personal reasons (religious prohibitions, family obligations, etc.) that would prevent them from actually acting on this desire. Although distinguishing between these subgroups may be important for some research questions, many important issues are best addressed by including both subgroups of patients with high desire for death (those who would and would not actually consider ending their lives).

Chochinov and colleagues[15] developed the first measure of desire for hastened death, the Desire for Death Rating Scale (or DDRS), which featured a series of semistructured questions and prompts to enable clinicians to rate patients along a 1–6 scale. Low scores on this measure reflect little or no interest in a hastened death, moderate scores reflect consideration or passive thoughts of a more rapid death, and high scores are assigned to patients who reveal a marked fixation or active desire for death. Although this study represented a significant advance in assisted suicide research, by both exploring the construct of desire for hastened death as well as providing a method for its measurement, the DDRS is not without its limitations. Because this measure is rated by clinicians, training raters and establishing inter-rater reliability are crucial, increasing the burden for potential investigators. More importantly, the restricted range of possible scores substantially limits the data analytic methods available (Chochinov et al.[15] resolved this problem by dividing subjects into those who had a "significant and pervasive" desire for death and those who did not).

In response to the limitations of the DDRS, Rosenfeld and colleagues[16,17] developed a 20-item self-report scale of desire for hastened death, the Schedule of Attitudes toward Hastened Death (SAHD). This true–false questionnaire, which has been validated in samples of patients with acquired immunodeficiency syndrome (AIDS) and cancer, has been used as the primary dependent variable in several recent and ongoing research studies.[18] The self-report format and avoidance of questions regarding actual behaviors which may be illegal circumvent many of the practical and ethical issues noted above and have obvious appeal for large-scale research studies.

Unfortunately, studies of desire for hastened death are also not without limitations. Most importantly, perhaps, is the absence of empirical evidence that this construct corresponds to actual requests for assisted suicide or suicide attempts.

It is certainly possible that one might have a high desire for hastened death yet have no interest in expediting the dying process (e.g., for religious or moral reasons, family obligations). Conversely, it is widely acknowledged that not all requests for assisted suicide or suicide attempts reflect a genuine desire for death. Instead, patients may use discussions of assisted suicide as a method to convey their distress to a physician or family member or to exert some control over their illness, rather than genuinely wanting a more rapid death. Thus, although desire for hastened death offers an important alternative to studying requests for assisted suicide, substantial differences may emerge between these alternative approaches.

As the preceding discussion demonstrates, the choice of dependent variables in assisted suicide research clearly has significant ramifications for the interpretation of results. Reliance on overly simplistic questions may reflect a desire, whether conscious or unconscious, to avoid asking more direct but obviously sensitive questions. Studies of desire for death or requests for assisted suicide, however, may offer more relevant information with which to guide ethical debates and policy discussions.

Whom to Study, When, and Where (Sampling Issues)

Another broad area of concern in end-of-life research involves the determination of what populations are relevant to study. Unlike many areas of psychological research, investigating the preferences or beliefs of undergraduate students in large, Midwestern universities has thankfully never been the norm. Much of the research addressing end-of-life issues has relied on samples of elderly, medically ill, or healthcare providers, all of whom have obvious relevance to the legal and clinical issues involved. Nevertheless, many empirical studies have utilized readily available populations ("convenience samples"), often resulting in idiosyncratic samples whose representativeness or appropriateness may be quite limited.

Sample representativeness

Concerns regarding sample representativeness are hardly unique to end-of-life research, but these issues have been unusually prominent in the rapidly growing literature on physician-assisted suicide and desire for death. One reason for the frequent reliance on samples of limited appropriateness is the sensitive nature of questions regarding end-of-life issues. Concern that patients may become upset by being asked sensitive questions no doubt leads many researchers to exclude patients perceived as psychologically vulnerable. While excluding patients who might become distressed by research procedures is certainly logical and researchers as well as hospital institutional review boards should certainly be concerned about the potential for distress induced by research studies, excessive prescreening is likely to yield samples with systematic biases (for example, by eliminating a large proportion of the most psychologically distressed or vulnerable subjects). An example of this methodology is the study by Emanuel and colleagues,[4] in which they mailed questionnaires to a sample of oncology outpatients who had been selected by their oncologists (who had presumably been informed that the study concerned attitudes toward euthanasia). This sampling methodology not only is likely to underestimate opposition to euthanasia, since patients strongly opposed to euthanasia are unlikely to have been selected for participation by their physicians, but also probably under-represented patients with a high degree of psychological distress. While investigators cannot ignore the potential for distress in the course of their research, studies of assisted suicide and other end-of-life issues are particularly vulnerable to these biases because of the sensitive nature of the topics. Moreover, given that distress and depression are often variables of interest to researchers studying end-of-life issues, methodologies that restrict the variance of these important variables hinder the ability to uncover relationships that may exist. In our own research, we have found adverse reactions to be quite rare, with many patients reporting that they perceived benefits from having the opportunity to discuss end-of-life issues.[19] Hence, the avoidance of inclusive sampling methodologies may be based more on fear than on the actual likelihood of adverse reactions.

A related issue concerns the potential for differences among different types of terminal illness. For example, desire for death or decision making regarding physician-assisted suicide may be influenced by different factors among patients with ALS versus cancer or AIDS. Patients with ALS may be much more concerned about their potential for becoming a burden to others or losing control over their ability to commit suicide without assistance, whereas patients with cancer may be more motivated by a fear of uncontrolled pain. Patients with AIDS, however, may have considerably higher expectations (than other terminally ill populations) regarding the likelihood that treatment advances will improve their prognosis and consequently may be much less likely to desire hastened death, even in advanced stages, than patients with, for example, metastatic lung cancer. Thus, researchers not only must tailor their methodology to the needs and issues of the population they propose to study but also should consider how their results might differ with different populations.

Study setting

Determining the most appropriate setting in which to conduct research on desire for death and other end-of-life issues often presents a substantial obstacle. It is perhaps self-evident that the optimal setting for many end-of-life research questions involves studying terminally ill individuals. Unfortunately, many practical difficulties exist when studying terminally ill patients. For instance, such studies are most easily conducted in inpatient settings as traveling to the homes of terminally ill patients is both time-consuming and intrusive and many home-care patients are unable to attend outpatient clinic appointments. However, hospitalized patients likely represent the most physically ill and disabled subset of terminally ill individuals. Moreover, financial resources may be somewhat more limited among hospitalized patients as wealthy individuals who can afford extensive home care are less likely to require hospitalization for end-of-life care. Thus, important differences may exist between terminally ill patients in hospital settings and those at home, which may translate into significant differences in correlates and predictors of desire for death or interest in assisted suicide.

Institutional factors may also influence the results of studies of desire for hastened death and must be considered, both clinically and empirically, when interpreting findings. For example, studies conducted in facilities with intensive palliative care services or comprehensive mental health treatment may reveal little influence of these factors on desire for hastened death or interest in assisted suicide because the number of patients with inadequately controlled pain or untreated depression will likely be relatively low. Obtaining a broad spectrum of patients from multiple institutions is clearly beneficial for both ensuring sample representativeness as well as analyzing the influence of institutional differences on desire for a hastened death.

Study timing

Another issue in studying terminally ill populations concerns the timing of data collection. As medical illnesses progress, the likelihood of cognitive dysfunction, including both gradual cognitive deterioration (dementia) and transient episodes of confusion (delirium), increases as well. Not only is the accuracy of data gathered from cognitively impaired individuals questionable, but at times this impairment may be sufficiently severe as to hinder a patient's ability to provide valid informed consent. Hence, cognitive screening of potential study candidates is necessary to determine whether patients have sufficient cognitive capacity to participate in research. While screening out cognitively limited individuals may have implications for sample representativeness (particularly if cognitive functioning is one of the issues to be studied),[20] this issue may be less problematic in other areas of end-of-life research. Many legal and policy issues, such as physician-assisted suicide and other end-of-life decisions, require that patients be competent to make treatment decisions on their own behalf. Thus, the subset of patients who are cognitively intact enough to participate in research includes patients for whom these issues are relevant.

The potential (or likely) cognitive limitations present in many terminally ill individuals also impact the feasibility of conducting longitudinal research. Many important end-of-life research questions are longitudinal in nature, such as the stability of desire for hastened death and the impact of palliative care interventions on this desire. But subjects who are capable of participating at the outset of a longitudinal study may deteriorate before follow-up assessments are completed. While many statistical techniques have been developed to deal with subject attrition,[21] the volume of attrition in studies of terminally ill populations may be quite large, necessitating initial samples of considerable size to maintain adequate statistical power. While this problem can be minimized using relatively brief intervals between follow-up assessments (to minimize attrition due to cognitive deterioration or death), the likelihood of observing changes in patients' psychological and/or medical condition may decrease as the time intervals decrease. Balancing the trade-off between high attrition rates and limited opportunity for clinical changes is a difficult task, which will probably (and should likely) result in different methodologies depending on the specific study questions.

Confounding Factors in Variable Measurement

Another set of methodological issues in end-of-life research concerns the influence of confounding factors on variable measurement. An extreme example of confounding influences is the potential for cognitive impairment, which often accompanies terminal illness and, as noted above, can render data meaningless. Many other factors, often more subtle than extreme cognitive dysfunction, can adversely impact the accuracy of desire for death and assisted suicide research. While many of these influences can be addressed quite readily, others are more problematic and cannot necessarily be resolved per se.

Measuring depression and psychological distress

Depression is the single most frequently studied predictor variable in studies of desire for death and interest in physician-assisted suicide; but when the population studied is severely ill, medical symptoms can confound the assessment of depression, anxiety, and other psychological or psychiatric conditions. Symptoms such as fatigue, difficulty sleeping or concentrating, gastrointestinal problems, and weight loss are common sequelae of advanced medical illness and can artificially inflate ratings of psychological symptom severity. Clinical guidelines for assessing depression in medically ill patients have been offered,[22–24] but they have rarely been operationalized into empirical measures of depression or psychological adjustment that are not confounded by "medical" symptoms. Instead, most researchers have relied on traditional measures, either ignoring this potential confound or simply omitting items which might be the result of a medical illness (that is, somatic symptoms).

However, the validity of abbreviated measures of depression or anxiety has rarely been systematically studied, and some researchers have questioned the practice of distinguishing "somatic" symptoms from other symptoms of depression.[25] In addition, studies that have compared results based on both complete and abbreviated depression scales have reported roughly comparable findings for each, suggesting that removing somatic items from these rating scales does little to resolve any potential biases.[26] One alternative would be to use clinician-rated instruments, in which etiological distinctions (such as whether a given somatic symptom is due to depression or medical illness) may be possible; but this option assumes that etiological distinctions can be made reliably and accurately, an issue that has been largely untested.

Perhaps the most difficult confound in studies of desire for death and depression is suicidal ideation. While thoughts of suicide are typically considered a symptom of depression, this assumption is problematic for researchers attempting to disentangle the two constructs (particularly if one assumes that not all individuals who have thoughts of death and suicide are depressed). This confound is perhaps best exemplified by the research of Brown and colleagues,[27] in their study of depression and desire for death in hospitalized terminally ill patients. They found that 10 of the 44 patients interviewed had a desire for death, and all 10 were diagnosed with major depression. However, not only did they consider suicidal ideation and desire for death to be equivalent, but the same clinical data were used to make both assessments. Since the expression of thoughts of death or suicide was quite likely influential in forming clinicians' opinions regarding depression, particularly in the absence of a structured diagnostic interview, the high degree of overlap is hardly surprising. Without independent ratings of depression and desire for death, the concordance between depression and desire for death is of limited significance. One solution to this problem lies in the use of self-report measures since items reflecting suicidal ideation can (and in this context should) be omitted from a depression measure, minimizing the overlap between desire for death and depression (that is, items reflecting thoughts of death or suicide which may be present in both rating scales).

Measuring demographic variables

Research on assisted suicide and desire for death has consistently demonstrated a strong influence from two demographic variables: race and religion.[2,28] While understanding cultural influences on desire for death and interest in (or even approval of) assisted suicide is clearly important, research on end-of-life care issues has typically employed simplistic methods to classify these variables. Most studies simply classify individuals according to racial category or religious affiliation, ignoring the possibility that important differences exist within members of any particular religion or race. For example, religiously conservative individuals may be more opposed to assisted suicide than less religious individuals regardless of which particular religion they represent. While many studies simply treat religion as a categorical variable and ignore differences within any particular religion, more meaningful information might be gleaned from studies of religiosity or spirituality. Breitbart and colleagues[18] found a high negative correlation between desire for death and spiritual well-being, but spiritual well-being overlapped considerably with other measures of psychological distress (depression and hopelessness in particular). Many scales exist to study both religiosity and spirituality, but these measures have been virtually absent from the desire for death literature.[29,30]

Similarly, simple racial classifications (white, black, Hispanic, Asian) ignore the potential for differences within these broad categories. Instead, all members of a given race are assumed (de facto) to be ethnically similar to one another. More meaningful data might be obtained by measures of acculturation and ethnic identity,[31,32] but these measures have also been absent from the literature on end-of-life care. Nevertheless, the importance of racial differences in attitudes toward assisted suicide highlights the need for more careful attention to these demographic variables if researchers are to better understand the influence of ethnicity and culture on end-of-life attitudes and behaviors.

Statistical Considerations

Few experienced researchers would dispute the truism that statistical concerns are inherent in all social science research. Nevertheless, a number of issues have arisen with some frequency in the assisted suicide literature and warrant brief review. Among the most obvious problems in statistical analysis is lack of adequate sample size. Particularly in assisted suicide research, where the frequency of interest in assisted suicide or hastened death is relatively low, the need to conduct large-scale investigations has become increasingly apparent. Empirical studies of terminally ill cancer and AIDS patients have typically found rates of elevated interest in desire for death ranging from 8% to 15%.[15–17] Of course, studies relying on less rigorous dependent variables (such as hypothetical interest in assisted suicide in the future) have reported substantially higher proportions of interested subjects, but such findings highlight the inadequacy of hypothetical interest as a dependent variable and, therefore, do not resolve the issue of sample size. In fact, very large samples of potential participants are likely necessary to obtain an adequate sample of patients interested in hastened death, and multi-center studies may be necessary to obtain sufficient subject pools. In the absence of sufficiently large samples, investigators have been forced to rely on simple univariate analyses, while the potentially interesting results that might emerge from studies using more sophisticated methods (for example, structural equation modeling, cluster analysis) have been ignored.

Another limitation in much of the assisted suicide literature, as in many empirical studies, is the difficulty establishing causal relationships from cross-sectional or correlational data. Despite the general awareness among researchers of the limitations in correlational data, discussions often ignore the well-known adage that correlation does not imply causality. What does help to establish causality is the use of experimental or longitudinal designs, which can help to disentangle the relationship between relevant variables at baseline and later. Unfortunately, most experimental methodologies are impractical in end-of-life research because of obvious ethical concerns, and longitudinal studies have been rarely used (perhaps because of the difficulties noted above). Not surprisingly, studies that have used longitudinal designs[33] have typically focused on relatively healthy subjects. Longitudinal designs are obviously difficult with terminally ill subjects since many individuals will die or become increasingly cognitively impaired during the course of the study. Nevertheless, important findings have emerged from this limited literature. Ganzini and colleagues[34] reported that the end-of-life treatment decisions of severely depressed elderly patients changed substantially after they were treated for their depression. With sufficiently large samples to allow for the high rate of attrition which may occur and cognitive assessments prior to data collection at each assessment point, short-term longitudinal studies of assisted suicide may be feasible even in terminally ill populations or palliative care institutions. In addition, long-term longitudinal studies focusing on medically ill but relatively healthy individuals (that is, beginning shortly after diagnosis) are crucial to understand how attitudes toward assisted suicide or hastened death evolve over the course of illness.

Conclusion

The challenges to assisted suicide research highlighted above are numerous but hardly insurmountable. Specialized instruments such as the SAHD and DDRS should facilitate research, as has the legalization of assisted suicide in Oregon. Legalization offers unique opportunities for researchers to study individuals who actually seek assisted suicide instead of the hypothetical preferences frequently studied, and this research promises to yield important data to guide future policy debates. The opportunity to improve assisted suicide research, however, will be underutilized unless researchers begin to incorporate more rigorous methodologies that are designed to address the relevant clinical and policy issues. Public debate and scientific interest in assisted suicide have escalated rapidly over the past decade, but the amount of new and relevant information generated has not kept pace. Future researchers must address these pressing questions, to improve clinical and legal decision making around end-of-life issues.

References

1. Rosenfeld B. Assisted suicide, depression and the right to die. Psychol Public Policy Law 2000; 6:529–549.
2. Breitbart W, Rosenfeld BD, Passik SD. Interest in physician-assisted suicide among ambulatory HIV-infected patients. Am J Psychiatry 1996; 153:238–242.
3. Owen C, Tennant C, Levi J, et al. Suicide and euthanasia: patient attitudes in the context of cancer. Psychooncology 1992; 1:79–88.
4. Emanuel EJ, Fairclough DL, Emanuel LL. Attitudes and desires related to euthanasia and physician-assisted suicide among terminally ill patients and their caregivers. JAMA 2000; 284:2460–2468.
5. Suarez-Almazor ME, Belzile M, Bruera E. Euthanasia and physician-assisted suicide: a comparative survey of physicians, terminally ill cancer patients, and the general population. J Clin Oncol 1997; 15:418–427.
6. Emanuel EJ, Fairclough DL, Daniels ER, et al. Euthanasia and physician-assisted suicide: attitudes and experiences of oncology patients, oncologists, and the public. Lancet 1996; 347:1805–1810.

7. Ganzini L, Johnston WS, McFarland BH, et al. Attitudes of patients with amyotrophic lateral sclerosis and their care givers toward assisted suicide. N Engl J Med 1998; 339:967–973.

8. Lee MA, Smith DM, Fenn DS, et al. Do patients' treatment decisions match advance statements of their preferences? J Clin Ethics 1998; 9:258–262.

9. Van der Maas PJ, van Delden JJM, Pijnenborg L, et al. Euthanasia and other medical decisions concerning the end of life. Lancet 1991; 338:669–674.

10. Chin AE, Hedberg K, Higginson GK, et al. Legalized physician-assisted suicide in Oregon—the first year's experience. N Engl J Med 1999; 340:577–583.

11. Sullivan AD, Hedberg K, Fleming DW. Legalized physician-assisted suicide in Oregon—the second year. N Engl J Med 2000; 342:598–604.

12. Ganzini L, Nelson HD, Schmidt TA, et al. Physician' experiences with the Oregon Death with Dignity Act. N Engl J Med 2000; 342:557–563.

13. Lee BC, Werth Jr JL. Observations on the first year of Oregon's Death with Dignity Act. Psychol Public Policy and Law 2000; 6:268–290.

14. Back AL, Gordon JR. Clinician responses to requests for physician-assisted suicide: what to do and what not to do. Presented at the annual meeting of the American Academy of Forensic Sciences, Seattle, WA, Feb 19–24, 2001.

15. Chochinov HM, Wilson KG, Enns M, et al. Desire for death in the terminally ill. Am J Psychiatry 1995; 152:1185–1191.

16. Rosenfeld B, Breitbart W, Stein K, et al. Measuring desire for death among the medically ill: the Schedule of Attitudes toward Hastened Death. Am J Psychiatry 1999; 156:94–100.

17. Rosenfeld B, Breitbart B, Galietta M, et al. The Schedule of Attitudes toward Hastened Death: measuring desire for death in terminally ill cancer patients. Cancer 2000; 88:2868–2875.

18. Breitbart W, Rosenfeld B, Pessin H, et al. Depression, hopelessness, and desire for death in terminally ill cancer patients. JAMA 2000; 284:2907–2911.

19. Pessin H, Galietta M, Rosenfeld B. Burden and benefit of end-of-life research in the terminally ill. Presented at the European Association of Palliative Care, Lyon, France, May 25–26, 2002.

20. Pessin H. The impact of cognitive functioning on desire for death in terminally ill patients with AIDS. Dissertation Abstr Int 2001; 62:2963.

21. Schafer JL, Olsen MK. Multiple imputation for multivariate missing-data problems: a data analyst's perspective. Multivar Behav Res 1998; 33:545–571.

22. Chochinov HM, Wilson KG, Enns M, et al. Prevalence of depression in the terminally ill: effects of diagnostic criteria and symptom threshold judgments. Am J Psychiatry 1995; 151:537–540.

23. Lynch M. The assessment and prevalence of affective disorders in advanced cancer. J Palliat Care 1995; 11:10–18.

24. Massie MJ, Gagnon P, Holland JC. Depression and suicide in patients with cancer. J Pain Symptom Manage 1994; 9:325–340.

25. Passik S, Lundberg J, Rosenfeld B, et al. Factor analysis of the Zung self rating depression scale in a large ambulatory sample of oncology patients. Psychosomatics 2000; 41:121–127.

26. Rosenfeld B, Breitbart W, McDonald M, et al. Pain in ambulatory AIDS patients—II. Impact of pain on psychological functioning and quality of life. Pain 1996; 68: 323–328.

27. Brown JH, Henteleff P, Barakat S, et al. Is it normal for terminally ill patients to desire death? Am J Psychiatry 1986; 143:208–211.

28. Blendon RJ, Szalay US, Knox RA. Should physicians aid their patients in dying? JAMA 1992; 267:2658–2662.

29. Brady MJ, Peterman AH, Fitchett G, et al. A case for including spirituality in quality of life measurement in oncology. Psychooncology 1999; 8:417–428.

30. Gorsuch R, McPherson S. Intrinsic/extrinsic measurement: I/E-revised and single-item scales. J Sci Study Religion 1989; 28:348–354.

31. Helms JE, Parham TA. The development of the Racial Identity Attitude Scale. In: Jones RL, ed. Handbook of Tests and Measurements for Black Populations. Hampton, VA: Cobb and Henry, 1996:167–174.

32. Landrine H, Klonoff EA. The African-American Acculturation Scale: development, reliability, and validity. J Black Psychol 1994; 20:104–127.

33. Wolfe J, Fairclough DL, Daniels ER, et al. Stability of attitudes regarding physician-assisted suicide and euthanasia among oncology patients, physicians, and the general public. J Clin Oncol 1999; 17:1274–1279.

34. Ganzini L, Lee MA, Heintz RT, et al. The effect of depression treatment on elderly patients' preferences for life-sustaining medical therapy. Am J Psychiatry 1994; 151:1631–1636.

VIII

RESEARCH IN
PRACTICE CHANGE

20

Changing Palliative Care Practice in Academic Medical Centers

DAVID E. WEISSMAN

Efforts to change the culture and practice of medical care at the end of life are undergoing a revolution in the United States. Although many U.S. medical schools and some residency programs now teach some aspects of "death and dying," most have been slow to develop clinical, education, and research programs in end-of-life care.[1,2] Findings from the Study to Understand Prognoses and Preferences for Outcomes and Risks of Treatment (SUPPORT), the Institute of Medicine analysis of end-of-life care in the United States, and the increasing public sentiment in favor of physician-assisted suicide have given new impetus for a comprehensive overhaul of end-of-life medical education in the United States.[3–5]

End-of-life care is increasingly referred to as the discipline of palliative medicine or palliative care.[6–10] Palliative care includes assessment and management of pain and other physical symptoms; psychosocial and disposition problems affecting dying patients and the patient–family unit; ethical issues and communication skills related to end-of-life care; application of specific treatment modalities such as hydration, nonoral feeding, blood products, or radiotherapy; and after-death care. Over the past 7 years, there has been increasing interest in improving end-of-life care within medical schools as demonstrated by a new training requirement, new undergraduate courses, clinical end-of-life training experiences, and development of academic palliative care programs.[11–29] Similarly, there have been recent improvements in postgraduate end-of-life physician education, most notably in internal and family medicine training programs.[30–35] Finally, new standards have been developed for end-of-life physician education, new materials have been developed for educators, and efforts are under way to include end-of-life content on certification examinations.[36–43]

Despite the recent flurry of activity, much work remains. In this chapter, we review the barriers and opportunities to changing end-of-life care within the medical school environment.

Opportunities for Palliative Care within the Academic Medical Center

Throughout the 1970s and 1980s, the only reliable source for good end-of-life care in the United States was within the hospice movement, a medical construct that has not been wholly embraced by either academic or community medicine. Similarly, there have been no sustained research efforts in end-of-life care and only nascent attempts at comprehensive physician end-of-life medical education. However, the opportunities for palliative care to expand and flourish within academic medicine are tremendous. First, the academic environment is principally known as the starting point for medical research based on the scientific method. The need for palliative care research is obvious as the current state of end-of-life medical practice is largely based on empirical findings rather than solid clinical research. The academic environment is well established to promote clinical and basic research aimed at answering the pressing issues of clinical end-of-life care.

Second, the academic environment is the home for physician education, as well as education for nursing, pharmacy, and other allied health professional schools. Although the non-physician schools have distinct curriculum and practice opportunities separate from their physician colleagues, sharing a campus offers the potential to develop integrated health professional education in end-of-life care. In regard to physician education, the academic environment is certainly where new paradigms for physician end-of-life education can be explored and tested through rigorous research. Key domains for physician education research in end-of-life care include symptom assessment and treatment skills, communication skills, practice behavior, and faculty development.

Third, the academic environment offers rich opportunities for providing interdisciplinary clinical care, bringing together the best elements of technology-based medicine and the principles and practice of palliative care. This latter point is critical for the evolution of palliative care as a legitimate medical domain within American medicine as clinicians, especially during their training years, need to see the clinical practice of palliative care integrated with traditional high-technology medicine.

Finally, the development of palliative care clinical services, education, and research can serve as an ideal bridge to community practice and education. The academic medical center should be viewed as a leader in community end-of-life care, helping to translate new advances to all sites of community healthcare practice. Academic medical centers should embrace their community home hospice partners, building collaborative relationships that strive to develop seamless transitions of care between hospital and home.

Barriers to Palliative Care within the Academic Medical Center

There are a host of barriers to the full integration of palliative care within academic medicine (Table 20.1). The first set of barriers relate to the current cohort

Table 20.1. Barriers to improvement in end-of-life care within academic medicine

Faculty physicians
- Negative value of end-of-life care as an academic discipline
- Poor end-of-life knowledge and clinical skills
- Lack of incentives for excellent teaching
- Poor financial resources for basic/clinical research in end-of-life care

Medical education
- Lack of opportunities for interdisciplinary education
- Little recognition of the "informal" curriculum[44]
- Little recognition of the importance of personal reflection as an educational domain
- Poor integration of nonhospital care sites into the educational environment
- Lack of rigorous methods for trainee evaluation of end-of-life knowledge and skills

Healthcare environment
- Lack of institutional standards for end-of-life care
- Public expectation of miracles
- Over-reliance on technology-based medical care
- Cumbersome relationships between medical schools and affiliated hospitals
- No funding mechanism for palliative care
- Confusion regarding hospice versus palliative care

of academic physician faculty. The current teachers of future physicians have poor training in end-of-life care and, at many medical schools, relatively few incentives to become excellent teachers. Until recently, the little research money in end-of-life care and the seemingly negative value placed on it as a valid domain of academic inquiry led few academic physicians to consider an academic career based around end-of-life care.

A second set of barriers relates to the current system of physician education. There is little interdisciplinary education with nonphysician health professionals, no recognition of the influence of the informal curriculum on attitudes toward end-of-life care, poor integration of nonhospital care sites such as the home or long-term care setting, little evaluation of trainee communication skills, and little emphasis placed upon personal reflection as a valid subject of medical education.[44,45]

A third set of barriers reflect the overall academic environment: public expectation that the academic medical center is where miracles happen, an over-reliance on high-technology and subspecialized care compared to primary care, cumbersome relationships between medical schools and affiliated academic hospitals that inhibit rapid changes in clinical care, and a lack of institutional (hospital) standards for end-of-life care.

Priority Areas for Change in Palliative Care

There are four critical areas for changes in end-of-life care that involve the academic medical center: faculty development, physician education, interdisciplinary care, and basic/clinical research. While not exclusive, these four elements are essential to establish palliative care as a recognized and respected entity within academia.

Faculty development

Helping faculty gain new knowledge, confidence, and education skills in end-of-life care is critical before there will be substantial improvements in physician education and clinical practice. Faculty generally do not know what they do not know and, when tested, have poor skills and confidence in their end-of-life clinical abilities.[46,47] Critical to faculty development in the clinical aspects of end-of-life care is the complementary need to improve faculty skills in end-of-life medical education. Since a large portion of end-of-life education involves understanding personal attitudes and values (both of patients and of clinicians), faculty must understand how to assist students with this aspect of care through role modeling, small group and individual discussion, and timely and constructive feedback. In particular, faculty need to better assess their students in the domains of care that relate to communication skills and personal reflection.

Physician education—curriculum and evaluation

Physician education is still largely hospital-based, emphasizing specialty care within a high-technology environment. To truly integrate end-of-life care into academic medicine, the structure of physician education needs to change to better reflect the needs of patients and families at the end of life. Key learning domains include the recognition of death as a normal life-cycle event, pain and symptom management, communication skills, after-death care, and personal reflection. These domains need to be taught and evaluated in both hospital and nonhospital settings, the latter to include the common sites of death, the home and long-term care facility. Such integration should be longitudinal across all years of medical school and postgraduate training; training should be experiential and include interdisciplinary experiences.

Beyond improving clinical care, all of these topics represent tremendous opportunities for medical education research, particularly in the realm of learner evaluation. We still know fairly little about how best to evaluate trainee performance in such areas as symptom assessment and management skills or end-of-life communication skills: giving bad news, discussing treatment withdrawal, performing a spiritual assessment, and discussing hospice referral.

Interdisciplinary care

A common theme in the discussion about how to improve end-of-life care is that physicians do not understand, or appreciate, the role of other health professionals. Nurses, social workers, therapists, chaplains, pharmacists, and others have distinct and vital contributions that can improve end-of-life care. However, there are distinct cultures and hierarchies that separate physician education from these disciplines, with little emphasis placed on physicians learning to function as a co-equal, rather than dominant, member of the healthcare team. A significant challenge of the coming years is to break down the walls that separate physicians from other disciplines in a manner that can improve the educational process for all.

Basic and clinical research

Many questions remain to be answered about how best to care for the dying. Pain and symptom management, grief and bereavement support, doctor–patient communication, and delivery systems for end-of-life care are a few of the areas in need of careful research. End-of-life care desperately needs to establish a solid foundation of basic and clinical research, both to improve clinical care and to become recognized as a valid domain of intellectual inquiry. Fortunately, the past 5 years have seen a surge of research money for end-of-life care. This needs to be continued and expanded to allow for the growth of programs in palliative care research within academic medical centers.

Making Change in Academic Medicine

There are two broad approaches to making change in academic medical centers. The first, a *top–down approach*, is to enlist the support of senior change agents, for example, deans, the president, hospital management, and department chairs. The second method, a *bottom–up approach*, is to work for change through colleagues, course and clerkship directors, clinic managers, etc. Both methods have their utility; and to accomplish the greatest degree of change, one should strive to work through both avenues. At the beginning of the change process, it is often easiest to work via colleagues using the bottom–up approach as small changes requiring minimal resources (such as introducing a new lecture) are typically easiest to accomplish through this approach. Major changes, in particular those requiring financial resources for new personnel, space, and dedicated faculty time, require more senior, top–down support. The latter will typically insist on documentation of the need for change. Compared to 10 years ago, this is now easier to accomplish given the national guidelines, position statements, and policy documents that support the need for change within academic medicine.[22,29,36–40] On the local level, it may still be necessary to document that a problem exists. This can be done via patient satisfaction surveys and tests of knowledge, attitudes, and skills among trainees and faculty.

Another approach to change in the academic medical center involves the development of a system that actively supports good end-of-life care. Improving the clinical setting in which training and faculty physicians work in a manner that encourages excellent end-of-life care can be a powerful step. This concept has been explored as a means to improve pain management and ethical decision making in acute-care hospitals and can be adapted for other elements of end-of-life care, such as advance care planning, hospice referrals, and bereavement support.[48–60] The essential elements of an institutional plan for improved care include the following:

- Facility commitment: a clear commitment from hospital administrators that end-of-life care is a priority and that resources (staff, time, money) will be directed toward improving clinical care
- Assessment: a hospital- or health system-wide program of end-of-life care assessment and documentation
- Responsibility: a system to ensure that poorly managed end-of-life care is identified in a timely manner and that the underlying causes for such problems are corrected
- Education: programs for new and existing staff, as well as patients and families to provide education about end-of-life care
- Standards: explicit standards of care which outline staff responsibilities and expected patient outcomes

The single most important first step in this process is to obtain a strong institutional commitment as this approach to change is time- and labor-intensive. Institutional change of this type can be conceptualized in three semidistinct phases. Depending on the specific issue and institutional culture, transition between phases may be rapid or occur at a seemingly glacial pace. Phase I is when there is a need to demonstrate that a problem exists, when "buy-in" must be established. This phase is truly daunting but crucial to validate that end-of-life care is important and needs inclusion in education and clinical care activities. This process is typically led by one or a small group of champion(s).[57] Phase II represents a time when an initial buy-in has been established and the change process is enlarged to include new individuals beyond the original champions. This is a time of pilot projects, action plans, educational initiatives, and identification of needed resources. Phase III is the crucial step of translating pilot projects into sustainable programs that impact on the depth and breadth of an institution. This is when prior commitments of time and money must be actualized into specific work duties and tangible resources. There is no question that this approach can take many years to actualize, but it is probably far more efficient to design a care environment that supports and encourages best practice, rather than to focus solely on physician education as a means to effect clinical practice change.

Summary

The academic medical center represents the pinnacle of modern medical achievement over the past 100 years. Unfortunately, until very recently academic medical centers have ignored death as a life-cycle event and the attendant education and clinical care issues and opportunities. The time is at hand to make major reforms in how physicians view end-of-life care, a view that must begin within the academic center. In particular, promoting faculty development, new education and evaluation initiatives, interdisciplinary education, and basic and clinical research has the potential to greatly improve end-of-life care. These changes will require commitment and vision on the part of medical center leaders, hospital administrators, and senior faculty.

Acknowledgments

Dr. Weissman is a recipient of the Open Society Institute Project on Death in American Faculty Scholars Award.

References

1. Billings JA, Block S. Palliative care in undergraduate medical education. JAMA 1997; 278:733–743.
2. Barzansky B, Veloski JJ, Miller R, et al. Education in end-of-life care during medical school and residency training. Acad Med 1999; 74:S102–S104.
3. Committee on Care at the End of Life, Division of Health Care Services, Institute of Medicine, National Academy of Sciences. Approaching Death: Improving Care at the End of Life. Washington DC: National Academy of Sciences, 1997.
4. SUPPORT Principal Investigators. A controlled trial to improve care for seriously ill hospitalized patients. JAMA 1995; 274:1591–1598.
5. Meier DE, Morrison RS, Cassel C. Improving palliative care. Ann Intern Med 1997; 127:225–230.
6. MacDonald N, ed. The Canadian Palliative Care Curriculum. Toronto: Canadian Committee on Palliative Care Education, 1991.
7. Twycross RG. Palliative cancer care and its implications for national cancer policy. Presented at the Second WHO Workshop on National Cancer Control Policy Development, Vienna, Austria, June 6–8, 1990.
8. World Health Organization. Cancer Pain Relief and Palliative Care: Report of a WHO Expert Committee. Technical Report Series 804. Geneva: WHO, 1990.
9. Block S, Billings JA. Nurturing humanism through teaching palliative care. Acad Med 1998; 73:763–765.
10. Billings A. What is palliative care? J Palliat Med 1998; 1:73–81.
11. Walsh TD. Continuing care in a medical center: the Cleveland Clinic Foundation Palliative Care Service. J Pain Symptom Manage 1990; 5:273–278.
12. Abrahm J, Callahan K, Rossetti L, et al. Impact of a hospice consultation team on the care of veterans with terminal cancer. Proc American Society of Clinical Oncology 1994; 13:451.
13. Weissman DE, Griffie J. The Palliative Care Consultation Service of the Medical College of Wisconsin. J Pain Symptom Manage 1994; 9:474–479.

14. Weissman DE. Consultation in palliative medicine. Arch Intern Med 1997; 157: 733–737.
15. Bascom PB. A hospital-based comfort care team: consultation for seriously ill and dying patients. Am J Hospice Palliat Care 1997; 14:57–60.
16. Von Gunten CF, Von Roenn JH, Neely KJ, et al. Hospice and palliative care: attitudes and practices of the physician faculty of an academic hospital. Am J Hospice Care 1995; 12:38–42.
17. Carlson RW, Devich L, Frank RR. Development of a comprehensive supportive care team for the hopelessly ill on a university hospital medical center. JAMA 1988; 259:378–383.
18. Pawling-Kaplan M, O'Connor P. Hospice care for minorities: an analysis of a hospital-based inner city palliative care service. Am J Hospice Care. 1989; 6 :13–21.
19. Weissman DE, Griffie J. Integrating palliative medicine at the Medical College of Wisconsin 1990–1996. J Pain Symptom Manage 1998; 15:195–201.
20. Meekin SA, Klein JE, Fleischman AR, et al. Development of a palliative education assessment tool for medical student education. Acad Med 2000; 75:986–992.
21. Ury WA, Reznich CB, Weber CM. A needs assessment for a palliative care curriculum. J Pain Symptom Manage 2000; 20:408–416.
22. Nelson W, Angoff N, Binder E, et al. Goals and strategies for teaching death and dying in medical schools. J Palliat Med 2000; 3:7–16.
23. Buss MK, Marx ES, Sulmasy DP. The preparedness of students to discuss end-of-life issues with patients. Acad Med 1998; 73:418–422.
24. Steen PD, Miller T, Palmer L, et al. An introductory hospice experience for third-year medical students. J Cancer Educ 1999; 14:140–143.
25. Linder JF, Blais J, Enders SR, et al. Palliative education: a didactic and experiential approach to teaching end-of-life care. J Cancer Educ 1999; 14:154–160.
26. Ross DD, O'Mara A, Pickens N, et al. Hospice and palliative care education in medical school: a module on the role of the physician in end-of-life care. J Cancer Educ 1997; 12:152–156.
27. Ross DD, Keay T, Timmel D, et al. Required training in hospice and palliative care at the University of Maryland School of Medicine. J Cancer Educ 1999; 14: 132–136.
28. Ogle KS, Mavis B, Rohrer J. Graduating medical students' competencies and educational experiences in palliative care. J Pain Symptom Manage 1997; 14: 280–285.
29. Liaison Committee on Medical Education Accreditation Standards. http://www.lcme.org/standard.htm, 2001.
30. Weissman D, Ambuel B, Mullan P, et al. Postgraduate physician education [abstract]. J Palliat Care 2000; 16:83.
31. Mullan PB, Weissman DE, von Gunten C, et al. Coping with certainty: perceived competency vs. training and knowledge in end of life care. J Gen Intern Med 2000; 15(Suppl):40 (abstract).
32. Mullan PB, Weissman DE, von Gunten C, et al. End-of-life care education in internal medicine residency programs: an inter-institutional study. J Palliat Med 2002 (in press).
33. Ferris TG, Hallward JA, Ronan L, et al. When the patient dies: a survey of medical housestaff about care after death. J Palliat Med 1998; 1:231–239.

34. Hallenbeck JL, Bergen MR. A medical resident inpatient hospice rotation: experiences with dying and subsequent changes in attitudes and knowledge. J Palliat Med 1999; 2:197–208.
35. Weissman DE, Mullan PB, Ambuel B. End-of-life curriculum reform: outcomes and impact in a follow-up study of internal medicine residency programs. J Palliat Med 2002 (in press).
36. Simpson D. National consensus conference on medical education for care near the end-of-life. J Palliat Med 2000; 3:87–91.
37. Steel K, Ribbe M, Ahronheim J, et al. Incorporating education on palliative care into the long-term care setting. J Am Geriatr Soc 1999; 47:904–907.
38. Weissman DE, Block SD, Blank L, et al. Incorporating palliative care education into the acute care hospital setting. Acad Med 1999; 74:871–877.
39. Block SD, Bernier GM, Crawley LM, et al. Incorporating palliative care into primary care education. J Gen Intern Med 1998; 13:768–773.
40. Danis M, Federman D, Fins JJ, et al. Incorporating palliative care into critical care education: principles, challenges, and opportunities. Crit Care Med 1999; 27: 2005–2013.
41. Bowles T. USMLE and end-of-life care. J Palliat Med 1999; 2:3–4.
42. Emanuel LL, von Gunten CF, Ferris FD, eds. The EPEC curriculum: education for physicians on end-of-life care. www.EPEC.net, 1999.
43. Simpson DE, Rehm J, Biernat K, et al. Advancing educational scholarship through the End of Life Physician Education Resource Center (EPERC). J Palliat Med 1999; 2:421–424.
44. Hafferty FW, Franks R. The hidden curriculum, ethics teaching and the structure of medical education. Acad Med 1994; 11:862–871.
45. Nowack DH, Suchman AL, Clark W, et al. Calibrating the physician: personal awareness and effective patient care. JAMA 1997; 278:502–509.
46. Weissman DE. A faculty development course for end-of-life care. J Palliat Med 1998; 1:35–44.
47. von Gunten CF, Von Roenn JH, Johnson-Neely K, et al. Hospice and palliative care: attitudes and practices of the physician faculty of an academic hospital. Am J Hospice Palliat Care 1995; 12:38–42.
48. Jacox A, Carr DB, Payne R, et al. Management of Cancer Pain. Clinical Practice Guideline 9. AHCPR Publication 94-0592. Rockville, MD: Agency for Health Care Policy and Research, U.S. Department of Health and Human Services, Public Health Service, 1994.
49. Greco PJ, Eisenberg JM. Changing physicians' practices. N Engl J Med 1993; 329: 1271–1274.
50. Weissman DE. Cancer pain education for physicians in practice: establishing a new paradigm. J Pain Symptom Manage 1996; 12:364–371.
51. Gordon DB, Dahl JL, Stevenson KK, eds. Building an Institutional Commitment to Pain Management. Madison: Wisconsin Cancer Pain Initiative, 1996.
52. Weissman DE. Educating home health professionals in cancer pain management. Home Health Care Consultant 1995; 2:10–18.
53. Weissman DE, Dahl JL. Update on the Cancer Pain Role Model Education Program. J Pain Symptom Manage 1995; 10:292–297.
54. Ferrell BR, Dean GE, Grant M, et al. An institutional commitment to pain management. J Clin Oncol 1995; 13:2158–2165.

55. Gordon DB. Critical pathways: a road to institutionalizing pain management. J Pain Symptom Manage 1995; 11:252–259.

56. Bookbinder M, Coyle N, Kiss M, et al. Implementing national standards for cancer pain management: program model and evaluation. J Pain Symptom Manage 1996; 12:334–347.

57. Weissman DE, Griffie J, Gordon DB, et al. A role model program to promote institutional changes for management of acute and cancer pain. J Pain Symptom Manage 1997; 14:274–279.

58. Solomon MZ, Jennings B, Guilfoy R, et al. Toward an expanded vision of clinical ethics education: from the individual to the institution. Kennedy Inst Ethics J 1991; 1:225–245.

59. Holloran SD, Starkey GW, Burke PA, et al. An educational intervention in the surgical intensive care unit to improve ethical decisions. Surgery 1995; 118:294–299.

60. Dowdy MD, Robertson C, Bander JA. A study of proactive ethics consultation for critically and terminally ill patients with extended lengths of stay. Crit Care Med 1998; 26:252–259.

21

Changing Pain Management Practices in Hospitals and Cancer Centers

MARILYN BOOKBINDER AND NESSA COYLE

Undertreatment of pain continues throughout the world. It is estimated that 34 million people in the United States suffer from chronic pain and that millions seek relief in hospitals, pain clinics, and cancer centers. Hospitalized patients with pain, however, continue to be inadequately managed, despite the availability of safe and effective treatments.[1,2] This chapter will familiarize the reader with the efforts of today's clinicians as they work toward achieving "best practices" in pain management. Whether the change in practice is targeted toward a small 200-bed community hospital or a large 800-bed comprehensive cancer center, the process of achieving best practices is similar: it requires champions, who build teams and use a systematic process to solve problems, seek evidenced-based solutions, and recognize the need for long-term evaluations.

The underpinning for this chapter is that through implementation of standards, such as the American Pain Society (APS) Quality Improvement Guidelines for the Treatment of Acute and Cancer Pain,[3] the Agency for Healthcare Research and Quality (AHRQ) Guidelines for Cancer Pain,[1,2] and new Joint Commission of Accreditation of Hospitals Organization (JCAHO) pain standards,[4] cancer centers and hospitals have the potential to improve pain management for all patients. We draw from the experience and knowledge of clinicians throughout the United States and around the world. We present three hospitals at varying levels of practice in implementing APS standards to illustrate the challenges and strategies faced by clinicians as they improve pain management at the point of service.

Examples of Three Hospitals' Pain Management Practices

In this section, we describe three hospitals at varying levels of implementing the five APS standards. Hospital 1 illustrates "exemplar" institutional practices. The

APS standards have been fully implemented and efforts continue to refine and improve pain control. Hospital 2 is "getting there" and struggling to put systems in place which will assure routine adoption of standards. Hospital 3 uses a "Band-Aid approach." There is minimal awareness of national standards, with pain improvement efforts driven by crisis events rather than a planned change approach.

Hospital 1: exemplar

Our exemplar hospital, described in Table 21.1, is the "gold standard." They have fully implemented the five APS standards: (1) pain is recognized and treated promptly, and levels have been established to trigger review; (2) information about analgesics is readily available; (3) patients are promised attentive analgesic care; (4) explicit policies have been defined for the use of advanced analgesic technologies; and (5) adherence to standards of care is monitored and patient satisfaction surveyed.[3]

Hospital 1 has an interdisciplinary team, which includes experts in the fields of pain, education, clinical practice, administration, pharmacy, and process evaluation. This hospital perceives itself as a "self-evaluating organization," that is, one that encourages performance improvement efforts that are driven by issues identified at the grass roots level and a high priority for quality patient care, in this case pain management. Implementation of the five APS standards is facilitated by administrative support (encouragement through validation of the team's progress) and assistance (providing essential resources, such as a designated Pain Clinical Nurse Specialist and educational efforts) coupled with multidisciplinary experts in pain management who are available to educate, implement, and reinforce new knowledge on a daily basis.

Challenges and strategies

Hold gain. The greatest challenge for the exemplar institution, once standards have become the "institutional norm"and integrated into routine care, is to keep the momentum and creative efforts of the program alive and well integrated, at both the hospital-team level and the unit level. The concept of holding gain is an important one because new unit priorities and other innovations will compete for the attention and energies of staff.

Qualities developed by the team at the exemplar institution are important to describe as they will contribute to future success. This team has learned the core elements of team building and has good meeting and delegating skills (for example, agenda setting, rules for decision making, keeping records of the process). They have developed educational materials for professionals, patients, and families and have a monitoring system with accountability in place to ensure that standards continue to be met. They have learned that routine pain assessment promotes early recognition and management of pain, as well as other symptoms affecting the patient's quality of life, such as depression or fatigue. Pain does not occur in isolation, and frequently there are multiple other symptoms that effect the patient's quality of life. Through the assessment of pain, a window opens, broadening the perspective of clinical assessment. The exemplar institution learns how to use the pain model as the template to address other symptoms.

One strategy to hold gain, used at a major cancer center, is described below. A continuous quality-improvement (CQI) pain team broadened its mission from pain to "pain and palliative care." Hospital administration acknowledged the team's achievements of (1) improving pain management institution-wide, (2) creating a benchmark for others to implement national pain standards, and (3) developing a template for improving other distressing patient symptoms, including those at the end of life.[5]

A second strategy to hold gain was to reassign pain Advanced Practice Nurses (APNs) at the point of service to maintain clinical expertise and quality patient care by educating, role modeling, and mentoring nursing staff. The APNs worked with unit managers to assure that quality thresholds were met and to develop other studies to improve symptom management and quality of life. The team was also asked to submit additional items related to pain to the hospital's patient satisfaction survey. Because of this, unit leaders were assured of a routine monitoring and feedback system about this important indicator of quality care used by accredited institutions.

The third and most important strategy for this interdisciplinary team to continue improvements was to expand the team's influence. Members became a steering committee for hospital-wide pain management and broadened their efforts to pain and palliative care. The team assumed leadership at the grass roots level by providing mentoring, support, coaching, and assistance to staff in developing their own unit-based projects related to pain. These projects, or "spin-offs," occur after hospital-wide standards are routine practice, are usually more focused, and examine well-defined groups. Staff selected areas to study that were relevant to their patient population and unit-specific problems with managing pain. These spin-off projects can make a vital difference in how pain is managed for individual patients.

In one spin-off study, patients' pain experiences were examined from the day of discharge to the first postoperative visit, 2 weeks later. Areas examined included patient's discharge instructions, level of pain on discharge, the analgesic prescribed, whether a follow-up system was in place to assess the adequacy of pain relief and the presence of side effects, and if used, the timeliness and effectiveness of the response.[6] In addition to learning that patients were undertreated for pain on discharge, clinicians found that few patients were prescribed treatment for constipation to accompany opioids.

Another example of a spin-off is a study related to procedural pain, inserting chest tubes in which pain and anxiety levels were significantly reduced following implementation of a standardized approach involving surgeons, nurses, and patients. The intervention involved addressing the patient's anxiety before, during, and after the procedure and addressing the pain incurred by the procedure.

Table 21.1. Three levels of implementation of the five American Pain Society quality improvement standards for acute pain and cancer pain: hospital 1, the exemplar

Standard 1a: Recognize and treat pain promptly: chart and display pain intensity and relief	Standard 1b: Establish levels to trigger review	Standard 2: Make information about analgesics readily available	Standard 3: Promise patients attentive analgesic care	Standard 4: Define explicit policies for the use of advanced analgesic technologies	Standard 5: Monitor adherence to standards: survey patient satisfaction
Routine screening done each shift (or outpatient visit) using a numeric (0 = no pain, 10 = worst) or categorical scale (none, mild, moderate, severe)	Red flags for pain intensity, relief, and distressing treatment side effects are agreed upon and algorithms developed to direct actions	Institutional commitment provides resources to educate all staff and a schedule for implementation and accountability	Pain assessed on admission and at each outpatient visit	New technologies, including neuroaxial interventions for acute and chronic pain syndromes, sought out and evaluated for use in specific populations; policies created for safe and effective use	An interdisciplinary team, including evaluation and quality improvement experts, routinely review hospital patient satisfaction data and disseminate findings to leadership teams at the unit level
Pain scales translated into the most common languages spoken by patients	Pain intensity ≥ 5 on two consecutive readings, inadequate relief of pain, or distressing side effects	Expert clinicians available at the unit level for consultation, education, and mentorship	Patients taught from admission that pain is an important aspect of care that needs to be treated and that staff will routinely ask if they have pain	A system is in place which ensures that necessary equipment is available to meet patient needs	Areas needing improvement identified at both the administrative and unit levels and more focused studies are developed
Pain intensity scores charted on vital signs sheet (or flow sheet)		Evidence-based educational programs attended by >80% of all staff	Patients taught how to communicate level of pain, effectiveness of treatment, duration of effect, and presence of distressing side effects		
Routine screening for analgesic side effects and level of		Multiple techniques used to increase dialogue about pain (videotape series, pain rounds, case-based teaching, focus groups, journal	Constipation addressed in all patients on chronic opioid therapy; patients given written information on discharge about their analgesic regimen, when and who to call, with the name of a		

associated patient distress

Comprehensive assessment and reassessment of pain, relief, and side effects charted in patient record (>90%)

clubs)

Ongoing continuing education provided for unit-specific needs and goals (improving pain control during chest tube insertion)

Internet access available for literature searches and website access

resource person to contact for assistance

Patients with chronic pain instructed to keep a daily diary on activities, level of pain, sleep; diaries used by clinicians to identify patterns of pain and interference with quality of life

Outpatient costs of analgesics considered in developing a discharge plan, and steps taken to ensure that medications and equipment are available and affordable to patients

Clinicians focus on pain relief while addressing known patient barriers (physical and psychological dependence, tolerance)

Patients at risk for poorly managed pain at home (elderly, cognitively impaired) routinely monitored through phone calls and appropriate referrals to the community

House staff were trained by the Thoracic Service to use a protocol including an-xiolytics before the procedure, the technique for inserting the chest tube, and the local and systemic analgesics to be given in preparation for the procedure. Nurses were taught anxiety-reducing techniques, including relaxation and the need for continuous communication and feedback from patients about comfort and distress. As a result of this spin-off study, standing orders for the insertion of chest tubes were developed for physicians and nurses and patients' pain and anx-iety levels averaged less than 3 on a 0 (no pain) to 10 (worst pain) rating scale.[7]

Disseminate knowledge gained. A second challenge for hospital 1 is to dis-seminate state-of-the-art pain management information to other professionals and the public both within and outside the institution. Strategies to meet this challenge include (1) offering observership and fellowship programs; (2) devel-oping web sites with state-of-the art information; (3) participating in pain spe-cialty organizations, universities and community initiatives at local, state, na-tional, and international levels to develop standards, position papers, curricula, and research programs; and (4) lecturing and publishing on topics which move the field of pain and symptom management forward.

Hospital 2: getting there

Hospital 2 is "getting there," and implementing the five APS standards is a strug-gle. In this large general hospital, the prevalence of pain has not been established and there is no professional group designated and accountable for addressing housewide pain issues. Reports from the hospital's quality improvement (QI) de-partment reveal less than adequate patient satisfaction with pain management and lower satisfaction scores than their regional and local counterparts. In hos-pital 2, standards for pain management are written into policy and procedure manuals; however, the consequences of not meeting expected levels remain un-clear, and enforcement of accountability at the unit level is inconsistent.

Table 21.2 shows that in hospital 2 nurses assess pain on admission, but re-assessment is inconsistent; also, no automatic action steps are in place to address inadequate pain relief. The focus of pain management activities has been on acute postoperative pain, with limited attention to the management of chronic pain, pain treatment side effects, and discharge planning for someone with chronic pain.

Challenges and strategies

Expand team effectiveness. The first challenge for this hospital is to examine the composition of their pain team and to expand it to one which is interdiscipli-nary in nature, emphasizing accountability at the grass roots level. While the structure of the team may vary based on purpose, objectives, goals, and available resources, research suggests that teams which originate from QI efforts, pain ser-vices, and educational programs have the greatest likelihood of improving pain management.

Table 21.2. Three levels of implementation of the five American Pain Society quality improvement standards for acute pain and cancer pain: hospital 2, getting there

Standard 1a: Recognize and treat pain promptly: chart and display pain intensity and relief	Standard 1b: Establish levels to trigger review	Standard 2: Make information about analgesics readily available	Standard 3: Promise patients attentive analgesic care	Standard 4: Define explicit policies for the use of advanced analgesic technologies	Standard 5: Monitor adherence to standards: survey patient satisfaction
Routine screening for pain is inconsistent (<60%) Routine screening for distressful side effects is rare Recording of initial pain assessment and side effects present but reassessment of effectiveness of intervention lacking	No consistent or agreed-upon guidelines for changing the course of action related to pain or side effect treatment Random reviews of effectiveness of pain and side effects usually occur when patient is in crisis	A commitment is made, but expertise in implementation is not available Agency for Health Care Policy and Research guidelines, pain education videotapes, and resource manuals are available but not used	Pain assessed on admission mission statements and Bill of Rights Patients taught how to communicate their pain intensity using a number scale or word descriptors Progress notes occasionally include effectiveness of treatment using intensity or word descriptors Minimal recognition of the need for a laxative regimen when patients are receiving chronic opioid therapy Discharge instructions give basic information about all medications and rarely individualize opioid therapy and the use of rescue doses according to the pattern of pain (such as the use of rescues to prevent activity-related breakthrough pain) Patients at risk for poorly managed pain at home (elderly, cognitively impaired) not routinely identified	Generic policies and procedures available for acute pain services and interventions only Use of advanced technology in chronic pain management rarely considered as an option	Patient satisfaction surveys routinely conducted by hospital administration, but no specific items address pain management Hospital espouses a performance improvement process but few staff are aware, of or use it

Determine the scope of the pain problem and where to begin. The second challenge for hospital 2 is to identify the scope of the problem of pain in the institution. An initial approach is to use the literature to identify specific disease groups and populations known to be at highest risk, to be most vulnerable, and to have the highest prevalence of pain. Populations include those with cancer, acquired immunodeficiency syndrome (AIDS), sickle cell disease, and other chronic debilitating illnesses; children; the elderly; the cognitively impaired; and the dying.

Results of the following studies show the value of QI work in reducing pain and raising standards of care. Grant et al.[8] identified the need for improved hospital policies related to discharge planning, analgesic prescribing, and resources once home. By implementing a Pain Resource Nurse program, the authors were able to significantly reduce admissions for uncontrolled pain within one year. In another study, pharmacy and nursing staff initiated a study team to examine the efficacy and use of fentanyl patches. The team produced a standardized protocol for patient care, educational materials for easier conversion of opioids, and a significant cost savings.[9]

Once patients are identified, the appropriate clinicians can be targeted. Because patients may be either scattered throughout the institution or on specific units, the team may need assistance from those with access to the hospital's information systems and databases. With this information, the team can select a population to target, such as those with AIDS, cancer, cognitive impairment, or sickle cell disease or those in pediatrics. Because patients, such as those with sickle cell disease, may be frequently admitted to several units (emergency departments, medical floors, obstetrics, and pediatrics), the team will need to bring representatives from all areas together and brainstorm about where to focus their work, in one, some, or all areas. Factors to be considered in making these decisions center around "readiness" and include (1) the extent of staff dissatisfaction with pain management, (2) the priority of pain relief in relation to other unit priorities, (3) the presence of a champion(s) or designated leader who can lead a change effort at the grass roots level, and (4) the extent of resources and administrative support available.

Implement pain standards. Once populations and staff champions are identified, the third challenge for this team is to devise strategies to implement the five APS standards in their respective populations. They will need to address the following: (1) Do standards currently exist? Where will assessment be recorded, how often, and by whom? What are the triggers for inadequate pain relief, who is accountable, and who will be called to assist in solving problems? (2) What staff education is needed and how will it be provided? (3) What patient and family education is needed and how will it be provided? (4) How will new technologies for pain management be integrated into practice, who will set policies and procedures, and how will competency be measured? (5) How will adherence to standards and patient satisfaction and other outcomes be monitored and measured?

Several well-recognized models are available for teams in this situation, such as the Pain Resource Nurse Program from Wisconsin,[10] and the Pain Management program using QI methods from Memorial Sloan-Kettering Cancer Center (MSKCC), New York.[11] Resources are also available from established resource centers funded by The Mayday Fund (mayday_pain@smtplinkcoh.org, mayday@ bethisraelny.org); these are national clearinghouses for pain information and excellent comprehensive resources for the team in developing a program.

Hospital 3: the Band-Aid approach

Hospital 3 uses a "Band-Aid" approach to solving hospitalwide pain management problems. At this large hospital, an acute pain service manages postoperative pain but may or may not be consulted in the management of other types of pain. Routine screening for the presence of pain and access to experts are inconsistent. The APNs may use APS or Agency for Health Care Policy and Research (AHCPR) pain management guidelines to address the needs of individual patients, but there is no standard for management of cancer pain or nonmaliganant pain syndromes or continuity of care among different settings or populations.

Systemwide and professional barriers may contribute to difficulties in implementing APS standards. For example, pain relief may not be given a high priority, routine screening for pain may not be an institutional standard, patient access to pain treatment may not be assured, ongoing pain education may not be available within the institution for clinicians (physicians and nurses), and lines of accountability for adequacy of pain relief and follow-through when relief is not acceptable may not be clearly stated. Further, concerns about potential problems associated with the use of opioid drugs, such as addiction, respiratory depression, and other side effects, may take priority with staff over that of achieving good pain relief. Finally, concerns about the scrutiny and regulation around controlled substances may influence pescribing habits[2] and create barriers to patients' right to pain relief.

Table 21.3 shows that in hospital 3 the routine systems for assessment, treatment, education, and evaluation of pain management are not in place. Although some clinicians attempt to improve pain management, this is done on a case-by-case basis, rather than through a systems approach. In the absence of a team, single clinicians, often APNs, have successfully championed efforts on one unit or with one population to improve pain management.[12]

Challenges and strategies

Take the lead. The first challenge for hospital 3 is for someone (such as a pain Clinical Nurse Specialist or physician) to take the lead in building a team and setting goals for each APS standard. The strategy to accomplish these goals, whether clinicians are lone champions or members of teams, is to use a systematic process to guide and evaluate any improvement efforts. Quality improvement

Table 21.3. Three levels of implementation of the five American Pain Society quality improvement standards for acute pain and cancer pain: hospital 3, the Band-Aid approach

Standard 1a: Recognize and treat pain promptly: chart and display pain intensity and relief	Standard 1b: Establish levels to trigger review	Standard 2: Make information about analgesics readily available	Standard 3: Promise patients attentive analgesic care	Standard 4: Define explicit policies for the use of advanced analgesic technologies	Standard 5: Monitor adherence to standards: survey patient satisfaction
No proactive screening to identify patients with pain intensity, relief, or side effects Pain assessment recorded only in patients known to have pain Recording of pain assessment inconsistent (<60%)	No guidelines to direct course of action related to pain or side effect treatment Review of effectiveness of pain and side effects primarily when patient is in crisis	Lack of awareness at the leadership level about the resources and expertise required to implement a hospital-wide pain program Pain clinicians available primarily for troubleshooting; unit-level mentorship rare Resource materials scant Pain education episodic and without implementation of continuing education for staff	Pain assessment included on admission history Patients not taught how to communicate their pain intensity, with a rare note on effectiveness of treatment Discharge instructions give basic information about scheduled analgesic doses Clinicians' fears about the addicting properties of drugs interfere with management and achieving pain relief	Policies available for acute postoperative pain management only	Patient satisfaction surveys not routinely conducted Quality improvement efforts aimed at meeting Joint Commission of Accreditation of Hospitals Organization minimal requirements Although no specified team is accountable for measuring patient outcomes related to pain, individual clinicians have Agency for Health Care Policy and Research guidelines and an expert team to guide best practice

methodologies, such as the FOCUS-PDCA,[13] and PDSA[14] have been effective at improving pain management practices within institutions.

Follow a systematic improvement process. The acronym *FOCUS-PDCA* represents a nine-step improvement method used by the authors at MSKCC. A similar approach, Plan-Do-Study-Act (PDSA), has been used extensively in regional QI collaboratives sponsored by the Institute for Healthcare Improvement (IHI) and the Center to Improve Care of the Dying.[14]

Although pain management has been identified by the clinician as a process for improvement, the segment of the pain process to be examined is not yet clearly delineated. Such delineation includes (*1*) the beginning and ending boundaries of the project (pain management from discharge from hospital to first clinic visit), (*2*) the population, (elderly or colon cancer), (*3*) outcomes (satisfaction with pain relief, reducing incidence of constipation, improving clinician knowledge), and (*4*) significance of the pain problem to the institution (no data available about adequacy of pain relief or associated side effects, improve patient satisfaction).

The clinician will need to recruit a team composed of staff who have knowledge about the process to be improved. Because pain is multidimensional and crosses departmental boundaries, an interdisciplinary team is needed. Members selected for the team should include not only those who understand the pain process but also those who can assist in data analysis and evaluating patient outcomes and are influential in changing the system. For example, to reduce the delay time in delivery of IV patient controlled analgesia (PCA) solutions to units, a team would need to include secretaries who transcribe medication orders, messengers who deliver drugs, and nurses.

The team will need to clarify what is currently known by gathering baseline data about the process. Several strategies for collecting data can be used. One approach is to use existing information from one of the hospital's databases. In our case above, the pharmacy might obtain the number and types of solution used for IV PCA by unit. These data could be used to determine if a par stock on key units could reduce one aspect of delays. Other approaches to gathering baseline data include conducting a 1-day cross-sectional "snapshot" of the prevalence of pain of all patients within the unit, auditing patient charts to assess the prevalence and characteristics of pain in oncology patients, and asking patients about their experience with pain and pain relief using survey or focus group techniques.

Flowcharting and brainstorming are useful techniques in understanding the underlying root causes of why variations in the process occur. For example, brainstorming the reasons why pain assessment is not recorded consistently may reveal multiple causes, directing the team to develop specific strategies. Causes may include lack of an agreed-upon pain rating scale, lack of a standardized pain flow sheet, and lack of communication with patients about an acceptable level of pain relief. In some situations, the team can develop immediate answers, known as "quick-fix" solutions. Longer-term solutions, however, which are the focus of this team, require continuing evaluation, the final step of the FOCUS-PDCA cycle, to standardize practices and reach improvement goals.

If the team has sufficient baseline data about the process to be improved, for example, 35% adherence to pain screening and reassessment on all shifts, an intervention can be developed and implemented and the PDCA cycle can be used to evaluate the effects. Interventions to improve pain screening and assessment include (1) selecting a pain rating scale that elicits patient self-report; (2) developing a standardized pain flow sheet; (3) educating staff and patients about the use of the tool; (4) setting a pain rating goal with patients that allows for comfort, sleep, and performance of activities that are important to daily life; (5) developing a plan for pain assessment that crosses the continuum of care (that is, through hospital, home care, ambulatory care, and nursing home care). At this point in the process, subcommittees may be needed to develop strategies for implementing each standard. For example, subcommittee 1 could address assessment and levels to trigger a review; subcommittee 2, the education of patients, families, and staff; subcommittee 3, policies and procedures, algorithms for pain relief, or care paths to establish standardization in using equipment and other aspects of pain care; and subcommittee 4, evaluation of standards. These authors suggest a fifth subcommittee, called "implementation," to design methods to assess the extent to which the intervention is being implemented as planned and address to barriers as they arise.

The four steps in the PDCA cycle, Plan-Do-Check-Act, also referred to as PDSA, Plan-Do-Study-Act, form the evaluative phase of the process. This phase is repeated until the desired end points are reached. Studies indicate that it takes 18 months on average to achieve adherence to pain screening standards of 90% in large (500- to 750-bed institutions). The team will need to develop a timeline for carrying out activities, a data collection tool, and a central database for compiling data and generating reports. They will plan for when, how, and who will collect data. The team will need to establish benchmarks for each outcome and decide at what threshold the team should reconvene and re-examine the process.

The motivating question "What can you do by Tuesday morning?" has been shown to accelerate the change process in the IHI collaboratives. In this model, teams are designated by administration, providing the initial buy-in and support for the effort. Teams are coached by an IHI faculty member for 1 year at three 1-day educational sessions, on-line discussion groups, on-site visits by faculty, and telephone conference calls on frequently discussed topics, such as advance directives and pain and symptom management. In the first part of the process, teams set aims, measure changes, and decide whether or not they represent a change.

Figure 21.1 shows the general approach to sequential PDSA cycles. Teams are encouraged to make small changes rapidly and, once met, to repeat the PDSA cycle with the next phase of the process or move to another process. This

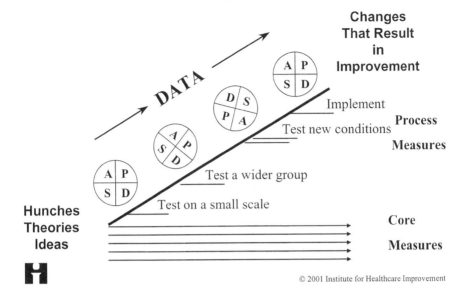

Figure 21.1. Measures and repeated use of the cycle.

method has helped many teams achieve positive results within weeks to months. Examples of studies can be found in *Improving Care for End-of-Life: A Source-book for Healthcare Managers and Clinicians*.[14] Encouraging teams to reach their targeted goals quickly reinforces team building and motivates them to examine other processes.

Link with peer groups. The third challenge for hospital 3 is to locate experts in the community who will provide ongoing knowledge and support during the process of change. Table 21.4 summarizes the challenges and strategies for the three hospitals implementing new standards. Table 21.5 offers examples of web-sites, listserves, and resources for those interested in pain and palliative care. Local assistance and materials can be found by joining professional organizations specializing in pain management, such as the Oncology Nursing Society, American Society for Pain Management Nurses, and the APS. More distant experts and resources can be located through the Internet and web pages such as www.stoppain.org and www.coh.org, where distance learning and teleconferences can provide specialized education, support, and access to pain resources. Yet another opportunity for clinicians can be found through private funders. For example, clinicians can receive one-to-one assistance for their initiative by applying to www.oncolink.org or www.stoppain.org for observerships and work-study programs. Awardees receive research and biostatistical assistance as they build a team to create changes in pain management practices.

Table 21.4. Challenges and strategies for three hospitals implementing American Pain Society quality improvement standards for the treatment of acute and cancer pain

Hospital	Challenges	Strategies
Hospital 1: the exemplar	Hold gain	Expand pain team to pain and palliative care
		Decentralize clinical expertise to unit level for quality control, role modeling, education, and mentoring
		Promote spin-off studies targeting specific populations/issues within settings
	Disseminate findings	Offer observerships, fellowships
		Participate in developing position papers, standards, curricula, and national policy committees
		Distribute resources through websites and access to expert materials
		Lecture, publish in field
Hospital 2: getting there	Expand team effectiveness	Examine composition of pain team and expand to multidisciplines
	Determine scope of pain problem and where to begin	Review related literature
		Access the hospital's databases
		Identify populations at high risk or problem-prone
		Identify champions to lead the effort
	Initiate parallel subcommittees to develop strategies for implementing American Pain Society standards	Team 1: Where will pain screening and assessment be recorded? Who is acountable?
		Team 2: What education is needed for staff, patients, families? Who will provide it?
		Team 3: How will new technologies/techniques in pain management be integrated? Who will develop new policies and procedures?
		Team 4: How will adherence to standards be monitored and patient outcomes measured?
	Evaluate results	Provide support and assistance to ensure successful implementation
Hospital 3: the Band-Aid	Take the lead	Decide to be a champion, find your own team
	Follow a systematic process to evaluate and improve pain management (FOCUS-PDCA)	**F**ocus on a pain management process which is feasible and targeted to a selected practice area
		Organize a team
		Clarify what is known (review literature, such as, guidelines, hospital patient satisfaction data)
		Understand the variation (brainstorm to identify barriers)
		Select an improvement (implementing the American Pain Society quality improvement standards)
		Plan/**D**o/**C**heck/**A**ct (gather baseline data through chart audit, prevalence study)
	Link with peer groups	Join national pain organizations and special interest groups, connect to internal and external experts for continued education and support
		Access pain education and experts through distance learning opportunities, teleconferences, listserves, and state coalitions

Table 21.5. Selected website resources in pain management and chemical dependence

1. Agency for Health Care Policy and Research
   http://www.ahcpr.gov
2. American Academy of Pain Management
   http://www.aapainmanage.org/index.html
3. American Chronic Pain Organization, Inc.
   http://www.coolware.com/health/medical_reporter/pain.html
4. American Council for Headache
   http://www.achenet.org/index.html
5. American Foundation for Pain Research (Interstitial Cystitis)
   http://www.social.com/health/nhic/data/hr2300/hr2313.html
6. American Pain Society
   http://www.ampainsoc.org
7. American Society for Action on Pain
   http://www.calyx.net/967Eschaffer/asap/asapain.html
8. American Society of Addiction Medicine
   http://www.asam.org
9. Arthritis Foundation
   http://www.arthritis.org
10. Cancer Pain Release
    http://www.biostat.weisc.edu/WHOcancerpain/contents.html
11. Cancer Pain Reviews
    http://www.132.183.171.10/mghpc/CancerReviews
12. Caregiver Network
    http://www.caregiver.on.ca:80/index.html
13. Caregiver Survival Resources
    http://www.caregiver911.com
14. Dee's Pain Management Site
    http://www.shack.com/dee
15. Drug and Alcohol Treatment Referrals
    http://www.DRUGHELP.org
16. Drug Enforcement Administration
    http://www.dea.gov
       Queries on physician registration or the Controlled Substances Act may be directed to:
          Drug Enforcement Administration
          Office of Diversion Control
          600 Army Navy Drive
          Arlington, VA 22202
17. International Association for the Study of Pain
    http://www.pslgroup.com/dg/1ff02.htm
    http://www.halcyon.com/iasp
18. Internet Medical Resources
    http://www.pslgroup.com/medres.htm
19. Latino Council on Alcohol and Tobacco
    No web resource given. Phone: 202-371-1186
20. Legal Action Center
    http://www.lacinfo@lac.org
21. Library Links to Journals
    http://www.www.graylab.ac.uk/cancerweb/library/journals/index.html
22. Mayday Pain Resource Center at the City of Hope
    e-mail: mayday_pain@smtplink.coh.org
23. Mayday Resource Center for Pain Medicine and Palliative Care (includes specific links for
       pain management and chemical dependence)
    http://www.stoppain.org
    e-mail: mayday@bethisraelny.org

(continued)

Table 21.5. Selected website resources in pain management and chemical dependence
—Continued

24. Medical Acupuncture Web Page
    http://www.med.auth.gr/~karanik
25. Medicare Rights Center
    http://www.medicarerights.org
26. Narcotics Anonymous
    http://www.wsoinc.com
27. National Alliance of Methadone Advocates
    http://www.methadone.org
28. National Asian Pacific American Families Against Substance Abuse, Inc.
    http://www.igc.apc.org/apiahf/napafasa
29. National Black Alcoholism and Addictions Council, Inc.
    No web resource given. Phone: 202-296-2696
30. National Clearinghouse for Alcohol and Drug Information
    http://www.health.org
31. National Center on Addiction and Substance Abuse at Columbia University
    http://www.casa.columbia.org
32. National Clearinghouse for Alcohol and Drug Information
    http://www.health.org
33. National Council on Alcoholism and Drug Dependence
    http://www.ncadd.org
34. National Family Caregivers Association
    http://www.nfcacares.org
35. National Headache Foundation
    http://www.headaches.org
36. National Institute on Drug Abuse
    http://www.nida.nih.gov
37. National Rehabilitation Information Center
    http://www.naric.com/naric
38. Office of Alternative Medicine, National Instititutes of Health
    http://www.altmed.od.nih.gov
39. Pain and Chemical Dependency List Serve
    http://www.pain_chem_dep@peach.ease.lsoft.com/scripts/
    wa.exe?SUBED1=pain_chem_dep&A=1
40. Pain Lecture Slide Show (Roxane)
    http://pain.roxane.com/index2.html
41. Pediatric Pain
    http://is.dal.ca/edpain/prohp.html
42. Purdue-Frederick
    http://www.partnersagainstpain.com
43. Reflex Sympathetic Dystrophy Association
    http://www.cyboard.com/rsds
44. Robert Wood Johnson Foundation
    http://www.RWJF.ORG/main.html
45. Roxane Laboratories Pain Institute
    http://pain.roxane.com/index2.html
46. Talarian Attachments, Pain Research
    http://www.stat.washington.edu/TALARIA/attachment.html
47. University of Wisconsin Pain and Policy Studies Group
    http://www.medsch.wisc.edu/painpolicy
48. USA Fibromyalgia Association
    ttp://www.w2.com/fibro1.html
49. Video Health Information Project
    http://www.sebridge.org/~vhip
50. Worldwide Congress on Pain
    http://www.pain.com

Used with permission from the Department of Pain Medicine and Palliative Care, Beth Israel Medical Center, New York.

Table 21.6. Common limitations in quality improvement studies

	Limitations	Strategies
1. Problem/ opportunity statements	Statements lack specificity (start and end points), variables lack definition	Define parameters of process and identify antecedents and covariates which may influence the process and outcomes
2. Intervention	Parameters of intervention (innovation) not well defined, nor is implementation monitored Evidence supporting the strength of the intervention not addressed	Define aspects of the intervention (structural changes, educational program), conduct process audits to monitor extent of implementation and institutional culture changes, identify best practices through literature and experts
3. Design	Lack experimental designs (control groups and randomization)	Strive for more rigor using quasi-experimental designs, conduct pilot studies to refine methods
4. Sample	Sample usually small, of convenience, and too varied (disease, age, ethnicity, and gender) Sampling procedures usually exclude weekends, evening, and night hours	Use systematic probability sampling techniques to increase sample size and maximize representativeness Strive for homogeneity and randomization techniques to minimize bias and systematic error
5. Instruments	Tools lack validity, reliability, and pretesting with study population Study procedures lack training for data collectors and consistency in use of tools Global measure (patient satisfaction, quality of life) frequently used as patient outcome without definition	Select tools with known validity and reliability in study population, pilot-test tools for feasibility and to minimize missing data Perform inter-rater reliability of tools with multiple auditors, strive for >90% consistency Define outcomes and select tools which measure the parameters of the study end point
6. Data analysis	Unit of analysis and level of data not defined, missing data not addressed, probability of Type II error high	Obtain biostatistical assistance to determine data analysis techniques
7. Results	Limitations not stated, conclusions not clearly reported, results not compared to previous findings	Include limitations and relationship of results to previous studies, provide clear statements of findings and implications for clinical practice Search the literature for benchmarks of ideal end points

Limitations of Quality Improvement Studies

Quality improvement is promoted by the JCAHO and other professional organizations as a viable approach to improving pain management in hospitals. Although QI frameworks offer clinicians substantial direction for carrying out change efforts, much variation exists within hospital QI departments as far as the number of resources available and level of formal training received by staff. The QI data and the adequacy of pain management will become increasingly important for hospitals seeking JCAHO accreditation. Table 21.6 lists common limitations noted in QI studies and suggests ways that clinicians can increase study rigor, strengthen results, and enhance applicability in practice. Adherence to new pain standards will remain a key quality outcome for surveyors to examine. For more information about pain standards, readers are referred to www.jcaho.org.

Summary

Three hospitals were used to illustrate the challenges faced by clinicians. We offer strategies for institutions to bring about positive changes in pain management and other areas. The 1995 APS Quality Improvement Guidelines for the Treatment of Acute and Cancer Pain continue to serve as a very useful guide to evaluate the quality of pain practices in hospitals and cancer centers. The cases presented can be used by clinicians to benchmark their own efforts and prepare for the tasks and issues that lie ahead.

It is hoped that clinicians who are successful at building teams and incorporating national standards into routine clinical practice will be better prepared to use their methodology as the template for future projects to improve other distressing symptoms. As a word of caution about changing practice cultures, it usually takes a longer time than anticipated and requires a planned approach, at least 1–2 years of sequential smaller studies that culminate into an institutional change. Those unaware of this finding may become easily discouraged and give up. The clinician's sense of isolation and discouragement can be lessened, however, by (1) gaining knowledge about the process and implementation of QI; (2) being part of a team which has acknowledged support, direction, and assistance; and (3) connecting with pain experts in the community, local or via Internet, who can provide mentorship and guidance during the change effort.

References

1. Acute Pain Management Guideline Panel. Acute Pain Management, Operative or Medical Procedures, and Trauma. Clinical Practice Guideline. AHCPR 92-0032. Rockville, MD: Agency for Health Care Policy and Research, Public Health Service, US Department of Health and Human Services, 1992.

2. Jacox A, Carr DB, Payne R, et al. Management of Cancer Pain. Clinical Practice Guideline. AHCPR 94-0592. Rockville, MD: Agency for Health Care Policy and Research, Public Health Service, US Department of Health and Human Services, 1994.
3. Max MB, Donovan M, Miaskowski C, et al. American Pain Society quality improvement guidelines for the treatment of acute pain and chronic pain. JAMA 1995; 274:1974–1880.
4. Joint Commission on Accreditation of Hospitals Organization. http://www.jcaho.org, 1999.
5. Bookbinder M, Coyle N, Kiss M, et al. Implementing national standards for cancer pain management: program model and evaluation. J Pain Symptom Manage 1996; 12:334–347.
6. Hennessey B. Pain Management: From Hospital to Home. A Quality Improvement Study. New York: Memorial Sloan Kettering Cancer Center, 1996.
7. Luketich JD, Kiss M, Hershey J, et al. Chest tube insertion: a prospective evaluation of pain management. Clin J Pain 1998; 14:152–154.
8. Grant M, Ferrell BR, Rivera LM, et al. Unscheduled readmissions for uncontrolled symptoms. A health care challenge for nurses. Nurs Clin North Am 1995; 30: 673–682.
9. Wakefield B, Johnson J, Kron-Chalupa J, et al. A research-based guideline for appropriate use of transdermal fentanyl to treat chronic pain. Oncology Nursing Forum 1998; 25:1505–1512.
10. Gordon DB, Dahl JL, Stevenon KK. Building an institutional commitment to pain management: The Wisconsin Resource Manual. 2d ed. The Resource Center of the American Alliance of Cancer Pain Initiatives, 2000.
11. Bookbinder M, Kiss M, Coyle N, et al. Improving pain management practices. In: McGuire D, Yarbro C, Ferrell B, eds. Cancer Pain Management, 2d ed. Boston: Jones and Bartlett, 1995:321–361.
12. Lavioe-Smith D, Whedon M, Bookbinder M. A multidisciplinary quality improvement approach to improve painful chemotherapy-induced peripheral neuropathy in patients receiving chemotherapy. Semin Oncol Nurs 2002; 18:36–43.
13. American Hospital Corporation. FOCUS-PDCA Methodology Sponsored by Medical Risk Management Associates, LLCHRM Consulting and Software Development Specialists. http://wwwsentinel-eventcom/focus-pdca_indexhtm, 1989.
14. Lynn J, Schuster JL, Kabcenell A. Improving Care for End-of-Life: A Sourcebook for Healthcare Managers and Clinicians. New York: Oxford University Press, 2000.

IX

RESEARCH ISSUES IN SPECIAL POPULATIONS

22

Current Status of Symptom Measurement in Children

JOHN J. COLLINS

The literature on symptom measurement in infants and children is largely confined to the measurement of pain. There is an enormous array of physiological, behavioral, and self-report pain measures for infants and children. Further, recent pain measurement research has begun studying two difficult pediatric patient populations: the preverbal and the cognitively impaired. With the exception of measures created for postchemotherapy nausea and vomiting and evolving measures of fatigue in children, few other measures of symptoms in children exist. Two new scales, the Memorial Symptom Assessment Scale (MSAS) 10–18[1] and the MSAS 7–12,[2] are multidimensional self-report scales designed to describe symptom prevalence, characteristics, and distress in children with cancer aged 10–18 and aged 7–12, respectively.

Measurement of Pain in Infants and Children

Physiological measures of pain

Considerable advances have been made in the investigation of physiological measures of pain in infants. These measures have included heart rate, vagal tone, respiratory rate, blood pressure, palmar sweating, oxygen saturation, transcutaneous oxygen tension, transcutaneous carbon dioxide tension, and intracranial pressure. The main problem with physiological measures is that not all of the variability they show can be related specifically to pain[3] and that few have been studied to test their response to analgesics. Most physiological measures have focused on the absence or presence of pain, rather than severity. As most of these measures have been studied in the setting of procedural pain or postsurgical pain, their applicability across different types of pain and chronic pain is unknown.[4]

Heart rate

Heart rate increases generally during pain and remains elevated after a painful stimulus. In one study of newborn infants,[5] heart rate increased slowly after heel lancing. It peaked, on average, 80 seconds after lancing at an average of 179 beats per minute and remained above the baseline heart rate for a mean of 3.5 minutes. Heart rate has decreased in response to analgesics in the setting of circumcision,[6–10] heel lancing,[11] and surgery.[12,13] Inconsistent changes in heart rate have been observed in connection with other measures used to calm, soothe, or distract persons during a painful stimulus.[14,15] When heart rate was measured in newborn infants during intensive care procedures, it showed no significant changes during heel-stick, physical handling, closed-system suctioning, and chest physiotherapy but a significant (4%) increase after standard suctioning, thus indicating that heart rate is not a specific measure of pain.[16]

Respiratory rate

The data on respiratory rate and pain are mixed, some studies indicating that respiratory rate increases in relation to pain,[17] and others indicating that it decreases.[18] The data on respiratory rate following administration of analgesics are similarly contradictory. For example, one study found that use of the eutectic mixture of local anesthetics (EMLA) cream during heel prick reduced variability in respiratory rate but not mean respiratory rate[3]; another study found that respiratory rate during infant circumcision did not differ significantly in infants who received a dorsal penile block versus no block.[9] Respiratory rate changes are associated more with painful versus nonpainful procedures.[19]

Blood pressure and oxygen saturation

Increases in blood pressure during and after painful episodes have been reported,[20] and changes to blood pressure are reduced following administration of analgesics.[12,13] Oxygen saturation decreases during a painful procedure, and these changes decrease when analgesics are administered.[6,10] Oxygen saturation may be related to other physiological measures of infant pain. In one study of very low birthweight premature infants undergoing real or sham heel pricks, maximum heart rate, heart rate standard deviation, minimum oxygen saturation, and intracranial pressure were significantly correlated.[21]

Transcutaneous oxygen and carbon dioxide tension

Transcutaneous oxygen levels decrease in response to pain related to circumcision[19] and during recovery from heel lancing.[18] There is conflicting evidence for the use of transcutaneous carbon dioxide tension as a measure of pain during procedures.[22] Levels of transcutaneous carbon dioxide vary with gestational age.[18]

Palmar sweating and skin blood flow

Palmar sweating increases in babies following a painful stimulus[23] and is measured by assessment of the gradient of water vapor pressure close to the skin's surface. Palmar sweating is proportional to the rate of water evaporation from the skin itself.[23] It is not specific to pain and may be a measure of other emotional states. Skin blood flow increases after a painful stimulus and decreases after administration of analgesics.[16] Skin blood flow may also increase after nonpainful stimuli[16] and is measured using laser Doppler technology.

Intracranial pressure

Intracranial pressure rises during painful procedures in infants[24] and is often associated with changes in other physiological parameters, such as maximum heart rate and oxygen saturation.[21] Intracranial pressure may be measured using a monitor placed over the anterior fontanelle.[21] Although impractical in a clinical sense, this method of pain measurement may be of value in research setting.[25]

Behavioral measures of pain

Almost all behavioral measures of pain have been developed and validated for short, sharp pain or for recovery from anesthesia.[26] Few behavioral measures have been evaluated for their response to analgesics, nor are there data on the levels of behavior significant enough to require intervention. Many of the behaviors caused by painful events in infants and children are not specific to pain and can be provoked by a broad range of states and situations.

Cry

There is an extensive literature on cry as a measure of pain in infants. Cry is not a specific pain signal but, rather, symbolic of generalized distress indicating pain, hunger, loneliness, or tiredness.[25] A wide variety of characteristics of cry have been examined in the setting of needle procedures, including frequency, latency, duration, phonation, and melody. The difficulties of using cry as a measure of pain include the fact that infants do not always cry when subjected to a noxious stimulus and the lack of specificity to the cry as a measure of pain: anger and fear cries cannot often be distinguished from pain cries. There are no data on the use of cry as a pain measure for chronic pain.[25]

Facial display of pain

Facial expression provides a valuable source of information concerning the nature and severity of pain.[27] The facial display during a painful experience evolved from behavioral and physical adaptations that have served to protect the individual from physical threat and to communicate distress to others who can benefit from this information.[27] Facial activity may be one of the most useful behavioral measures of pain. Facial response to pain, for example, is more consistent across infants than qualities of cry, heart rate, or body movements.[28] Facial activity contributes more to adult judgments of pain than cry.[29]

The most objective, detailed, and comprehensive studies of facial activity during painful events have used either the Facial Action Coding System (FACS)[30] or its adaptation to the study of facial activity in infants.[27] These are anatomi-cally based measurement systems requiring observers to be trained to identify the presence or absence, intensity, and temporal features of 45 well-defined, discrete facial actions using filmed facial recordings. These measures are best suited to research applications, rather than the clinical management of patients.

The Neonatal Facial Coding System (NFCS)[31] was based on FACS, and trained coders use videotaped recordings of a child's behavior during procedural pain. The immediacy of the child's response and the rapid resolution have per-mitted coding of relatively brief spans of time, ranging from 30 seconds to sev-eral minutes. Studies of response to surgical procedures require longer record-ing intervals and time sampling procedures. The facial reaction in infants can be generally characterized as brow bulge, eyes squeezed shut, deepening of the nasolabial furrow, open lips, mouth stretched vertically, and a taut tongue in a raised, cupped form. The presence of a protruding tongue seems to indicate an absence of pain.[27]

The Children's Facial Coding Scale, adapted from both NFCS and FACS, similarly captures facial activity in toddlers through school-aged children to pro-vide an index of pain when self-report may be unreliable. It is designed to cap-ture both acute and chronic pain expressions.[27] A measure of pain in premature infants, the Premature Infant Pain Profile,[32] utilizes facial activity in combination with behavioral state, physiological activity, and information about the develop-mental state of the infant.

At least three clinical studies have used facial activity as an outcome measure of analgesic efficacy. Two have been used in the study of the EMLA for circum-cision pain[33] and for intramuscular injections[27]; another study showed that preterm infants displayed less facial activity when receiving morphine analgesia during heel lancing for blood sampling.[18]

Composite behavior measures of pain

The categories of information available to observers include speech and other purposeful actions, vocalizations (crying, screaming), facial activity, posture, and limb and torso movements. These scales have been validated in the setting of postoperative pain or procedural pain. The Children's Hospital of Eastern Ontario Pain Scale (CHEOPS), which is responsive to the effects of intravenous opioids and procedural pain but not long-term pain, is widely used. The Neonatal Infant Pain Scale is a neonatal version of the CHEOPS based on nurses' reports of changes in behavior with pain and has been used for short, sharp pain. The Observational Scale of Behavioral Distress (OSBD)[34] has been used predominantly in children with cancer undergoing medical procedures, and the Gauvain-Piquard rating scale[35] is an observation scale designed for the as-sessment of chronic pain in oncology patients aged 2–6 years.

Measurement of pain by self-report

Self-report scales are a form of communication about pain intensity and other dimensions of pain in children with sufficient cognitive and language development. Most children older than 5 years can reliably use visual analogue scales (VASs) and faces scales to rate their pain intensity.[36,] Verbal rating scales can be used with children 12 years or older, but simple versions may be useful for younger children. Many younger children, 2–4 years old, can use simple, concrete, categorical scales adequately, for either clinical or research purposes.

Faces scales

The ability of children to perceive degrees of facial expression of pain appears to be established by the age of 6 years.[37] A variety of faces scales have been created; however, the Faces Pain Scale[37] incorporates the following properties[36]: the faces were derived from drawings done by children, it represents a continuum of the universal reaction to pain, it achieves strong agreement among 6- to 8-year-old children in the rank ordering of pain, it indicates approximate ratio scale properties (with the first face approximating 0 and the intervals between consecutive faces being close to equal), it does not show tears or anchor "no pain" with a smiling face, it exhibits test–retest and inter-rater reliability, and it displays change over time in response to analgesia. Faces scales may present younger children with too many options. Children younger than 5 years have difficulty with more than four or five choices.

Pain measurement in cognitively impaired children

There is little literature on the assessment of pain in cognitively impaired children. One scale was developed based on 22 items that physicians thought were indicative of pain in this population.[26] These items included crying and painful expressions during physical examination, guarding of a painful area, and difficulty sleeping. Each behavior was rated on a five-point scale during the examination of 100 patients aged 2–33 years. A major difficulty in the development of this scale was the wide diversity of responses by individuals.

A recent study evaluated the psychometric properties of the Noncommunicating Children's Pain Checklist—Postoperative Version (NCCPC-PV) when used on children with severe intellectual disabilities.[38] The caregivers of 24 children with severe intellectual disabilities (aged 3–19 years) took part. Each child was observed by one caregiver and one researcher for 10 minutes before and after surgery. They independently completed the NCCPC-PV and made a VAS rating of the child's pain intensity for those times. A nurse also completed a VAS for the same observations.

The NCCPC-PV was internally reliable (Cronbach's α = 0.91) and showed good inter-rater reliability. A repeated-measures analysis of variance indicated that NCCPC-PV total and subscale scores were significantly higher after surgery and did not differ by observer. Postoperative NCCPC-PV scores correlated with VAS ratings provided by caregivers and researchers but not with those of nurses. In summary, the NCCPC-PV displayed good psychometric properties when used for the postoperative pain of children with severe intellectual disabilities and has the potential to be useful in a clinical setting. The results suggest that familiarity with an individual child who has intellectual disabilities is not necessary for pain assessment.

Measurement of symptoms in children with cancer

Although numerous symptom assessment instruments have been developed and validated for adults in a variety of clinical settings, there is a paucity of symptom assessment tools for children with cancer. In particular, there is no pediatric symptom assessment tool which assesses multiple symptoms in a multidimensional manner. The few validated symptom assessment tools in pediatrics have focused on two common symptoms, pain and nausea. In contrast to instruments measuring nausea and vomiting, instruments measuring pain in children have largely been validated in predominantly the noncancer setting.

Instruments for the assessment of pain in children with cancer

Unidimensional self-report measures. Self-report measures of pain in children have largely focused on the assessment of pain severity. Generally the data support the use of VASs or numerical rating scales for children over the age of 5 years. The VAS design has been used in the assessment of pediatric cancer pain; they frequently have anchors of "no pain" and "worst pain possible." To use such scales, children must understand the concept of proportionality, be able to conceptualize their pain experience along a continuum, and be able to translate that understanding to the visual representation of the line and the anchors.

Similar strategies, such as Likert scales with anchor points of 1 ("no pain") and 5 ("extreme pain"), have been used to assess pain in children with cancer.[39] However, research on the use of verbal rating scales with children (9 years and older) has not clearly established the utility of this approach over the VAS.[40] Other investigators have used visual cues, such as different pictures of a child's face graded from neutral or happy expressions (no pain) to sad/distressed expressions (extreme pain).[41,42]

Behavioral observation measures. The subjective distress of acute pain, particularly after traumatic medical procedures, often manifests itself in certain facial expressions and verbal and motor responses. Behavioral methods for assessing pain in children require independent raters recording the physical behaviors of children in pain, as well as the frequency of their occurrence.[34] Behavioral measures of pain in children consist of observation checklists in which a trained observer records the occurrence of certain pain-related behaviors. The frequency and duration of the behaviors that occur during the medical procedures are scored to produce a numerical value, which represents the child's overall distress. This value is an integrated index of a child's anxiety, fear, distress, and pain; but children's behavioral scores have been interpreted as their global pain scores.[43]

Observation methods have generally been used to obtain data on specific treatment-related pain/distress reactions in infants (for example, following heel lancing or circumcision) or children (for example, bone marrow aspiration, lumbar puncture, postoperative pain). Four observational distress scales have been elaborated in the setting of pediatric oncology. Three have been used during lumbar puncture or bone marrow aspiration to quantify the occurrence, intensity, and range of a child's pain and distress. The fourth was developed to measure chronic pain in children with cancer.

The Procedure Behavioral Rating Scale (PBRS)[44] was developed to assess pain associated with lumbar puncture and bone marrow aspiration in children aged 8 months to 18 years. Observers noted the occurrence of 13 behaviors prior to, during, and following the medical procedure. Based in part on the PBRS, Jay et al.[34] developed the OSBD.

The OSBD permits continuous sampling throughout the medical procedure, with 15-second recording intervals. Eleven operationally defined behaviors are included (such as crying, screaming, muscular rigidity), with a weighting system based on severity (screaming = 4.0, muscular rigidity = 2.5, and information seeking = 1.5). A between-observer reliability of 0.98 was reported, and interobserver agreements for each of the 11 behaviors ranged from 67% to 100%, with a mean of 84%[45]; however, correlations with psychophysiological measures (heart rate and blood pressure) were unstable and in the low range (0.30–0.40).[46] The OSBD and a revision of the PBRS have been applied to coding children's distress during venipuncture.[45]

The Procedure Behavior Checklist (PBCL)[44] utilizes an eight-category observation system and allows the observer to code intensity levels for each action recorded (from 1, very mild, to 5, extremely intense). Validity data indicate that the scores are significantly correlated with children's self-rated pain and with observer ratings of pain and anxiety.

The Gauvain-Piquard rating scale[35] is an observation scale designed for the assessment of chronic pain in pediatric oncology patients aged 2–6 years. It consists of 17 items, seven of which are related to pain assessment (antalgic rest position, spontaneous protection of painful areas, somatic complaints, pointing out painful areas, antalgic behavior during movement, control exerted by child when moved, emotional reactions to medical examination of painful regions), six to depression (child retires "into his shell," lack of expressiveness, lack of interest in surroundings, slowness and rarity of movements, signs of regression, social withdrawal), and four to anxiety (nervousness/anxiety, ability to protest, moodiness/irritability, tendency to cry). Each child was observed for 4 hours and scored at the same time by four independent observers (two nurses and two aides). Kappa statistics analyzing the correlation between observers were low, ranging 0.24–0.60.

Factorial correspondence analyses indicated that both pain and depression items contributed to the first factor, accounting for 51% of the variance, whereas anxiety items contributed to the second factor, accounting for 13% of the variance. The lack of operational definitions and the low kappa coefficients call into question the reliability of this scale.

Instruments for the assessment of nausea in children with cancer

A rating scale for nausea and vomiting employing verbal descriptors was used in a series of assessment studies of children with cancer aged 5–18.[46–50] Children younger than 10 years had faces included above numbers on the scale. There was 80% agreement between parent and child ratings when assessed independently.

Child and parent ratings of children's nausea and emesis symptoms were compared in a study of 33 children (aged 1.7–17.5 years, median 4.7 years) with acute lymphoblastic leukemia receiving identical chemotherapy.[51] The measures utilized nausea and vomiting vignettes designed to assess the frequency and severity of nausea and emesis symptoms as reported by children and their parents based on the previous chemotherapy experience of the child. The vignettes, based on the work of Zeltzer et al.,[52] consisted of 12 questions separately assessing nausea and emesis at three time intervals: prior to, during, and after chemotherapy. A five-point Likert-type rating scale, ranging from "not at all" to "all the time" for the frequency items and from "not bad" to "real bad" for the severity items, was employed. A composite nausea/vomiting score was determined by calculating the mean of the 12 frequency and severity items. Children younger than 5 years were not asked to complete this measure because of their difficulty understanding the instructions. This study demonstrated a significant correlation between child and parent ratings of nausea. Significant inter-rater correlations for nausea frequency and severity, but not for emesis frequency or severity, were found.

Memorial Symptom Assessment Scales for children

The measurement of symptoms is one aspect of quality-of-life (QOL) assessment. All recently developed validated measures of cancer-specific QOL for adults assess a selected group of prevalent symptoms within a broader assessment of physical, social, and psychological functioning.[53–56] Understanding symptom prevalence and characteristics in children with cancer has been hampered by the lack of symptom assessment tools validated in this population. Neither of the two QOL measures developed for children with cancer, the single-item observer-rated Play Performance Scale for Children[57] and the 21-item parent-rated Pediatric Quality of Life Scale,[58] measures symptoms. Symptom-specific scales available for children with cancer either evaluate pain using self-report[39,41,44,45,59] or observer ratings[46,60] or assess chemotherapy-related nausea and vomiting using self-report.[50,51] Without the means to comprehensively measure symptoms, the epidemiology of symptoms in childhood cancer is poorly characterized and symptom intervention trials, other than those evaluating anti-emetics for postchemotherapy nausea and vomiting,[61-65] are lacking.

The MSAS 10–18 is a 30-item patient-rated instrument adapted from a previously validated adult version to provide multidimensional information about the symptoms experienced by children with cancer.[1] This instrument was administered to 160 children with cancer aged 10–18 years (45 inpatients, 115 outpatients). To confirm the instrument's reliability and validity, additional data about symptoms were collected from both the parents and the medical charts and retesting was performed on a subgroup of inpatients.

The scale was easily completed by patients in a mean time of 11 minutes. The analyses supported the reliability and validity of the MSAS 10–18 subscale scores as measures of physical, psychological, and global symptom distress. Symptom prevalence ranged from 49.7% for lack of energy to 6.3% for problems with urination. The mean ($\pm$SD) number of symptoms per inpatient was 12.7 $\pm$ 4.9 (range 4–26), significantly more than that per outpatient (6.5 $\pm$ 5.7, range 0–28). Patients who had recently received chemotherapy had significantly more symptoms than patients who had not received chemotherapy for more than 4 months (11.6 $\pm$ 6.0 versus 5.2 $\pm$ 5.1), and patients with solid tumors had significantly more symptoms than patients with either hematological or central nervous system malignancies. The most common symptoms (prevalence >35%) were lack of energy, pain, drowsiness, nausea, cough, lack of appetite, and psychological symptoms (feeling sad, feeling nervous, worrying, feeling irritable). Of the symptoms with prevalence rates >35%, those that caused high distress in more than one-third of patients were feeling sad, pain, nausea, lack of appetite, and feeling irritable. Subscale scores demonstrated large variability in symptom distress and could identify subgroups with high distress.

The prevalence, characteristics, and distress associated with physical and psychological symptoms could be quantified in older children with cancer using the MSAS 10–18. The data confirm a high prevalence of symptoms overall and the existence of subgroups with high distress associated with one or multiple symptoms. Symptom distress is relatively higher among inpatients, children with solid tumors, and children undergoing antineoplastic treatment.

A revised MSAS was created for the assessment of symptoms in children with cancer aged 7–12 years.[2] Validity was evaluated by comparison with the medical record, parental report, and concurrent assessment on VASs for selected symptoms. The data provided evidence of the reliability and validity of the MSAS 7–12 and demonstrated that children with cancer as young as 7 years could report clinically relevant and consistent information about their symptom experience. The completion rate for the MSAS 7–12 was high, and the majority of children completed the instrument in a short period of time and with little difficulty. The instrument appeared to be age-appropriate and may be helpful to older children unable to independently complete the MSAS 10–18.

Systematic symptom assessment using a validated questionnaire may be useful in future epidemiological studies of symptoms and in clinical chemotherapeutic trials. Symptom epidemiology may also provide a focus for future clinical trials related to symptom management in children with cancer.

Future Directions

The literature on symptom measurement in infants and children is largely confined to the measurement of pain and has been validated in the setting of postoperative and procedural pain. With the exception of measures of postchemotherapy nausea/vomiting and pain, few other measures of symptoms in children exist. Symptom epidemiological data underscore the need for controlled clinical trials of therapies for symptoms in children with cancer. These trials will require the development of novel study designs applied to common symptoms, such as pain. The value of these epidemiological data will be realized only when further studies of symptom control therapies are directed at the most prevalent and distressing symptoms of children with cancer.

References

1. Collins JJ, Byrnes ME, Dunkel I, et al. The Memorial Symptom Assessment Scale (MSAS): validation study in children aged 10–18. J Pain Symptom Manage 2000; 19:363–367.
2. Collins JJ, Devine TB, Dick G, et al. The measurement of symptoms in young children with cancer: the validation of the Memorial Symptom Assessment Scale in children aged 7–12. J Pain Symptom Manage 2002; 23:10–16.
3. McIntosh N, van Veen L, Brameyer H. The pain of heel prick and its measurement in preterm infants. Pain 1993; 52:71–74.
4. Hester NO. Assessment of pain in children with cancer. In: Chapman CR, Foley KM, eds. Current and Emerging Issues in Cancer Pain: Research and Practice. New York: Raven Press, 1983:219–245.
5. Owens ME, Todt EH. Pain in infancy: neonatal reaction to heel lance. Pain 2002; 20:77–86.
6. Benini F, Johnston CC, Faucher D, et al. Topical anesthesia during circumcision in newborn infants. JAMA 1993; 270:850–853.
7. Arnett RM, Jones JS, Horger EO. Effectiveness of 1% lidocaine doral penile nerve block in infant circumcision. Am J Obstet Gynecol 1990; 163:1074–1080.
8. Holve RL, Bromberger PJ, Groveman HD, et al. Regional anesthesia during newborn circumcision. Clin Pediatr (Phila) 1983; 22:813–818.
9. Williamson PS, Williamson ML. Physiologic stress reduction by a local anesthetic during newborn circumcision. Pediatrics 1983; 71:36–40.
10. Maxwell LG, Yaster M, Welzel RC. Penile nerve block reduces the physiologic stress to the newborn. Anesthesiology 1986; 65:A432.
11. McIntosh N, van Veen L, Brameyer H. Alleviation of the pain of heel prick in preterm infants. Arch Dis Child 1994; 70:F177–F181.
12. Robinson S, Gregory GA. Fentanyl-air-oxygen anesthesia for ligation of patent ductus arteriosus in preterm infants. Anesth Analg 1981; 60:331–334.

13. Yaster M. The dose response of fentanyl in neonatal anesthesia. Anesthesia 1987; 66:433–435.
14. Campos RG. Soothing pain-elicited distress in infants with swaddling and pacifiers. Child Dev 1989; 60:781–792.
15. Field T, Goldson E. Pacifying effects of non-nutritive sucking on term and preterm neonates during heelstick procedures. Pediatrics 1984; 74:1012–1015.
16. McCulloch KM, Ji SA, Raju TNK. Skin blood flow changes during routine nursery procedures. Early Hum Dev 1995; 41:147–156.
17. Howard CR, Howard FM, Weitzman ML. Acetaminophen analgesia in neonatal circumcision. Pediatrics 1994; 93:641–646.
18. Craig KD, Whitfield MF, Grunau RVE, et al. Pain in the preterm neonate: behavioral and physiological indices. Pain 1993; 52:299.
19. Rawlings DJ, Miller PA, Engel RR. The effect of circumcision on transcutaneous pO_2 in term infants. Am J Dis Child 1980; 134:331–334.
20. Durand M, Ssangha B, Cabal LA, et al. Cardiopulmonary and intracranial pressure changes related to endotracheal suctioning in preterm infants. Crit Care Med 1989; 17:506–510.
21. Johnston CC, Stevens BJ, Yang F, et al. Differential responses to pain by very premature neonates. Pain 1995; 61:471–479.
22. Porter F, Miller JP, Coles FS, et al. A controlled trial of local anesthesia for lumbar punctures in newborns. Pediatrics 1991; 88:663–669.
23. Harpin VA, Rutter N. Development of emotional sweating in the newborn infant. Arch Dis Child 1982; 57:691–695.
24. Stevens BJ, Johnston CC. Physiological responses of premature infants to a painful stimulus. Nurs Res 1994; 43:226–231.
25. Sweet SD, McGrath PJ. Physiological measures of pain. In: Finley GA, McGrath PJ, eds. Measures of Pain in Infants and Children. Seattle: IASP Press, 1998:59–81.
26. McGrath PJ. Behavioral measures of pain. In: Finlay GA, McGrath PJ, eds. Measurement of Pain in Infants and Children. Seattle: IASP Press, 1998:83–102.
27. Craig KD. The facial display of pain. In: Finlay GA, McGrath PJ, eds. Progress in Pain Research and Management. Seattle: IASP Press, 1998:103–121.
28. Johnston CC, Strada ME. Acute pain response in infants: a multidimensional description. Pain 1986; 24:373–384.
29. Hadjistavropoulos HD, Craig KD, Grunau RVE, et al. Judging pain in newborns: facial and cry determinants. J Pediatr Psychol 1994; 19:305–318.
30. Ekman P, Oster H. Facial expressions of emotion. Annu Rev Psychol 1970; 30:527–554.
31. Grunau RVE, Craig KD. Pain expression in neonates: facial action and cry. Pain 1987; 28:395–410.
32. Stevens BJ, Johnston CC, Petryshen P, et al. Premature Infant Pain Profile: development and initial validation. Clin J Pain 1996; 12:13–22.
33. Taddio A, Stevens BJ, Craig KD, et al. The efficacy and safety of lidocaine-prilocaine cream for neonatal circumcision. N Engl J Med 1997; 336:1197–1199.
34. Jay SM, Ozolins M, Elliott C, et al. Assessment of children's distress during painful medical procedures. J Health Psychol 1983; 2:133–147.
35. Gauvain-Piquard A, Rodary C, Rezvani A, et al. Pain in children aged 2–6 years: a new observational rating scale elaborated in a pediatric oncology unit: a preliminary report. Pain 1987; 31:177–188.

36. Champion GD, Goodenough B, von Baeyer CL, et al. Measurement of pain by self-report In: Finlay GA, McGrath PJ, eds. Measurement of Pain in Infants and Children. Seattle: IASP Press, 1998:123–160.
37. Bieri D, Reeve RA, Champion GD, et al. The Faces Pain Scale for the self-assessment of the severity of pain experienced by children: development, initial validation, and preliminary investigation for ratio scale properties. Pain 1990; 41:139–150.
38. Breau LM, Finley GA, McGrath PJ, et al. Validation of the Non-communicating Children's Pain Checklist—Postoperative Version. Anesthesiology 2002; 96: 523–526.
39. LeBaron S, Zeltzer L. Assessment of acute pain and anxiety in children and adolescents by self-reports, observer reports and a behavior checklist. J Consult Clin Psychol 1984; 52:729–738.
40. Savedra M, Gibbons P, Tesler M, et al. How do children describe pain? A tentative assessment. Pain 1982; 14:95–104.
41. Kuttner L, Bowman M, Teasdale M. Psychological treatment of distress, pain and anxiety for children with cancer. Dev Behav Pediatr 1988; 9:374–381.
42. Manne SL, Bakeman R, Jacobsen P, et al. Adult and child interaction during invasive medical procedures: sequential analysis. Health Psychol 1992; 11:241–249.
43. Shacham S, Daut R. Anxiety or pain: what does the scale measure? J Consult Clin Psychol 1981; 49:469.
44. Katz ER, Kellerman J, Siegal S. Behavioral distress in children with cancer undergoing medical procedures: developmental considerations. J Consult Clin Psychol 1980; 48:356–365.
45. Manne SL, Redd WH, Jacobsen P, et al. Behavioral intervention to reduce child and parent distress during venipuncture. J Consult Clin Psychol 1990; 58:565–572.
46. Elliott C, Jay SM, Woody P. An observational scale for measuring children's distress during medical procedures. J Pediatr Psychol 1987; 12:543–551.
47. Zeltzer L, Kellerman J, Ellenberg L, et al. Hypnosis for reduction of vomiting associated with chemotherapy and disease in adolescents with cancer. J Adolesc Health Care 1983; 4:84.
48. Zeltzer L, LeBaron S, Zeltzer PM. A prospective assessment of chemotherapy related nausea and vomiting in children with cancer. Am J Pediatr Hematol Oncol 1984; 6:5–16.
49. LeBaron S, Zeltzer L. Behavioral intervention for reducing chemotherapy-related nausea and vomiting in adolescents with cancer. J Adolesc Health Care 1984; 5:182.
50. Zeltzer L, LeBaron S. Effects of the mechanics of administration on Doxorubicin induced side effects: a case report. Am J Pediatr Hematol Oncol 1984; 6:212–215.
51. Tyc VL, Mulhearn RK, Fairclough D, et al. Chemotherapy induced nausea and emesis in pediatric cancer patients: external validity of child and parent ratings. Dev Behav Pediatr 1993; 14:236–241.
52. Zeltzer L, LeBaron S, Richie DM, et al. Can children understand and use a rating scale to quantify somatic symptoms? Assessment of nausea and vomiting as a model. J Consult Clin Psychol 1988; 56:567–572.
53. Cella DF, Tulsky DS, Gray G. The Functional Assessment of Cancer Therapy Scale: development and validation of the general measure. J Clin Oncol 1993; 11: 570–579.

54. Aaronson NK, Ahmedzai S, Bergman B. The European Organization for Research and Treatment of Cancer QLQ-C30: a quality of life instrument for use in international clinical trials in oncology. J Natl Cancer Inst 1993; 85:365–376.

55. Schipper H, Clinch J, McMurray A, et al. Measuring the quality of life in cancer patients: the Functional Living Index—Cancer. Development and validation. Qual Life Res 1992; 1:19–29.

56. Ganz PA, Schag CAA, Lee JJ. The CARES: a generic measure of health-related quality of life for patients with cancer. Qual Life Res 1992; 1:19–29.

57. Lansky SB, List MA, Lansky LL, et al. The measurement of performance in childhood cancer patients. Cancer 1987; 60:1651–1656.

58. Goodwin DA, Boggs SR, Graham-Pole J. Development and validation of the Pediatric Quality of Life Scale. Psychol Assess 1994; 6:321–328.

59. Jay SM, Elliott C, Katz E, et al. Cognitive, behavioral, and pharmacologic interventions for children's distress during painful medical procedures. J Consult Clin Psychol 1987; 55:860–865.

60. Jay S, Elliott C. Behavioral observation scales for measuring children's distress: the effects of increased methodological rigor. J Consult Clin Psychol 1984; 52: 1106–1107.

61. Graham-Pole J. Anti-emetics in children receiving cancer chemotherapy: a double-blind prospective randomised study comparing metoclopramide with chlorpromazine. J Clin Oncol 1994; 4:1110–1113.

62. Hahlen K, Quintana E, Pinkerton R, et al. A randomized comparison of intravenously administered granisetron versus chlorpromazine plus dexamethasone in the prevention of ifosfamide-induced emesis in children. J Pediatr 1995; 126:309–313.

63. Mehta P, Gross S, Graham-Pole J, et al. Methylprednisolone for chemotherapy-induced emesis: a double-blind randomized trial in children. J Pediatr 1986; 108: 774–776.

64. Relling MV, Mulhearn RK, Fairclough D, et al. Chlorpromazine with and without lorazepam as antiemetic therapy in children receiving uniform chemotherapy. J Pediatr 2002; 123:812–816.

65. Alvarez O, Freeman A, Bedros A. Randomized double-blind cross-over ondansetron–dexamethasone versus ondansetron–placebo study for treatment of chemotherapy induced nausea and vomiting in pediatric patients with malignancies. J Pediatr Hematol Oncol 1995; 17:145–150.

23

Research in Pediatric Palliative Care

BETTY DAVIES, ROSE STEELE,
KELLI I. STAJDUHAR, AND ANNE BRUCE

The World Health Organization (WHO) defines palliative care as the active total care of patients whose disease is not responsive to curative treatment. Control of pain, other symptoms, and psychological, social, and spiritual problems is paramount. The goal of palliative care is to achieve the best quality of life for patients and their families.[1]

Implicit in the last sentence of the definition is the notion that palliative care, including pediatric palliative care, is a philosophy or an approach that encompasses the whole person. However, the reference to "control of symptoms" has sometimes narrowed the clinical and research focus to symptom management strategies. Thus, attention in adult palliative care has often been directed primarily toward development and measurement of the outcome of those strategies. Randomized control trials (RCTs) have achieved considerable status as the best method for evaluating outcomes, but they are limited by numerous ethical and practical difficulties, particularly in pediatric palliative care. Moreover, they rely heavily on objective measures. However, all symptoms and child/family needs occur within the context of each child and family's biography, so understanding the child's whole experience is integral to providing optimal pediatric palliative care. Subjective measures, consequently, take on increasing importance in gaining this more comprehensive understanding.

Even when the adult patient's subjective experience has been taken into account, many researchers have continued to apply objective criteria and perspectives that can only partially capture subjective phenomena. Instead, multiple perspectives, obtained through a variety of research methods, are necessary to provide a greater understanding of the whole person. In pediatric palliative care, where systematic knowledge development is only in its infancy, such perspectives become even more critical. In this chapter, we will identify extant research in pediatric palliative care and suggest additional methods or approaches for gaining these multiple perspectives.

Setting the Context

Unlike adult palliative care, where most patients have cancer and palliative care is provided for a relatively short period of time, children typically have a wide range of diseases and require palliative care for many years.[2] Most of the children's care is provided at home by their families, who need intermittent relief from the constant demands of providing care. Respite care, therefore, along with end-of-life and bereavement care, is an integral component of pediatric palliative care.[2]

Families play a unique role in pediatric palliative care. Although the WHO[1] definition implies that the family is the unit of care, this focus is particularly critical in pediatric palliative care because the child is inseparable from the family. Families influence their children, and the children in turn influence their families.[3] Moreover, not only do families provide the majority of care, but parents are usually surrogate decision makers for their child. Perceiving the family as the unit of care involves more than merely thinking about the family as the object of care. It means working with families to solve problems and make decisions.[4] It also means incorporating families into pediatric palliative care research. When the family is viewed as the unit of care, researchers must investigate the individuals in a family, the family as a whole, and the reciprocal child–family interactions. Family-level research presents its own unique challenges, which are beyond the scope of this chapter. However, one cannot assume that the perspective of one individual reflects the perspective of the family as a whole.[5]

Children are not miniature adults. They are physiologically and developmentally different from adults. Their age and developmental level affect both their comprehension and ability to communicate verbally. Therefore, these factors must be taken into account when designing and conducting pediatric palliative care research. In addition, research that focuses on vulnerable populations, such as those who are dying or children, is often perceived as ethically challenging and difficult.[6] As a result, adults often impose barriers to conducting research with children when, in fact, many children are capable of understanding the purpose of the research and of consenting to participate. This difficulty is further compounded when research involves children who are dying because they are seen as especially vulnerable and in need of protection. Yet, although children may not have the legal capacity to consent, this does not negate their right to assent to participate in research if that is their wish.[7] Research, however, must be meaningful and provide answers to relevant questions without imposing harm on the participants.

Overview of Research in Pediatric Palliative Care

There is relatively little research in pediatric palliative care. Many of the available studies have been conducted on children who have cancer. Much of the literature reflects theoretical perspectives based on clinical practice and individual experience rather than on systematic research. Thus, authors often have only clinical articles to cite in their own publications. However, pediatric palliative care is a recent entity. Adult palliative care has developed markedly over the past 30 years, yet research efforts among children have intensified only in the last 10 years. Thus, the paucity of research in pediatric palliative care reflects the early stage of its development rather than a lack of interest.

Despite the temptation to transfer findings from research on adults to children, the growing body of knowledge in adult palliative care cannot be applied uncritically to a pediatric population. For example, the presentation of symptoms may be different between children and adults. Moreover, children vary in their ability to describe their symptoms. As a result, tools designed for assessment of adult symptoms seldom work with children. Treatment protocols that have been established as safe and effective for adults may not necessarily be so for children. Furthermore, many of the diagnoses in pediatric palliative care, such as certain congenital disorders, are unique to children. Consequently, it is impossible to investigate issues arising from these diagnoses without focusing on the children themselves.

Extant Research in Pediatric Palliative Care

Similar to adult palliative care, the field of pediatric palliative care is complex and multi-dimensional. While there are many aspects that could be explored, this chapter will focus on four areas critical for developing state-of-the-art research in this field: (1) pain and symptom management, (2) psychosocial and spiritual care, (3) location of care, and (4) education. Taking these four areas into account, the existing research will first be reviewed and the gaps identified. Priorities for research will then be formulated, and appropriate methods for conducting this research will be discussed.

Pain and symptom management

Textbooks on palliative care have few references on pain and symptom management in children. Most of the available studies focus on pain management in children with cancer who are receiving active treatment, and even these studies are limited.[8] As well, little information is available about the pharmacodynamic properties of the drugs used to treat pain and other symptoms in the pediatric palliative care population. Thus, drug protocols are usually based solely on clinical experiences with dying children and often on experiences in general pediatrics or adult palliative care.

While some tools have been developed for children to document their pain, there has been little instrument development for other symptoms. Moreover, the available tools have not been validated in the pediatric population.[9] Symptoms are subjective phenomena, yet children are often not asked about them. Even if they are asked, many are unable to talk or otherwise communicate. Therefore, there is a need to develop ways of collecting information that allow nonverbal children to give their input and that are creative enough to provide information about noncommunicative children.

Hardly anything is known about the child's or family's perception of symptoms. The prevalence of symptoms has been documented in several studies, but these were limited by the setting, the small number of participants, and the retrospective nature of data collection.[10-15] Research is required to identify the prevalence of symptoms and to determine which are the most troublesome to children and their families. While Levy et al.[16] prospectively identified troublesome symptoms in terminally ill children on a neurosurgical unit, they examined only nine cases. Little research has examined the impact of pain and other symptoms on the child. Researchers have only recently begun to determine the impact of a child's cancer pain on the family.[17,18] Much work is needed to identify this impact. Existing protocols for management of symptoms must be identified and evaluated to form a sound research base.

Further, research studies are needed to identify the characteristics of symptoms, how people manage the symptoms, and what helps or interferes with symptom management. In many cases, family and staff need to identify symptoms for a child who cannot communicate. Studies are particularly needed to determine how staff and family identify symptoms in such cases, how they manage the symptoms, and how they evaluate the outcomes of their management strategies. The increasing use of alternative or complementary therapies (ACTs) in the general population suggests that there may be a similar increase in the pediatric palliative care population. No studies were found that addressed this issue. However, a large-scale, population-based study of children with cancer reported that 42% of patients used ACTs.[19] Research is needed to assess the prevalence of ACTs for symptom management, to identify the ones that families use, to determine reasons for using ACTs, and to evaluate their effectiveness.

Provision of psychosocial and spiritual care

Research in the psychosocial/spiritual realm focuses primarily on the impact of a child's illness and death on parents,[20-24] especially mothers.[25] Very little research includes other family members, such as the ill child, siblings, and grandparents, or the family unit as a whole. This limited research tends to focus on siblings and has demonstrated that siblings may have more problems than the ill child.[26,27] After a child's death, siblings adapt better when they are included and valued by their parents and other significant adults in their lives.[28] Studies in families following the death of a child give some indication of what helps families cope with terminal illness and subsequent bereavement.[29] Families who are more open; share thoughts, feelings, and opinions; and are more expressive, open-minded, and tolerant seem to cope better. However, these studies are limited in both number and scope.

Published research has historically focused on the impact of cancer, but more recent studies have begun to explore the impact of other diagnoses, such as cystic fibrosis or acquired immunodeficiency syndrome (AIDS).[23,24,30–34] These findings suggest that a child's illness and death have wide-ranging implications for families (emotionally, spiritually, financially, and structurally) as a result of the progressive and terminal nature of the illness. Results consistently show that families want to be as fully informed as possible. For example, parents want to know what to expect during the entire illness trajectory, how to deal with issues that arise, and how to prepare for their future without the child, yet they are often given insufficient information. In addition, families want to participate in caring for their child.[27,30,31,35–37]

The long-term trajectory of progressive, life-threatening illnesses in children means that their psychosocial and spiritual needs, as well as those of their families, are not static but continually changing during the respite component of pediatric palliative care. Little research has been directed toward children and families who require respite care. One recent study[36] characterized how families' emotions and needs varied over time and in response to their changing situation as "navigating uncharted territory." For example, when a child with a neurodegenerative disorder developed pneumonia, parents' uncertainty and grief intensified until they learned how to deal with this new situation and the crisis was finally resolved. In another recent study, parents whose children were receiving respite care in a children's hospice program appreciated staff's responsiveness to their families' changing needs.[35]

Few studies focus directly on the end-of-life stage of illness, yet end-of-life issues are significant. One of the first such studies[27] focused on families cared for at Helen House, the first free-standing children's hospice in the world. In one study of parents whose children were human immunodeficiency virus (HIV)–infected, the experience of parents changed when their child became extremely debilitated and they realized that their child's death was imminent.[38] James and Johnson[39] also focused specifically on the end-of-life phase in their study about the needs of parents whose children had cancer. They and others[35] identified the needs of parents to have their child recognized as special, to have caring and connectedness with health professionals, and to retain responsibility for parenting their dying child.

Though spiritual issues are integral to palliative care, little is known about children's spirituality and even less about the spiritual needs of children in palliative care. However, children do respond spiritually to illness, and seriously ill children exhibit thoughts and feelings about prayer and a deity.[40] In hospitalized adolescents, the significance of spiritual and religious issues increases directly with the seriousness of illness.[41] Recent guidelines have been developed for approaching spiritual issues with families in pediatric palliative care.[42] Many questions arise concerning the spiritual nature of children in palliative care, the impact of spiritual issues on quality of life, the relationship between spirituality in ill children and their parents, the assessment of spirituality in children, and whether or not and how spiritual care can be evaluated in pediatric palliative care.

Location of care

In North America, one of the primary goals of palliative care is to support people dying in the comfort of their own home.[43–46] As such, many palliative care practitioners hold death at home as a "gold standard."[47] While there are no pediatric studies that have asked dying children their preferences about location of care, it is believed that most children would prefer to be at home.[48]

The importance to families of the location of care and the assumed preference for home versus hospital care is generally supported in the literature. A preference for home care was demonstrated in three studies involving children with terminal illnesses.[49–52] Results suggested that many families want their ill child at home as much as possible. Overall satisfaction with the various palliative care programs was strongly related to being able to care for the child at home with the support of professionals. While the illness was very disruptive for parents, home care reduced this disruption and allowed parents to have more control. Parents also valued being constantly near their child.

Currently, no data are available to support the cost–effectiveness of pediatric palliative home care. Even though home care may be the preferred choice for some families, Schweitzer and colleagues[53] noted that the cost of nonreimbursed expenses may be enough to exclude many families from participation in a home-based program. The limited research has identified high cumulative, monetary costs incurred by families who participate in home-based palliative care.[27,54,55] In addition, researchers have described indirect costs that may result in a loss of family income at the same time that financial costs are increasing.[56] For example, parents with health insurance may be unable to change jobs because new insurance companies may not cover them. Even when families have insurance coverage, either by private coverage as they do in the United States or through government health plans as in Canada, families may still incur great financial costs when a child is ill.

There is little debate that death at home can contribute significantly to the overall well-being of children and families. However, little research has been conducted to explore the attitudes and cultural practices among different populations. While the advantages of supporting families and children dying at home may seem obvious, there are many issues to consider when plans are made for a home death. Of primary importance are the pressures imposed on families over the trajectory of the illness and the subsequent implications of home death for families. There is a paucity of research that examines families' experiences at home when caring for a child with a terminal illness. Although it appears that some families want to have their child at home, we have only a cursory understanding of the cultural, social, and economic factors that influence this preference. Further research is required to better understand the preferences of children and the impact on family life of caring for a terminally ill child at home. Evaluative research that examines both the global costs of palliative home care services and the costs for families over time is also needed to support policy decisions related to reimbursement and access to services.

Education

Clinicians have described their experiences and the challenges they face in providing pediatric palliative care.[57] Again, research studies are rare. Only three projects have been reported.[55,58,59] All concluded that staff are better able to care for dying children and their families when the organizational climate facilitates open communication and shared decision making among colleagues. Further, reciprocal support moderates the personal impact of working in this field. As a result, the education of healthcare professionals must include strategies for enhancing communication and interdisciplinary teamwork, in addition to knowledge about child development, child psychology, cultural and religious influences, pathophysiology of disease, and therapeutics and pain control. Literature on adult palliative care supports the value of education as a mechanism for improving the provision of palliative care,[60,61] though the majority of studies simply outline the necessary elements required to prepare professionals to care for dying adults.[62–66] There is a dearth of research that addresses educational needs for professionals when a child is dying.[67,68] There remains a need for research about the kind of education required in pediatric palliative care, the most appropriate ways of providing it, and the impact it makes on the provision of care.

Even less is known about the educational needs of families. Studies are required to ensure that the education provided to families is appropriate, is applicable to their situation, and best meets their learning styles. In addition, outcomes of educational programs need to be evaluated.

Critique of Extant Research

Much of the extant research in pediatric palliative care has been retrospective, often after the child's death. Thus, memories of the palliative care experience may have been influenced by the passage of time. While some qualitative work has been done, there is little evidence of theory testing or continuous building of beginning theories. The quantitative research is mostly characterized by small sample sizes. When standardized instruments have been used, they were usually developed for other purposes and not for these families. Reliability and validity evidence for instruments used in this population are severely lacking. There has been very little research with the children themselves, while the perspective of parents, often only the mother, or professionals has usually been sought. Little is known about fathers, siblings, and other family members such as grandparents. In many cases, the limited information has been obtained from retrospective chart reviews. Most of the research is descriptive and dated, using data obtained from retrospective chart reviews; few studies have been reported in recent years.

The long-term goals of clinical research in this field are to understand the experiences of children and their families who are receiving pediatric palliative care and to promote optimal quality of life. To date, little is known about the many dimensions of families' experiences. One area requiring research attention is identifying how families make choices about the services they use. For example, what do families consider when deciding on treatment options such as repeated surgeries? How do families decide when to discontinue active treatment? A related area involves families' perceptions of the effect of various types of program and service. Little is known about the kinds of service that contribute to their well-being or their perceptions of the care they have received. Answers to such questions would provide information about the kind of support families need and would give direction for program development.

Children in palliative care present with many different diagnoses. While it appears that there are similarities in the needs of these children and their families, differences have also been noted, for example, between children with cancer and those with neurodegenerative illnesses. Research into these similarities and differences is imperative so that results can eventually be pulled together to find commonalities across diagnoses and to provide optimal, disease-specific care. Families requiring pediatric palliative care reflect the cultural pluralism of our society. However, most participants in the limited research studies are Caucasian. Cross-cultural aspects of pediatric palliative care are severely understudied. Much remains to be discovered about how families of various cultures perceive death, especially the death of a child. Clinicians suggest that culture affects families in areas such as the preferred location of death, decision making, and participation in services. However, very little is known about the extent of cultural influences. Finally, there is a need to study research issues. For example, the tendency to protect children from research ought to be explored. Children themselves could be asked whether or not they want to participate in research. Questions about how it was for the child to participate in a project could be included in various studies. Experiences with such issues could be described for the purposes of sharing information and to alleviate some of the difficulties encountered in conducting research with dying children.

It is important to uncover what is happening with families during the various phases of the illness trajectory. How can we best understand palliative care, including respite, end-of-life care, and bereavement, from the perspective of those most directly affected? Descriptions and theoretical formulations about families' experiences are needed as a basis for further assessment, to determine the prevalence of various symptoms and dimensions of the experience, for tool development, and to plan interventions and subsequent evaluations.

The priorities for research in these four areas suggest questions for future research. These questions, although not exhaustive, can be found in Tables 23.1 through 23.4.

Methodologies

Depending on the research question, valuable information may be gained not only from cross-sectional, retrospective studies but also from longitudinal and prospective designs. The purpose of this section is to identify various research methods that may be used to obtain multiple perspectives and to gain a greater understanding of the whole person and family. Multiple methods add to the completeness and validity of results but are considerably more demanding of time and other resources. Given the complexity of using multiple methods, the relatively small numbers of children requiring palliative care, and the diversity of their illnesses, collaborative multisite research programs may be required to ensure development of a sound research base.

Research designs and methods must be appropriate for the existing level of knowledge and for answering the research question. When little is known

Table 23.1. Developing state-of-the art research in pediatric palliative care: critical questions in pain and symptom management

- What are the most appropriate ways to collect symptom information from children?
- What is the prevalence of various symptoms in pediatric palliative care?
- What is the child's, family's, and staff's experience with symptoms?
- How do children with differing diagnoses differ in their experiences with symptoms?
- Which symptoms are the most troublesome?
- How are these symptoms assessed?
- How are these symptoms managed?
- How is management of these symptoms evaluated?
- What helps with symptom management?
- What interferes with symptom management?
- What is the prevalence of alternative and complementary therapy (ACT) use in pediatric palliative care?
- Which ACTs are used?
- Why are these ACTs used?
- How effective are these ACTs?
- Do available instruments need validity and reliability testing?
- Is instrument development required on other symptoms, such as dyspnea, nausea, and vomiting?

Table 23.2. Developing state-of-the art research in pediatric palliative care: critical questions in provision of psychosocial and spiritual care

- What is the impact of the child's illness on the ill child?
- What is the impact of the child's illness on other family members (siblings, parents, grandparents)?
- What is the impact of the child's illness on the family unit?
- Do these experiences differ based on diagnosis?
- How do these experiences change over time as the illness trajectory changes?
- What are the needs of children, parents, siblings, other family members, and staff during the respite, palliative, and bereavement components of pediatric palliative care?
- How do children, parents, siblings, other family members, and staff cope with the illness experience during the respite, palliative and bereavement components of pediatric palliative care?
- What do families consider when deciding on treatment options such as repeated surgeries?
- How do families decide when to discontinue active treatment?
- How effective are parent and sibling support groups at various periods throughout the illness trajectory and during bereavement?
- What are the experiences of children and families who come from differing cultural and ethnic backgrounds?
- How important is the concept of spirituality in pediatric palliative care?
- How is spirituality expressed?
- How can spirituality be assessed?
- How can healthcare professionals support a child's and family's spirituality?
- Is instrument development required regarding psychosocial needs and spirituality?

about an area or a different perspective is sought, qualitative methods are often more appropriate than traditional quantitative approaches. Given the dearth of research and the importance of gaining the child and family perspective, qualitative methods should play a central role in pediatric palliative care research.

A variety of qualitative methods may be appropriate, depending on the research question. A phenomenological approach would be useful when trying to elicit the essence of experiences or examine the meaning of an individual's experiences. Data would be collected through audiotaped conversations with people who are having or have had the experience in question or by written anecdotes from them about their personal experiences.

Descriptive questions about values, beliefs, and practices of a cultural group suggest the use of ethnographic methods where unstructured interviews, participant observation, and field notes provide the sources of data. Grounded theory methods, particularly tape-recorded interviews with participants who are undergoing the experience, are especially suitable for process questions, such as those exploring experiences or changes over time.

Table 23.3. Developing state-of-the art research in pediatric palliative care: critical questions in location of care

---

- What is the child's preference for location of care?
- How do families make choices about the location of care?
- How do families make choices about the services they use?
- How do the services that are currently provided to children and their families meet their needs?
- What is the experience of families and health-care professionals who provide care to children as they die at home?
- What is the experience of families and health-care professionals who care for children who die at home?
- What are the implications of home death for families?
- What are the cultural practices of different populations at home?
- What are the direct and indirect costs of home-based palliative care?
- What are the financial implications to the family of keeping children at home for palliative care?
- Does cost play a factor in whether or not families keep their children at home?
- Is instrument development required regarding location of care?

There are relatively few studies in which qualitative methods have been used with children. While the methods are suitable for children, they need to be refined to ensure that results are not misinterpreted. Children often attach meanings to situations that are different from the meanings of an adult. It is crucial, therefore, that interpretation is up-front and central with children, to ensure credibility of the data. Children also like to communicate in their own way, often with art or play. Interpretation of these sources of data must also be verified with the children at the time of data collection.

Table 23.4. Developing state-of-the art research in pediatric palliative care: critical questions in education

---

- What education is needed to support families, children, and staff?
- Who requires education in pediatric palliative care?
- What are the most appropriate ways of delivering education about pediatric palliative care?
- Who should deliver this education?
- What impact does education have on care provision?
- What impact does education have on families' and staff's experiences?
- What are the ethical and research issues in pediatric palliative care?
- Is instrument development required regarding education in pediatric palliative care?

Quantitative methods strive to answer research questions or test hypotheses with the minimum amount of bias or contamination. Maintaining control over the setting, subjects, sample size, instruments, and conditions under which data are collected is critical. Control is maximized through randomization of subjects to groups, homogeneity of the sample, consistency in data collection procedures, and manipulation of independent variables. Pragmatic issues that will affect the scope and breadth of a study include the time required to complete a project, subject availability, financial and equipment resources, and ethical concerns.

While RCTs allow for maximal control, the pragmatic issues may preclude, or at least severely restrict, the use of RCTs and quasi-experimental studies in pediatric palliative care research. For example, longitudinal studies may be limited because the children are dying, so mortality becomes an issue; or the child's condition may deteriorate to the point where continued participation in an experiment is impossible. Further, the availability of subjects is restricted because of the relatively low numbers of children requiring palliative care and because of the diversity of their diseases. Finally, researchers should not place unethical demands on subjects, yet increased ethical difficulties arise when working with dying children and their families. In addition, randomization becomes an ethical concern when one is giving a potentially useful treatment to one group and not to another when all of the children are dying.

Nonexperimental studies, such as correlational or descriptive designs, are more feasible in pediatric palliative care. They are efficient and effective ways of collecting large amounts of data about a problem in a realistic setting and allow for the investigation of complex relationships among variables. While these designs consider concepts of control as much as possible, strict controls are not as critical as in experimental research.

Data can be collected through a number of means in quantitative research, such as observation, biological and physiological measurements, interviews and questionnaires, or records of available data. However, many of these measures are obtained objectively and do not access the subjective perspective of the individual. Further, chart audits and use of available records are limited to the information that has been collected. Much information is never documented and much of what is available is subjective from the perspective of the healthcare professional.

Interviews (verbal, face-to-face, or telephone) and questionnaires (written, face-to-face, or mailed) are the most appropriate tools to allow children and families to express their own ideas. Open-ended questions, to which subjects respond in their own words, and closed-ended questions, which have a fixed number of alternative responses, are both suitable. However, young children will be unable to answer some questions. They may require assistance, and interviews with open-ended questions are often easier than questionnaires with fixed responses. Creative ways of collecting data include pictorial descriptors instead of words on questionnaires and the use of drawings to allow children to express what they know. Parents are an extremely valuable source of information too, especially when the child is unable to communicate verbally, because they know their child well and can recognize and interpret the child's cues.

Quantitative methods lend themselves to answering many of the questions identified as priorities for pediatric palliative care research, such as questions about the prevalence of various symptoms, the coping strategies used by children and families, and evaluation research. In contrast to quantitative research, qualitative research explores the social world with the assumption that day-to-day realities change and are both variable and complex. Qualitative methods are particularly suited to describing, explaining, and interpreting experiences of children, their families, and their caregivers; their perceptions of and satisfaction with care; and the meanings they attach to their experience with the various aspects of pediatric palliative care. Conceptualizations, and sometimes even theory development, about everyday experiences, starting with the subjective perspectives of participants, are the major products of qualitative research. Qualitative approaches can often complement quantitative findings; in addition, they reflect the complexity of care, which is not possible with other methods. The strengths of qualitative methods in pediatric palliative care research are seen in the flexibility and responsiveness of data collection. Qualitative approaches acknowledge the uniqueness of each child and family and attempt to tailor care to match individual needs within the context of the numerous factors that affect the quality of life of those in need of pediatric palliative care. Pediatric palliative care emphasizes a holistic, individualized, and collaborative approach to the child and family and respects the varying ways in which children and their families perceive and interpret their experience and make meaning. Such also are the underlying principles of qualitative research. A qualitative approach, therefore, is imperative, along with more traditional methods, to the development of research in pediatric palliative care.

References

1. World Health Organization. Cancer Pain and Palliative Care. Technical Report Series 804. Geneva: World Health Organization, 1990.
2. Davies B, Howell D. Special services for children. In: Doyle D, Hanks G, MacDonald N, eds. Oxford Textbook of Palliative Medicine, 2d ed. Oxford: Oxford University Press, 1998:1084–1095.
3. Leonard K, Enzle S, McTavish J, et al. Prolonged cancer death. A family affair. Cancer Nurs 1995; 18:222–227.
4. Davies B, Steele R. Families in pediatric palliative care. In: Portenoy RK, Bruera E, eds. Topics in Palliative Care, vol 3. New York: Oxford University Press, 1998: 29–49.
5. Davies B, Reimer J, Brown P, et al. Fading Away: The Experience of Transition in Families with Terminal Illness. Amityville, NY: Baywood Publishing Company, 1995.
6. Davies B, Steele R. Challenges in identifying children for palliative care. J Palliat Care 1996; 12:5–8.

7. Masri C, Farrell A, Lacroix J, et al. Decision making and end-of-life care in critically ill children. J Palliat Care 2000; 16(Suppl):S45–S52.

8. Collins J. Pharmacologic management of pediatric cancer pain. In: Portenoy RK, Bruera E, eds. Topics in Palliative Care, vol 3. New York: Oxford University Press, 1998:7–28.

9. Levetown M. Treatment of symptoms other than pain in pediatric palliative care. In: Portenoy RK, Bruera E, eds. Topics in Palliative Care, vol 3 New York: Oxford University Press, 1998:51–69.

10. Chambers E, Oakhill A, Cornish J, et al. Terminal care at home for children with cancer. BMJ 1989; 298:937–940.

11. Hain R, Patel N, Crabtree S, et al. Respiratory symptoms in children dying from malignant disease. Palliat Med 1995; 9:201–206.

12. Hirschfeld S, Moss H, Dragisic K, et al. Pain in pediatric human immunodeficiency virus infection: incidence and characteristics in a single-institution pilot study. Pediatrics 1996; 98:449–452.

13. Hunt A. Child care: open house. Nurs Times 1986; 82:53–57.

14. Hunt A. A survey of signs, symptoms and symptom control in 30 terminally ill children. Dev Med Child Neurol 1990; 32:341–346.

15. Hunt A. Medical and nursing problems of children with neurodegenerative disease. Palliat Med 1995; 9:19–26.

16. Levy M, Duffy C, Pollock P, et al. Home-based palliative care for children. Part 1: The institution of a program. J Palliat Care 1990; 1:11–15.

17. Ferrell B, Rhiner M, Shapiro B, et al. The experience of pediatric cancer pain. Part I: Impact of pain on the family. J Pediatr Nurs 1994; 9:368–379.

18. Rhiner M, Ferrell B, Shapiro B, et al. The experience of pediatric cancer pain. Part II: Management of pain. J Pediatr Nurs 1994; 6:380–387.

19. Fernandez C, Stutzer C, MacWilliam L, et al. Alternative and complementary therapy use in pediatric oncology patients in British Columbia: prevalence and reasons for use and nonuse. J Clin Oncol 1998; 16:1279–1286.

20. Spinetta J, Swarner J, Sheposh H. Effective parental coping following the death of a child from cancer. J Pediatr Psychol 1981; 6:251–263.

21. Klass D. Parental Grief: Solace and Resolution. New York: Springer, 1988.

22. Segal S, Fletcher M, Meekison WG. Survey of bereaved parents. CMAJ 1986; 134: 38–42.

23. Davies BYH. Living with dying: families coping with a child who has a neurodegenerative genetic disorder. Axon 1996; 18:38–44.

24. Gravelle A. Caring for a child with a progressive illness during the complex chronic phase: parents' experience of facing adversity. J Adv Nurs 1997; 25:738–745.

25. Davies B, Deveau E, deVeber B, et al. Experiences of mothers in five countries whose child died of cancer. Cancer Nurs 1998; 21:301–311.

26. Spinetta J. The sibling of the child with cancer. In: Spinetta J, Deasy-Spinetta P, eds. Living with Childhood Cancer. St. Louis: Mosby, 1981:133–142.

27. Stein A, Forrest G, Woolley H, et al. Life threatening illness and hospice care. Arch Dis Child 1989; 64:687–702.

28. Davies B. Putting sibling bereavement into perspective. In: Davies B, ed. Shadows in the Sun: Experiences of Sibling Bereavement in Childhood. Philadelphia: Brunner/Mazel, 1999:195–220.

29. Davies B. Family functioning: impact on siblings. In: Davies B, ed. Shadows in the Sun: Experiences of Sibling Bereavement in Childhood. Philadelphia: Brunner/Mazel, 1999:149–170.
30. Bluebond-Langner M. In the Shadow of Illness: Parents and Siblings of the Chronically Ill Child. Princeton, NJ: Princeton University Press, 1996.
31. Cohen M. The stages of the prediagnostic period in chronic, life-threatening childhood illness: a process analysis. Res Nurs Health 1995; 18:39–48.
32. Ievers CE, Drotar D. Family and parental functioning in cystic fibrosis. Dev Behav Pediatr 1996; 17:48–55.
33. Lesar S, Moldonado Y. Parental coping strategies in families of HIV-infected children. Child Health Care 1996; 25:19–35.
34. Mastrogiannopoulou K, Stallard P, Lewis M, et al. The impact of childhood non-malignant life-threatening illness on parents: gender differences and predictors of parental adjustment. J Child Psychol Psychiatry 1997; 38:823–829.
35. Davies B, Collins J, Steele R, et al. Final Report: Family Voices—An Evaluation of the Impact of the Canuck Place Children's Hospice Program on Families. Vancouver, B.C.: British Columbia Health Research Foundation, 1999.
36. Steele R. Navigating Uncharted Territory: Experiences of Families when a Child has a Neurodegenerative Life Threatening Illness. Vancouver: University of British Columbia, 1999, Dissertation.
37. Vickers JL, Carlisle C. Choices and control: parental experiences in pediatric terminal home care. J Pediatr Oncol Nurs 2000; 17:12–21.
38. Wiener L, Theut S, Steinberg S, et al. The HIV-infected child: parental responses and psychosocial implications. Am J Orthopsychiatry 1994; 64:485–492.
39. James L, Johnson B. The needs of parents of pediatric oncology patients during the palliative care phase. J Pediatr Oncol Nurs 1997; 14:83–95.
40. Pehler S. Children's spiritual response: validation of the nursing diagnosis of spiritual distress. Nurs Diagn 1997; 8:55–66.
41. Silber TJ, Riley M. Spiritual and religious concerns of the hospitalized adolescent. Adolescence 1985; 20:217–224.
42. Davies B, Brenner P, Orloff S, et al. Addressing spirituality in pediatric hospice and palliative care. J Palliat Care 2002; 18:59–67.
43. Fraser K. Comforts of home: home care for the terminally. Can Fam Physician 1990; 36:977–981.
44. Mor V, Hiris J. Determinants of site of death among hospice cancer patients. J Health Soc Behav 1983; 24:375–384.
45. Ramsay A. Care of cancer patients in a home-based hospice program: a comparison of oncologists and primary care physicians. J Fam Pract 1992; 34:170–174.
46. Stajduhar K, Davies B. Death at home: challenges for families and directions for the future. J Palliat Care 1998; 14:8–14.
47. Field D, James N. Where and how people die. In: Clark D, ed. The Future for Palliative Care: Issues in Policy and Practice. Philadelphia: Open University Press, 1993:6–29.
48. Kopecky EA, Jacobson S, Joshi P, et al. Review of a home-based palliative care program for children with malignant and non-malignant disease. J Palliat Care 1997; 13:28–33.
49. Duffy C, Pollock P, Levy P, et al. Home based palliative care for children. Part 2: The benefits of an established program. J Palliat Care 1990; 6:8–14.

50. Lauer M, Camitta B. Home care for dying children: a nursing model. J Pediatr 1980; 997:1032–1035.

51. Martinson I. Hospice care for children: past, present and future. J Pediatr Oncol Nurs 1993; 10:93–98.

52. Martinson I, Moldow D, Armstong G, et al. Home care for children dying of cancer. Res Nurs Health 1986; 9:11–16.

53. Schweitzer S, Mitchell B, Landsverk J, et al. The costs of a pediatric hospice program. Public Health Rep 1993; 108:37–44.

54. Birenbaum L, Clarke-Steffen L. Terminal care costs in childhood cancer. Pediatr Nurs 1992; 18:285–288.

55. Stein A, Woolley H. An evaluation of hospice care for children. In: Baum J, Dominica F, Woodward R, eds. Listen: My Child Has A Lot of Living to Do. New York: Oxford University Press, 1990:66–90.

56. Parker M. Families caring for chronically ill children with tuberous sclerosis complex. Fam Community Health 1996; 19:73–84.

57. Sumner L, Hurula J. Pediatric hospice nursing: making the most of each moment. Nursing 1993; 23:50–55.

58. Davies B, Clarke D, Connaughty S, et al. Caring for dying children: nurses' experiences. Pediatr Nurs 1996; 22:500–507.

59. Papadatou D, Papazoglou I, Petraki D, et al. Mutual support among nurses who provide care to dying children. Illness Crisis Loss 1999; 7:37–48.

60. Ferrell B, Grant M, Ritchey K, et al. The pain resource nurse training program: a unique approach to pain management. J Pain Symptom Manage 1993; 8:549–556.

61. Copp G. Palliative care nursing education: a review of research findings. J Adv Nurs 1994; 19:552–557.

62. Brockopp D. Palliative care: essential concepts in the education of health professionals. J Palliat Care 1987; 2:18–23.

63. Degner L, Gow C. Preparing nurses for care of the dying: a longitudinal study. Cancer Nurs 1988; 11:160–169.

64. Degner L, Gow C, Thompson L. Critical nursing behaviors in care for the dying. Cancer Nurs 1991; 14:246–253.

65. Yuen K, Barrington D, Headford N, et al. Educating doctors in palliative medicine: development of a competency-based training program. J Palliat Care 1998; 14: 79–82.

66. MacDonald N. Priorities in education and research in palliative care. Palliat Med 1993; (Suppl 1):65–76.

67. Charlton R. Medical education—addressing the needs of the dying child. Palliat Med 1996; 10:240–246.

68. Liben S. Pediatric palliative medicine: obstacles to overcome. J Palliat Care 1996; 12:24–28.

24

Palliative Care Research in Human Immunodeficiency Virus/Acquired Immunodeficiency Syndrome: Clinical Trials of Symptomatic Therapies

KRISTINA JONES AND WILLIAM BREITBART

With the widespread introduction of highly active antiretroviral therapies (HAARTs), mortality rates among patients with advanced human immunodeficiency virus (HIV) disease have declined dramatically.[1] While media attention continues to focus on the encouraging advances in treatment, the fact remains that acquired immunodeficiency syndrome (AIDS) kills many young Americans. There were an estimated 21,000 deaths from AIDS in the United States in 1997. This is a sharp contrast to 1995, during which over 49,000 deaths were reported.[2] While death rates from AIDS have been halved by the introduction of HAART, AIDS remains a disease without a definitive treatment. Clinical data are being generated by following populations of patients being treated with increasingly complex arrays of new medication. Although early results for some patients are encouraging, a proportion of patients will be considered treatment failures when, despite aggressive salvage regimens, viral load measures rise, CD4 counts decline, and AIDS progresses. For these patients, it is essential that the clinician be aware of state-of-the-art palliative interventions.

Research into symptom control from palliative care specialists must be applied to new clinical realities: a substantial proportion of patients require aggressive symptom management of side effects to enable them to continue antiretroviral treatment. With prolonged survival comes the challenge of providing symptom control over longer periods of time. Interestingly, the boundary between active and palliative treatment may be blurred, with patients choosing to continue only those medications they can tolerate and clinicians managing patients who may elect to continue only one or two new medications while also requiring symptom control for irreversible conditions, such as peripheral neuropathy.

Palliative care and quality of life in patients with advanced AIDS continue to be important areas of clinical care and investigation.[3] Significant progress has been made in extending a palliative care and quality of life research agenda to the clinical problems of patients with AIDS.

New research into quality of life for AIDS patients shows a high prevalence of symptoms and symptom distress. Vogl et al.[4] used the Memorial Symptom Assessment Scale, a validated measure of physical and psychological symptom distress, to evaluate 504 AIDS outpatients. The mean number of symptoms was 16. The most prevalent symptoms were worrying (86%), fatigue (85%), sadness (82%), and pain (76%). Other common symptoms included feeling irritable (75%), difficulty sleeping (73%), feeling nervous (68%), dry mouth (67%), difficulty concentrating (64%), shortness of breath (62%), drowsiness (61%), cough (60%), numbness and tingling in hands and feet (58%), itching (56%), and sweats (55%). Patients with Karnofsky performance scores less than 70 had more symptoms and higher symptom distress than patients with higher Karnofsky scores. Both the number of symptoms and symptom distress were highly associated with psychological distress and poorer quality of life. Neither gender nor CD4 or T-cell count was associated with symptom number or distress. This empirical evidence amply illustrates that AIDS patients experience many distressing physical symptoms and a high level of distress. Research into symptom assessment provides information that is valuable in evaluating AIDS treatment regimens and defining strategies to improve quality of life. Supportive care and palliative care principles and practices can address symptoms with evidence-based interventions to ensure high quality of life for those living longer with AIDS.

This chapter will review the major areas of research in AIDS palliative care (Table 24.1) and begins with research addressing the important issues of pain and fatigue. Studies dealing with the major neuropsychiatric syndromes of delirium and dementia will be discussed in detail. This is followed by an overview of the research focusing on major psychiatric illnesses, including depression, anxi-

Table 24.1. Major areas of research

Pain
Fatigue
Delirium
Dementia
Psychiatric disorders: depression, anxiety, psychosis
Wasting/anorexia
Endocrinopathies: hypogonadism, lipodystrophy
End-of-life issues I: physician-assisted suicide
End-of-life issues II: desire for death

---

ety, and psychosis. Intervention trials for endocrinopathies and AIDS-related cachexia will be described. The chapter concludes with a brief look at two complex end-of-life issues: physician-assisted suicide and desire for death in the terminally ill. A discussion of research methodology in HIV palliative care and suggestions for further areas of inquiry is presented at the end of the chapter.

Major Areas of Research

Pain

Despite advances in AIDS therapies, pain continues to be a major issue.[5] The following discussion will be limited to the specific area of clinical trials. Pain is highly prevalent, diverse, and varied in syndromal presentation. Research illustrates that pain is associated with significant psychological and functional morbidity and is alarmingly undertreated.[6]

Prevalence studies
Estimates of the prevalence of pain in HIV-infected individuals have ranged from 30% to over 90%, with the occurrence of pain increasing as the disease progresses. In a prospective cross-sectional survey of 438 ambulatory AIDS patients in New York City, the prevalence of pain increased significantly as HIV disease progressed, with 67% of those with Centers for Disease Control (CDC) category C disease reporting pain.[7] Patients were also more likely to report pain if they had other concurrent HIV-related symptoms (such as fatigue, wasting), had been treated for an opportunistic infection, or had not been receiving antiretroviral medication.[7] Those cared for by hospice workers at home had prevalence rates and intensity ratings that were comparable to, and even exceeded, those of cancer patients.[8]

Pain syndromes
Pain syndromes in AIDS are diverse in nature and etiology; the most common pain syndromes include sensory peripheral neuropathy, extensive Kaposi's sarcoma, headache, oral and pharyngeal pain, abdominal pain, chest pain, arthralgias and myalgias, and dermatological conditions. Among palliative care patients with low $CD4^+$ counts, pain of a neuropathic nature (polyneuropathies, radiculopathies, toxic neuropathies) comprises a large proportion of pain syndromes, with up to 40% of patients reporting this type of pain. In studies conducted by the Memorial Sloan-Kettering group, over 50% of pain syndromes were classified as rheumatological in nature, including various forms of arthralgia and myalgia.[9]

World Health Organization guidelines
Empiric treatment using standard pain medications for all pain syndromes (including the neuropathies) which are derived from treating diseases other than

AIDS is common practice, though hard data on actual effectiveness are lacking. The Word Health Organization (WHO) guidelines for the analgesic management of cancer pain (the WHO analgesic ladder) have been recommended by clinical authorities in the field of pain management in AIDS. The WHO guidelines have been endorsed for use in AIDS pain by the federal Agency for Health Care Policy and Research.[10] Because of widespread clinical use and general efficacy in cancer and other illnesses, validation studies of opioids in AIDS hospice settings are unlikely to be conducted; instead, case reports and clinical practice patterns are described in the literature.[11]

Opioids: clinical trials

Opioids are the mainstay of pharmacotherapy for pain of moderate to severe intensity in the patient with HIV disease, and there are several reports of safe and effective use of opioids for HIV-related pain. Kaplan and colleagues[12] conducted a multicenter open-label prospective study in which 44 patients with moderate to severe AIDS-related pain were treated with sustained-release oral morphine for up to 18 days. In the patients who were fully evaluated, pain intensity decreased by 65%, quality of life was "good" in 80% of patients, and 78% rated the acceptability of treatment as "excellent." Side effects occurred in 62% of those treated but were resolved in 92% of patients with standard clinical management techniques. Morphine dose remained stable during the study, even for a subgroup with a history of intravenous (IV) drug abuse.[12]

Lefkowitz and Newshan[13] studied 35 AIDS patients in an open-label comparison of oral opioids versus transdermal fentanyl patch. Twice as many patients had total pain relief using fentanyl patches, and 89% said they preferred the patch to oral opioid during the clinical study period.[13] Nonenteral routes of administration for pain medication clearly deserve further investigation: in a study on patient-related barriers to pain management in AIDS, the vast majority of subjects endorsed a pain intervention that would require taking a minimal number of additional pills.[14]

Anticonvulsants may prove useful as an adjuvant to opioids for pain in AIDS patients. Caraceni et al.[15] suggested that gabapentin was useful as an "add-on" therapy in 22 cancer patients with neuropathic pain only partially responsive to opioids. Their open-label study found that gabapentin decreased mean pain scores, decreased lancinating pain, and was very useful in allodynia.

Neuropathic pain

Neuropathic pain remains a challenging clinical issue for almost half of the HIV/AIDS population, related both to the virus itself and to neuropathic toxicities of HAART.[16] Since opioids alone are rarely satisfactory in treating neuropathic pain, adjuvant analgesics such as antidepressants and anticonvulsants are widely used.[17] For a recent review of adjuvant drugs for neuropathic cancer pain, see Hewitt and Portenoy.[18] While studies of the analgesic efficacy of antidepressants (including both selective serotonin reuptake inhibitors [SSRIs] and tricyclic antidepressants) in AIDS patients have not yet been conducted, such agents are widely applied clinically, using the models of diabetic and postherpetic neuropathies.

Antidepressant studies. Amitriptyline is the tricyclic antidepressant most studied and has been proven effective as an analgesic in a large number of clinical trials addressing a wide variety of chronic pain syndromes, including neuropathy.[19,20] While many AIDS patients find the anticholinegic effects of tricyclics intolerable, for some, particularly those with chronic diarrhea, the same side effects may be clinically useful.

Paroxetine is widely used in clinical practice for AIDS neuropathy based on research evidence for effectiveness as an analgesic in a controlled trial for the treatment of diabetic neuropathy.[21] While well tolerated in terms of side effects, clinicians must be aware of the potential P-450 interaction with protease inhibitors such as ritonavir.[22]

Anticonvulsant studies. Selected anticonvulsant drugs appear to have analgesic effect in the lancinating dysesthesias that characterize diverse types of neuropathic pain.[17] While many pain and palliative care physicians prefer to begin with carbamazepine because of its efficacy in trigeminal neuralgia, this drug must be used with some caution in AIDS patients with thrombocytopenia and those at risk for marrow failure. Estimates of risk of serious adverse effects, such as Stevens-Johnson syndrome, have not been made for AIDS populations.[23]

Research evaluating the newer anticonvulsants is appearing in the literature and may be generalizable to the AIDS population. Backonja et al.[24] used gabapentin in a large sample of patients with diabetic neuropathy. They studied 165 patients in a randomized double-blind control trial for 8 weeks and found that gabapentin improved pain, sleep, mood, and quality of life. Gabapentin also had significant positive results in a large group of patients with postherpetic neuralgia. Rowbotham and colleagues[25] conducted a multicenter randomized double-blind placebo-controlled trial with 229 postherpetic neuralgia patients. Patients were given a maximum of 3,600 mg/day of gabapentin over 8 weeks, resulting in significant improvement in pain, sleep disturbance, quality of life, and mood. Clearly, trials of gapabentin and the newer anticonvulsants are needed in a large AIDS sample. Initial clinical impressions, open-label studies, and case reports suggest that there may be some use not only for gabapentin but for valproate, phenytoin, and clonazepam as well.[17]

Tramadol. Tramadol is a centrally acting, binary analgesic that is neither an opiate-derived nor a nonsteroidal anti-inflammatory drug, which was approved for use in the United States in 1995. It is a cyclohexanol derivative with mu-agonist activity, which also inhibits norepinephrine reuptake and stimulates serotonin release. Results of a double-blind randomized trial of tramadol for diabetic neuropathy in 65 patients indicated that at an average dose of 210 mg/day it was significantly more effective than placebo for treating the pain of diabetic neuropathy.[26] Trials of tramadol in AIDS-related peripheral neuropathies are not available. Important safety considerations must be given to the potential for serotonin syndrome if tramadol is coadministered with serotonergic antidepressants.[27,28]

Peptide T, amitriptyline, and mexiletine. The burden of suffering for patients with neuropathic pain is severe: research into new primary and adjuvant drugs is ongoing. Simpson et al.[29] conducted a multicenter, double-blind, randomized 12-week trial of intranasal peptide T in HIV neuropathy. While there were no significant adverse effects, the study regimen of 6 mg/day of intranasal peptide T failed to show any significant change in pain intensity scores or improvement on clinical exam. The study revealed no positive change on neuropsychological measures or serial nerve conduction studies. In another study, the AIDS Clinical Trial Group investigated amitriptyline versus mexiletine for pain in HIV neuropathy. They enrolled 137 patients in a multicenter, double-blind randomized, placebo-controlled trial. While no major toxicities were reported, results were disappointing, with no significant difference in mean decrease in Gravely pain scores (amitriptyline = 0.36, mexiletine = 0.35, placebo = 0.26 unit improvements).[30]

It is clear from the survey of research into pain in AIDS that, though data are lacking for many clinical interventions currently in use, new interventions are being actively investigated. While continued efforts in pain medication research are essential, there are unique issues that face the clinical population of patients with AIDS-related pain which also deserve notice. Research has demonstrated a dramatic undertreatment of pain in AIDS: in one cohort of ambulatory AIDS patients, 18% of patients with "severe" pain were prescribed no analgesics whatsoever, 40% were prescribed nonopioid analgesics, and only 22% were prescribed a "weak" opioid (such as acetaminophen in combination with oxycodone).[31] This degree of undermedication of pain in AIDS (85%) far exceeds published reports of undermedication of pain in cancer patient populations.[32]

Barriers to pain control

Research on a cohort of 200 ambulatory AIDS patients revealed a number of AIDS-specific barriers to pain management, specifically that 66% of these patients try to limit their overall intake of medication ("pills") or to use nonpharmacological interventions for pain, 50% cannot afford a prescription for analgesics or have no access to pain specialists, and about 50% are reluctant to take opioids for pain out of a concern that family, friends, and physicians will assume they are misusing or abusing these drugs.[14]

Barriers to effective pain management also exist on the side of AIDS care providers. In a survey of approximately 500 AIDS care providers (primarily physicians and nurses), 51.8% endorsed a lack of knowledge regarding pain management, 51.5% were reluctant to prescribe opioids, and 50.9% reported lack of access to pain specialists. There were concerns regarding drug addiction and/or abuse in 50.5% of the sample, and finally, 43% of providers reported that lack of psychological and drug abuse treatment services interfered with providing effective pain management.[31] Clinicians' fears that AIDS patients with a history of substance abuse might over-report their pain or that patients currently using substances would over-report their pain in order to obtain drugs for illicit use or diversion were not borne out by empirical research. A study of 516 ambulatory AIDS patients found little difference in pain reporting among substance users versus non-users. The study did reveal a dramatic undertreatment of those with drug abuse histories.

Impact of pain on quality of life

Pain in patients with HIV disease has a profound negative impact on physical and psychological functioning, as well as on overall quality of life. In a study addressing the impact of pain on quality of life and on psychological functioning in ambulatory AIDS patients, depression was correlated significantly with the presence of pain.[33] In addition to being markedly more distressed, depressed, and hopeless, those with pain were twice as likely to have suicidal ideation (40%) than those without pain (20%). Patients who were HIV-positive and in pain were more functionally impaired. Larue and colleagues[8] noted that HIV-infected patients with pain intensities greater than 5 (on a 0–10 numerical rating scale) reported significantly poorer quality of life during the week preceding the survey than patients without pain. Pain intensity had an independent negative impact on HIV patients' quality of life.

Fatigue

Fatigue is an overlooked, under-reported, and undertreated symptom in the palliative care of AIDS patients.[34,35] Breitbart and colleagues[36] completed a prospective cross-sectional survey of 427 ambulatory AIDS patients and found that 54% endorsed fatigue based on their responses to fatigue items on the Memorial Symptom Assessment Scale. The study found a higher prevalence of fatigue in women and that patients who reported homosexual contact as their transmission risk factor were significantly less likely to report fatigue than those reporting injection drug use or heterosexual contact. The presence of fatigue was significantly correlated with the number of current AIDS-related physical symptoms, current treatment for HIV-related medical disorders, pain, anemia, and physical debilitation. Fatigue was also associated with poorer quality of life and psychological distress as measured by the Brief Symptom Inventory, Beck Depression Inventory (BDI), Beck Hopelessness Scale, and Functional Living Inventory for Cancer (modified for AIDS).

General perceptions concerning fatigue, including the view that its etiology cannot be determined, that it is an inevitable manifestation of illness that must be endured, or that few interventions are available, need to be challenged by good research evidence that there are recognizable causes for fatigue for which interventions can be beneficial. For a comprehensive approach to fatigue, see Cella et al.[37] Fatigue can be treated directly, or the underlying cause can be treated; in both cases, patient and family education is important, as is the management of the consequences of fatigue, such as deconditioning or decline in occupational functioning.[37] Specific interventions can be targeted at anemia,[38] hypogonadism,[39] myopathy,[40] wasting,[41] pain,[42] HIV dementia or central nervous system (CNS) infection,[43] and depression or other psychiatric illness.[36]

Psychostimulants

Despite the prevalence and clinical significance of fatigue in HIV/AIDS patients, there are few published sources of quality regarding treatment. The pharmacological intervention that has shown the most promise in patients with cancer and multiple sclerosis is the use of psychostimulants: to date, there have been few controlled studies of these medications.[44]

Two controlled trials of psychostimulants in non-HIV populations have included fatigue as one of several outcome variables. Bruera and colleagues[45] demonstrated the utility of psychostimulants for treatment of fatigue in a controlled trial of methylphenidate as an adjuvant analgesic for the treatment of cancer pain. Weinshenker et al.[46] reported positive results from a controlled trial of pemoline (Cylert) for fatigue in patients with multiple sclerosis. The utility of psychostimulants for the treatment of fatigue in patients with AIDS was suggested by Fernandez and colleagues,[47] who administered stimulants to patients with AIDS dementia.

In the first well-designed study of its kind, Breitbart and colleagues[48] conducted a randomized, double-blind placebo-controlled trial of two psychostimulants for the treatment of fatigue in ambulatory patients with HIV disease. Subjects were randomized to receive methylphenidate, pemoline, or placebo. The average age of the 109 subjects was 40 years, with a mean CD4 count of 314. Seventy percent of the patients met the 1992 CDC criteria for a diagnosis of AIDS. Subjects were screened using the Folstein Mini-Mental State Exam (MMSE), the Structured Clinical Interview for Diagnosis, and a neuropsychological battery designed to screen for HIV dementia. Evidence of cognitive impairment on either the MMSE (scores below 22) or on the neuropsychological battery (performance more than 1 standard deviation below normative data) excluded patients from the study. Patients were also excluded if they were diagnosed with a major depressive episode or tested positive for current substance abuse. Subjects were included if they rated their fatigue greater than 5 on a 0–10 numeric rating scale and were administered two self-report measures of fatigue: the Piper Fatigue Scale (PFS) and the Visual Analogue Scale for Fatigue Severity (VAS-F).[49] Subjects were randomized to three groups and assessed in person on a weekly basis, with intensive telephone contact between visits over 6 weeks. The maximum doses allowed by the protocol were 60 mg/day of methylphenidate, 150 mg/day of pemoline, and 8 capsules/day of placebo.

Methylphenidate and pemoline were equally effective, and both were significantly superior to placebo at decreasing fatigue severity with minimal side effects. A multivariate analysis of variance assessing the impact of psychostimulant treatment on improvement in the various measures of fatigue demonstrated an overall significant effect for the total scores on the PFS. The Affective and Sensory subscales yielded significant improvement, while there were no significant differences on the Cognitive and Severity subscales. Methylphenidate and pemoline were equally effective on the PFS subscales that showed improvement in fatigue. Results using the VAS-F yielded no significant differences between the psychostimulants and placebo, on either total score or the Fatigue subscale. However, changes in the Energy subscale of the VAS-F did differ significantly across the three groups.

   Improvement of fatigue was significantly associated with improved quality of life and with decreased levels of both depression and psychological distress. Measurement of fatigue is clearly a complex and difficult task: the degree of improvement was not uniform across all measures. The strongest, most consistent, and statistically significant group differences were evident on the PFS, which is an extensively validated, multidimensional self-report scale. Fatigue contributes independently to physical limitation and disability in AIDS patients.[50] It is a frequently neglected part of the symptom management of AIDS patients, which deserves greater attention and study.

Delirium

Delirium is a common and often serious medical complication in the patient with advanced illness. Cognitive disorders, and delirium in particular, have enormous relevance to symptom control and palliative care. Delirium is highly prevalent in cancer and AIDS patients with advanced disease, particularly in the last weeks of life, with prevalence rates ranging 25%–85%.[51] The prevalence of delirium in the hospitalized medically ill generally ranges 10%–30%.[52,53] At greater risk for delirium are the elderly, postoperative, cancer, and AIDS patients.[54–56] Approximately 30%–40% of medically hospitalized AIDS patients develop delirium, and as many as 65%–80% develop some type of organic mental disorder.[57,58]

Morbidity
Delirium is associated with increased morbidity in the terminally ill, causing distress in patients, family members, and staff.[59] (Delirium can interfere dramatically with the recognition and control of other physical and psychological symptoms, such as pain.[60])

Clinical features
The clinical features of delirium are quite numerous and include a variety of neuropsychiatric symptoms that are also common to other psychiatric disorders, such as depression, dementia, and psychosis.[61] In the palliative care setting, delirium can be manifested by nonspecific prodromal symptoms, such as restlessness, anxiety, sleep disturbance, and irritability.

   The *Diagnostic and Statistical Manual*, edition IV (DSM-IV) diagnostic criteria for delirium include symptoms in four different domains: disturbances of consciousness, attention, cognition, and perception. The DSM-IV criteria are defined as follows: (1) disturbance of consciousness (reduced clarity of awareness of the environment) with reduced ability to focus, sustain, or shift attention; (2) a change in cognition (such as memory deficit, disorientation, language disturbance) or development of a perceptual disturbance which is not better accounted for by a preexisting, established, or evolving dementia; (3) the disturbance develops over a short period of time and tends to fluctuate during the course of the day; (4) evidence from the history, physical examination, or laboratory findings that the disturbance is caused by the direct physiological consequences of a general medical condition.[62]

Perceptual disturbances in delirium commonly include loosely organized delusions, often of a suspicious type; illusions; misperceptions; and less commonly, visual hallucinations.[63] Further symptoms include increased or decreased psychomotor activity, disturbance of sleep–wake cycle, and affective symptoms (emotional lability, sadness, anger and euphoria).[64]

Delirium assessment research instruments

The quality of research into delirium is improving as more investigators employ DSM-IV criteria and screening instruments are based on either the DSM-IV or the International Classification of Diseases (ICD) criteria. Smith and colleagues[65] have critically reviewed instruments used to detect, diagnose, and rate delirium. They note that both the DSM-IV and the ICD-9 and ICD-10 criteria are valid for diagnosis but not for severity of delirium. They reviewed the reliability and validity of a wide range of instruments, including the Delirium Symptom Interview (DSI), Confusion-Assessment Method, Confusion-Rating Scale, NEECHAM Confusion Scale, Delirium Scale, Global Accessibilty Rating, Saskatoon Delirium Checklist, Delirium Rating Scale (DRS), and Memorial Delirium-Assessment Scale (MDAS). They note that in studies of efficacy of treatment for delirium, the MDAS would be particularly useful as it is specifically designed to measure the changes in severity of delirium over time.[66]

Management

The standard approach to the management of delirium in the medically ill includes specific interventions directed at elucidating and correcting the underlying causes and more nonspecific interventions directed at controlling the symptoms of delirium. Important nonspecific interventions include psychosocial and environmental approaches, such as frequently orienting the patient, arranging visits by family members, providing a clock, and giving brief and simple commands. The mainstay of symptomatic treatment involves the use of pharmacotherapies, including neuroleptic drugs, benzodiazepines, and other sedatives.[67,68]

The literature on the pharmacological management of symptoms commonly associated with delirium in the medically ill includes an early series of controlled intervention trials that compared haloperidol to thioridazine and thioridazine to diazepam in the treatment of "agitation and psychotic symptoms" related to dementia (often with superimposed delirium) in geriatric populations.[69–72]

Two additional controlled trials compared haloperidol to droperidol in "agitated and combative" emergency room patients with a variety of undefined organic mental and functional disorders and paraldehyde to diazepam in medically hospitalized patients with alcohol withdrawal and delirium tremens.[73,74] While these studies suggest a role for neuroleptics, benzodiazepines, and other sedatives in the management of symptoms such as those seen in delirium, it is not clear that they were, in fact, conducted in delirious populations. Rather, the groups studied appear to be heterogeneous cohorts of demented, delirious, and psychotic patients. None of the studies used the validated rating scales described above.

A common strategy in the management of symptoms related to delirium is to add parenteral lorazepam to a regimen of haloperidol, for example, lorazepam 0.5 mg to 1.0 mg q 3–4 hours PO or IV, along with haloperidol, typically 0.5 mg to 1.0 mg (PO, IV, intramuscularly, or subcutaneously), using a low daily total dose of 1.0–3.0 mg, unless the patient manifested physical agitation or combativeness, in which case up to 10 mg/day or more could be employed.[75] (In general, doses need not exceed 20 mg of haloperidol in a 24-hour period; however, there are those who advocate high doses of intravenous Haldol in selected cases.[76])

Delirium study

In the only study of its kind to date, Breitbart and colleagues[77] conducted a double-blind, randomized comparison trial of haloperidol versus chlorpromazine versus lorazepam in hospitalized AIDS patients. Of the 244 patients entered into the trial, 30 developed delirium. This study demonstrated that lorazepam alone, in doses up to 8 mg in a 12-hour period, was ineffective in the treatment of delirium and, in fact, contributed to worsening delirium and cognitive impairment. Both neuroleptic drugs, however, in low doses (approximately 2 mg of haloperidol equivalent per 24 hours), were highly effective at controlling the symptoms of delirium, as measured by the DRS. Haloperidol and chlorpromazine also improved cognitive function, as illustrated by a dramatic improvement in Folstein MMSE scores. Both haloperidol and chlorpromazine significantly improved the symptoms of delirium in both the "hypoactive" as well as the "hyperactive" subtypes of delirium. This important study provides empirical evidence to guide clinical management and can be generalized to non-AIDS populations of delirious patients.

Novel antipsychotics

Several new antipsychotic agents with less or more specific dopamine-blocking effects, carrying less risk of extrapyramidal side effects, are now available and include clozaril, risperidone, and olanzapine. Risperidone had been clinically useful in the treatment of delirium, dementia, and psychosis in AIDS patients at doses of 1–6 mg/day, suggesting that it might be safe for use in patients with delirium.[78,79]

While lacking a randomized controlled trial of novel antipsychotics versus traditional neuroleptics, palliative care clinicians are increasingly using risperidone in low doses (0.5–1.0 mg BID PO) in the management of both dementia and delirium in terminally ill patients who have a demonstrated intolerance to the extrapyramidal side effects of the standard neuroleptics.[80] Currently, a limitation of the use of these new agents is their lack of availability in parenteral formulations.

Terminal delirium

While neuroleptic drugs such as haloperidol are most effective at diminishing agitation, clearing the sensorium, and improving cognition in delirious patients, neuroleptics alone are not always fully effective in the delirium that complicates the last days of life. Processes causing delirium may be ongoing and irreversible during the active dying phase. Independent research groups report that a significant proportion of terminally ill patients (10%–20%) experience delirium that can be controlled only by sedation to the point of significantly decreased consciousness.[81,82] The goal of treatment with such agents as midazolam, propofol, and to a lesser extent methotrimeprazine is quiet sedation only. Midazolam, given by subcutaneous or IV infusion in doses of 30–100 mg/day, can be used to control agitation related to delirium in the terminal stages.[83] Propofol, a short-acting anesthetic agent, has also begun to be employed as a sedating agent for terminal delirium. In several case reports of its use in terminal care, an IV loading dose of 20 mg was followed by continuous infusion, with initial doses ranging from 10 mg/hour to 70 mg/hour and titration up to a maximum of 400 mg/hour over a period of hours to days for severely agitated patients.[84] Propofol has an advantage over midazolam in that the level of sedation is more easily controlled and recovery is rapid upon decreasing the rate of infusion.

Controversies in the management of terminal delirium

Delirium is viewed by some as a natural part of the dying process, which should not be altered. In particular, some clinicians view hallucinations and delusions as an important element in the transition from life to death. This is particularly the case when patients speak of seeing or hearing dead relatives or souls communicating with them, possibly welcoming or calling them to heaven, or giving them permission to die. Clearly, there are some patients who experience these welcoming hallucinations during delirium as comforting, so it may be questionable whether to intervene. Another concern is that these patients are so close to death that aggressive treatment is unnecessary. Parenteral neuroleptics or sedatives may be mistakenly avoided because of exaggerated fears that they might hasten death through hypotension or respiratory depression. It is often wrongly assumed that because the underlying pathophysiology of hepatic or renal failure cannot be altered, no improvement can be expected in the patient's mental status. There is often the fear that neuroleptics or benzodiazepines may worsen a delirium by making the patient more sedated and therefore more confused.

Clinical experience in managing delirium suggests that the use of neuroleptics in the management of agitation, paranoia, hallucinations, and altered sensorium is safe, effective, appropriate, and of comfort to the dying patient. Management of delirium on a case-by-case basis seems wisest. The agitated, delirious dying patient should probably be given neuroleptics to help restore calm. A "wait-and-see" approach to neuroleptics with some patients who have a lethargic delirium or who find hallucinations comforting may be adopted. This must be tempered with the knowledge that neuroleptics relieve both *hyperactive* (agitated) and *hypoactive* (quiet) delirium. Additionally, neuroleptics should be withheld only in the setting of constant observation of the patient; it is important to remember that comforting hallucinations and delusions during terminal delirium can quickly become menacing and terrifying and that somnolence and agitation, as with other key symptoms of delirium, are unstable and fluctuate over time.

Dementia

Although the neuropsychological impairment associated with HIV is often subtle, it can affect day-to-day life and is associated with earlier mortality. It is not clear whether milder forms of neurocognitive disturbance necessarily presage advanced dementia. Current data suggest a two-factor model: a subacute relapsing–remitting condition that can occur at any stage of HIV disease and a progressive fulminant HIV dementia.[85] New regimens involving protease inhibitors need to be evaluated in terms of benefit to the CNS because many drugs of this class do not penetrate the blood–brain barrier efficiently.[86] The difficulty of measuring CNS viral load and the lack of correlation between magnetic resonance imaging findings and clinical symptoms present difficulties in evaluating dementia and assessing trials of interventional medication. Cerebral metabolite ratios and concentration in the frontal lobe and basal ganglia were measured using proton ^{1}H magnetic resonance spectroscopy in patients on HAART in the early stages of dementia, and it was found that HAART improved HIV cognitive–motor complex in a small sample of 12 patients.[87]

Numerous pharmacological agents are under investigation as treatment for HIV dementia, including nucleoside and non-nucleoside reverse transcriptase inhibitors, pentoxifylline, nitroglycerin, memantine, nimodipine, and peptide T.[88] Zidovudine is the most thoroughly investigated medication, with patients developing HIV dementia less frequently and showing improvement on neuropsychological, cerebrospinal fluid, and neuropathological evaluations. Zidovudine has been tested in placebo-controlled trials, which found that 2000 mg was more effective at improving cognitive deficits than 1000 mg. Clinically, this higher dose was not tolerated by large numbers of patients due to nausea, diarrhea, and fatigue.[89] Sustained response to zidovudine lasts 6 months to 1 year, and optimal response is achieved at the higher but less-tolerated dosages. Zidovudine was also found in a large retrospective study to increase survival, as well as to improve symptoms of dementia.[90] Recommendations for other medications cannot be made at this time, due to a lack of research data.[91]

In the palliative care setting, the clinician will be faced with the challenge of managing advanced AIDS dementia patients. Dementia in HIV is characterized by a triad of disturbances in cognition, motor performance, and behavior. Acquired cognitive abnormalities include deficits in attention, concentration, abstraction, memory, learning, speech, and language. Psychiatric and behavioral manifestations of AIDS dementia include apathy, inertia, irritability, emotional lability, impaired judgment, disinhibition of sexual or aggressive impulses, and socially inappropriate behavior.

There are no clinical trials concerning the management in behavioral disturbances in HIV dementia. For the psychomotor slowing, apathy, and inertia, many clinicians use methylphenidate, though seizure precautions should be observed when initiating medication.[92] Some improvement may be seen in patients with mood lability using anticonvulsants such as divalproex sodium or gabapentin, though this is based on clinical impressions of efficacy and not on clinical trials. Lastly, more severe behavioral disturbance is best managed with antipsychotics, such as olanzepine 2.5–5.0 mg PO QHS. Benzodiazepines should be avoided in patients suffering from dementia as they can cause further disinhibition.

Psychiatric Disorders: Depression, Anxiety, Psychosis

Early descriptions of psychopathology in people with HIV/AIDS, published until the late 1980s, reported alarmingly high rates of depression and suicide.[93] This led to the initiation of several large community cohort studies, for which results began to appear around 1990. These studies compared HIV-positive and HIV-negative communities and used the Structured Clinical Interview for DSM-III-R (SCID). Despite geographic and demographic differences, the findings were similar: substantially elevated rates of lifetime major depression and substance use were consistently observed. Rates of current mood disorder among non-IV drug–using HIV-positive men were not significantly different from rates of matched comparison groups included in the same studies. Rates of current major depression were in the 5%–9% range.[94]

Prevalence studies of psychiatric disorders

Rabkin et al.[94] conducted a cross-sectional, controlled study of 112 AIDS patients, the results of which are summarized below. They found no statistically significant differences between patients in their sample who were HIV-negative or HIV-positive or who had AIDS. They found that 3.0% of patients with AIDS met the criteria for depression using SCID, the Hamilton Rating Scale for Depression (HAM-D), and the BDI. This contrasted with current prevalence rates of 5.0% for HIV-positive subjects and 8.0% for HIV-negative gay men. These rates are higher than the Environmental Catchment Area (ECA) study's current depression prevalence of 2.2% in the general population.[95] The Rabkin study found no difference in the rate of depressive disorder as a function of HIV-illness stage. For none of the psychiatric disorders that they assessed were rates significantly higher among men with AIDS than among either the HIV-negative or the HIV-positive group. However, rates of *dysthymia* (mild chronic depression) were higher among men with CD4 counts between 200 and 500.

For any anxiety disorder (including panic disorder, generalized anxiety disorder, and social or simple phobias) Rabkin et al.[94] found rates of 8.0% for HIV-negative men and 13% for AIDS patients, which were not statistically significantly different and were comparable to ECA rates.

Rates of current alcohol-use disorder for groups of HIV-negative, HIV-positive, and AIDS patients were approximately the same as the total population rate of 6.2% found in the ECA study. Current drug-use disorder rates were substantially higher: 14.0% of AIDS subjects met criteria for a drug-use disorder, as did 17.0% of HIV-positive subjects, though this was not statistically significantly different from the 10.0% rate for HIV-negative subjects. This is in stark contrast to the 2.3% rate found in the ECA study.

Percentages of subjects taking antidepressant or anxiolytic medication were 32.0% for AIDS patients, 34.0% for those with CD4 counts between 200 and 500, and 14.0% for those with CD4 counts above 500. Data for antidepressant and anxiolytic use were not collected for the HIV-negative control group.

Depression

A thorough diagnostic assessment for depressed mood, which carefully differentiates between depression, fatigue, and wasting syndrome, should be undertaken in each patient presenting with depressed mood. Hormone levels, including thyroid and testosterone, should be measured in the workup for depression. Once organic factors in the patient's presentation have been evaluated, conventional antidepressants or psychostimulants may be used for biological treatment, along with psychotherapy or psychosocial intervention.

Rabkin and colleagues[94] (Table 24.2) conducted a randomized, placebo-controlled trial of fluoxetine, which included 120 patients, 51.0% of whom had AIDS. Patients were assessed using the Clinical Global Impression Scale and the HAM-D and followed for 8 weeks. This sample was predominantly male, and two-thirds white and included only 6.0% who had IV drug use as a risk factor. In an intention-to-treat analysis, 57.0% of fluoxetine patients and 41.0% of placebo patients were responders. Six patients dropped out due to side effects (one with a possible allergic rash), 16 did not return for follow-up appointments, and nine were removed from the study because of AIDS-related conditions. Among pa-

Table 24.2. Clinical trials in depression

Study	Design	Drug	Outcome
Rabkin et al.[94]	RPCT (n = 120, 51% subjects with AIDS)	Fluoxetine	74% positive response 41% placebo response
Elliott et al.[95]	RPCT (n = 75, 45% subjects with AIDS)	Paroxetine vs. imipramine	Both comparably effective, imipramine dropouts 48% due to side effects
Ferrando et al.[96]	Open label (n = 33, 80% subjects with AIDS)	Sertraline vs. Paroxetine vs. Fluoxetine	83% positive response, 27% dropout due to side effects Reduced somatic complaints
Elliot et al.[97]	Open label (n = 15, 60% subjects with AIDS) 50% on HAART	Nefazodone	73% response decrease Hamilton Anxiety Scale scores
Wagner et al.[98]	Meta-analysis (n = pooled)	All antidepressants Psychostimulants Testosterone	70%–74% response rate 93% response rate 81% response rate

RPCT, randomized, placebo-controlled trial; AIDS, acquired immunodeficiency virus; HAART, highly active anti-retroviral therapy.

tients who completed the study, 74% responded to fluoxetine and 47% to placebo; this difference was statistically significant. Severity of immunosuppression was not related to antidepressant response, attrition, or side effects; and fluoxetine was not associated with change in CD4 cell count.

Elliott and colleagues[95] conducted a randomized, placebo-controlled trial of paroxetine versus imipramine in 75 depressed outpatients with HIV/AIDS. Of their sample, 45% met the criteria for AIDS; the sample was predominantly white gay males. Patients were given paroxetine, imipramine, or placebo for 12 weeks. The mean dose of paroxetine was 33.9 mg and that of imipramine, 162.5 mg, both of which were significantly more effective than placebo. There were significantly more dropouts for imipramine (48%) than from both paroxetine (20%) and placebo (24%). Statistically significant improvements were shown on the Hamilton Depression Scale and on the Hamilton Anxiety Rating Scale (HAM-A) for paroxetine and imipramine. There was no apparent relationship between response to antidepressants and HIV status, symptom severity, lifetime psychiatric history, or chronicity of depression.

Ferrando et al.[96] conducted an open-label trial with 33 moderately to severely depressed HIV patients, the majority of whom met CDC criteria for AIDS. Patients were treated with sertraline, paroxetine, or fluoxetine. They assessed whether treatment of depression resulted in a reduction in both affective and somatic symptoms. Nine of the 33 subjects dropped out within the first 3 weeks of treatment because of adverse effects, mostly agitation, anxiety, and insomnia. Of the 73% of subjects who completed the trial, 83% were considered clinical responders. This was true for scores on the HAM-D and BDI scales, as well as for the HIV Symptom Scale, which inquires about 31 physical symptoms of HIV and their severity. Subjects who completed the 6 weeks of SSRI treatment experienced significant reductions in both affective and somatic symptoms, many of the latter having been attributed to HIV rather than depression. These results indicated that, even in later stages of HIV illness, the contribution of depression to perceived somatic symptoms may be significant and that these symptoms improve with antidepressant treatment.

Elliot et al.[97] conducted an open-label trial of nefazodone with 15 depressed HIV/AIDS patients. Sixty percent of their sample met the criteria for AIDS, and the sample had an average CD4 cell count of 266 cells/mm^3. Seventy-three percent of patients completed the study, and all of these had at least a 50% reduction in HAM-D scores. Scores on the HAM-A declined from 26.4 ± 5.6 at baseline to 8.2 ± 7.2 at week 12. Half of this sample were taking triple-drug therapy (two nucleoside reverse transcriptase inhibitors, NRTIs) plus a protease inhibitor or two nucleoside reverse transcriptase inhibitors plus a non-nucleoside reverse transcriptase inhibitor (NNRTI). These patients did not have any greater incidence of dropout or side effects than those not taking this regimen.

Wagner et al.[98] conducted a comparative analysis of the data pooled from antidepressant and psychostimulant trials in HIV patients. Response rates for standard antidepressants ranged from 70%–74%, with similar or higher response rates found in trials of dextroamphetamine (93%) and testosterone (81%). All of the treatments showed evidence of strong efficacy and relatively unique benefits, which gives valuable options to clinicians when addressing the individual needs of patients.

Psychostimulants for depression
In the palliative care setting, clinicians and patients may feel that the several weeks' delay between starting SSRIs and evidence of symptomatic improvement is unacceptable. In this instance, psychostimulants may be a viable treatment option for depression and the psychomotor slowing which often accompanies mood disorders in the last 6 months of life.

Caution must be exercised in patients with any demonstrable brain lesions, a history of seizures, intermittent delirium, or CNS infection since psychostimulants can precipitate seizures in neurologically vulnerable patients. Ritalin can be started at 2.5–5.0 mg at breakfast and lunch and titrated upward to 20–50 mg BID to clinical effect. Psychostimulants can also vastly improve sedation secondary to opioids and allow the patient periods of alertness, increased activity, and increased well-being.

Wagner et al.[99] reported findings from an open trial of dextroamphetamine in the treatment of 19 AIDS patients (with a CD4 count of less than 200 cells/mm^3) and a DSM diagnosis of depression. Ninety-five percent of patients who completed 6 weeks of treatment with dextroamphetamine at a maximum dose of 30 mg PO BID demonstrated substantial improvement with regard to mood and energy at a median dose of 10 mg BID/day. Both HAM-D scores as well as measures of fatigue were improved dramatically. This group noted the limitations of their study design and concluded that their results call for a larger, controlled trial.[99]

Anxiety

The prevalence of anxiety disorders in palliative AIDS patients is not well studied. Atkinson et al.,[100] before the era of protease inhibitors, reported that 36.4% of AIDS patients experienced sufficient symptoms to qualify for a National Institute of Mental Health Diagnostic Interview Schedule diagnosis of an anxiety disorder compared to HIV-positive men (17.6%) and seronegative gay men (9.1%). Rabkin et al.[101] investigated the association between mood status and progression of HIV illness in a 4-year prospective study. Using the HAM-A, HIV-positive men had slightly more anxiety throughout the study than HIV-negative men, but there was no increase in rates of anxiety over the 4 years despite substantial illness progression. Rates of psychiatric disorders in AIDS patients from non-Western countries, where the AIDS pandemic affects predominantly heterosexuals, including large numbers of women (as in Africa, Latin America), and of depression are significantly higher in symptomatic AIDS groups (20%–35%).[102]

Death anxiety

Death anxiety was studied by Catania et al.,[103] who operationally defined "death anxiety" by an item of the Brief Symptom Inventory (BSI) that assesses how much discomfort respondents experienced in the previous months related to "thoughts of death or dying." Mean levels of death anxiety were significantly different among all three cohorts studied, with HIV-negative men reporting the lowest level, HIV-positive asymptomatic men reporting moderate levels, and HIV-positive symptomatic men reporting the highest levels. This study might yield very different results if it were repeated in the current post-HAART era. It is our clinical impression that in the psychiatric palliative care of AIDS patients who are in hospice or hospitalized settings, low-dose neuroleptics, particularly the novel neuroleptic olanzapine (2.5 mg PO QHS), can be used to calm death-related anxiety, which patients frequently report at night, causing insomnia. This approach prevents the delirium that can follow upon the use of benzodiazepines in this population.

Assessing anxiety in AIDS patients, particularly in the hospice setting, should include inquiries about uncontrolled pain, careful history to elicit withdrawal states, investigations for abnormal metabolic states, and a review of medication which may reveal agents such as corticosteroids or sympathomimetics (bronchodilators) that can have anxiety as a side effect. For those patients with primary anxiety disorders not related to a general medical conditions and who do not show evidence of significant dementia, standard psychopharmacological therapy can be applied. This usually includes an SSRI given at higher doses than used for depression, supplemented by a low-dose benzodiazepine in the early phases of treatment. There are no randomized controlled trials of SSRIs for anxiety disorders in HIV/AIDS patients: clearly, this is an area where empirical research is needed.

Psychosis

Although of an epidemiologically much smaller magnitude, psychosis does present in HIV/AIDS patients, though the phenomenology is not well studied and the pathophysiology not well understood. According to Sewell,[104] estimates of new-onset psychosis in patients with HIV-spectrum illness range between 0.2% and 15% and may increase as the stage of HIV illness progresses. While many affected by HIV are of the age group during which schizophrenia presents, many patients have no risk factors or family history. Regardless of which illness came first, the co-occurrence of psychosis and HIV appeared to be associated with higher morbidity and mortality than would be expected by either illness alone. Psychosis can sometimes complicate late-stage HIV dementia and require treatment with antipsychotic medication for behavioral control.

Sewel and the University of California San Diego group[105] conducted a rater-blinded randomized study of neuroleptic treatment of HIV psychosis. Thirteen subjects had no history of psychosis prior to infection with HIV, and none of the subjects had psychosis attributable to delirium or non-HIV-related organic factors. Patients were treated with either haloperidol or thioridazine, up to a dose of 124 mg chlorpromazine equivalents. Both neuroleptics produced modest but significant reduction in overall level of psychosis in positive symptoms but not in negative symptoms. All of the haloperidol-treated patients developed extrapyramidal symptoms requiring anticholinergic medication, whereas only three of the five thioridazine-treated patients developed noticeable side effects.[105]

Wasting/anorexia

Severe anorexia and wasting are common problems in patients with advanced HIV infection. Weight loss of greater than 10% of body weight is the index diagnosis for almost one-fifth of AIDS cases. Many possible etiologies for cachexia exist in AIDS, including malabsorption secondary to gastrointestinal parasites (cryptosporidium or microsporidium), viruses (cytomegalovirus), neoplasms (Kaposi's sarcoma), or the pathogenic and hypermetabolic effects of HIV itself. Lesions secondary to opportunistic infection, such as *Candida albicans*, are common, as is the nausea secondary to HAART.

Nutritional issues have traditionally been a low priority for clinical researchers.[106] Published trials of interventions have therefore focused on the appetite stimulants megestrol and dronabinol and on anabolic agents such as testosterone and growth hormone.

Appetite stimulants: megesterol and dronabinol

Von Roenn et al.[107] performed a randomized, double-blind, placebo-controlled trial of megestrol acetate (Megace) in 270 patients. Patients were given 800 mg/day for 12 weeks. Results were positive, with 64.2% of patients gaining 2.27 kg (5 lb) or more compared to only 21.4% of subjects in the placebo group. There was significant improvement in appetite, mean weight gain, lean body mass, caloric intake, and overall well-being. Megestrol is commonly used in both supportive care and palliative care settings.

Beal et al.[108] performed a randomized, double-blind, placebo-controlled trial of dronabinol as a treatment for anorexia associated with weight loss in 139 patients with AIDS. Trial participants were predominantly gay white males who had lost at least 2.3 kg (5 lb) from normal body weight, with an average mean loss of ~10 kg, or 13% of body weight. The CD4 count at the time of the trial for both placebo and study subjects was about 50 cells/mm^3. Subjects were given capsules of dronabinol 2.5 mg BID 1 hour before lunch and supper. Patients rated appetite, mood, and nausea using a VAS three times per week over 12 weeks. Dronabinol was associated with increased appetite above baseline in 38% versus 8% for placebo and with decreased nausea (20% versus 7%). Weight was stable in dronabinol patients, while in the placebo group, patients had a mean loss of 0.4 kg. Of the dronabinol patients, 22% gained more than 2 kg compared to only 10.5% of placebo patients.

Mood effects for dronabinol were small: improvement in mood was noted by 7% of patients treated with dronabinol and 2% of patients treated with placebo. Nausea decreased 20% by end point in the dronabinol group and 7% in the placebo group. Side effects were mostly mild to moderate in severity and included euphoria, dizziness, thinking abnormalities, and somnolence. These adverse effects were experienced by 35% of the dronabinol group versus 9% of the placebo group. There was no clinically significant interaction between dronabinol and either opioid analgesics or bezodiazepines in term of adverse events.

Nandrolone decanoate and oxandrolone

Nandrolone decanoate, an anabolic steroid, was found to be safe and well tolerated and to result in modest weight gain in 6- and 12- week trials without adverse changes in immunological markers of HIV viral load.[109] However, there are to date no randomized controlled trials of nandrolone or oxandrolone in HIV-wasting syndrome. While there are some benefits from both nandrolone decanoate and oxandrolone, both require further research to assess efficacy.[110]

Endocrinopathies

Hypogonadism

Hypogonadism, as measured by low serum total and free testosterone, occurs in HIV/AIDS patients and increases in frequency as CD4 counts decline.[111] Symptoms of low testosterone can include loss of appetite and or weight, low energy, low mood, diminished libido, and decreased sexual functioning. While there is some epidemiological evidence that hypogonadism and wasting are less common in the era of HAART, for the palliative care physician, hypogonadism and its myriad symptomatic manifestations should be investigated and treated.[112]

Intramuscular injections of testosterone were studied by Wagner and Rabkin[113] in an open-label study, which did not include a placebo arm. Twenty-three men with AIDS (average CD4 cell count 150) but normal-range testosterone (at least 500 ng/dl) were given biweekly intramuscular injections of testosterone cypionate. Diminished libido was an inclusion criterion, and each patient had to have at least one additional symptom: low mood, low energy, loss of appetite, and/or weight. Response rates were very positive, with 89% of subjects reporting libido response, 67% reporting improved mood, 71% improved energy, and 67% increased appetite. Average weight gain was 2.3 kg, with a 1.8 kg increase in body cell mass and no change in body mass.

A randomized, double-blinded study using 200 mg of testosterone cypionate given intramuscularly every 2 weeks for 3 months to 40 AIDS patients with weight loss was conducted by Coodley et al.[114] Their end point was weight gain. Unlike other studies, they found that treatment with testosterone cypionate compared to placebo did not result in significant weight gain. They did, however, note that testosterone supplementation appeared to produce improved overall sense of well-being and possibly some increase in muscle strength.

Lipodystrophy

A unique and unexpected syndrome consisting of metabolic abnormalities (hyperlipidemia and insulin resistance) and body fat redistribution (central adiposity and peripheral fat wasting) has been reported with increasing frequency in HIV patients, most of whom are receiving HAART including HIV-1 protease inhibitors.[115] The catalytic region of HIV-1 protease, to which protease inhibitors bind, has approximately 60% homology to regions within two proteins that regulate lipid metabolism.[116] Clinicians need to be aware of symptoms of endocrine disturbance in patients and of emerging guidelines for management of serious adverse effects of HAART at every stage of HIV illness.

End-of-Life Issues

Physician-assisted suicide

Breitbart and colleagues[117] conducted a study of 378 ambulatory HIV-infected patients, 90% of whom met CDC criteria for AIDS. Sixty-three percent of the patients supported physician-assisted suicide, and 55% acknowledged considering physician-assisted suicide as an option for themselves. The strongest predictors of interest in physician-assisted suicide were high scores on measures of psychological distress, specifically depression, hopelessness, suicidal ideation, and overall psychological distress, as well as experience with terminal illness in a family member or friend. For example, among the 117 patients with high levels of depressive symptoms (BDI score of 21 or more), 67% ($n = 78$) considered physician-assisted suicide as an option, whereas 50% ($n = 131$) of the 261 less depressed subjects considered physician-assisted suicide as an option.

Patients who reported suicidal ideation were also significantly more likely to consider physician-assisted suicide (72% versus 49%). Other strong predictors were Caucasian race, infrequent or no attendance at religious services, and perceived low level of social support. Importantly, interest in physician-assisted suicide was not related to severity of pain, pain-related functional impairment, physical symptoms, or extent of HIV.

The authors concluded that HIV-infected patients supported physician-assisted suicide at rates comparable to those in the general public. Patients' interest in physician-assisted suicide appears to be more a function of psychological and social factors than physical factors. This study highlights the importance of psychiatric and psychosocial assessment and intervention in the care of patients who express interest in or request physician-assisted suicide.[117]

Desire for death

Despite years of public debate regarding assisted suicide and euthanasia, medical and psychiatric practitioners continue to face many unanswered questions in understanding why terminally ill patients occasionally desire a hastened death. One central issue concerns the role of depression and physical symptoms in driving a patient's expressed desire for hastened death. Understanding the complex, inter-related issues of depression, pain, disease stage, and existential factors has been limited by a lack of valid measures for assessing desire for hastened death.

Rosenfeld et al.[118] published preliminary validation data for a new self-report instrument: the Schedule of Attitudes towards Hastened Death (SAHD). This self-report instrument consists of 20 items which the patient rates as true of false, such as "Dying seems like the best way to relieve the pain and discomfort my illness causes" and "I am seriously considering asking my doctor for help in ending my life."

The SAHD was validated on 195 patients, 47 of whom had been recently admitted to a facility for end-of-life care. The total score for all study subjects was significantly correlated with measures of depression and psychological distress. For example, the total score was significantly correlated with scores on the BDI, the Global Severity Index of the BSI, and the HAM-D. Patients with a history of psychiatric treatment had significantly higher mean scores on the SAHD than patients without a history of prior psychiatric treatment (3.90 versus 2.16).

Rosenfeld et al.[118] found that their instrument designed to measure patients' attitudes toward hastened death demonstrated high reliability. It was statistically significantly correlated with an existing instrument, the Desire for Death Rating Scale.[97,119] For the 47 palliative AIDS patients assessed by Rosenfeld et al.,[118] half had scores of 0 on the Desire for Death Rating Scale. Scores on this clinician-rated measure ranged from 0 to 6, with 0 representing no desire for death. Seven patients in the sample (15%) received ratings of 3 or greater, defined by Chochinov and colleagues[119] as reflecting a "serious and pervasive" desire for death. The remaining 17 patients were given ratings of 1 or 2, reflecting mild or moderate desire for death, respectively. Results of this sample of AIDS patients resemble those from Chochinov et al.'s[119] sample of terminally ill cancer patients. Specifically, Chochinov and colleagues[119] reported that 18% of their 200 subjects expressed a significant desire for hastened death. Additionally, 44.5% had at least occasional wishes that death would come sooner. Of the patients with significant desire for death, 10 of 17 (58.8%) met research diagnostic criteria for depression. The study did not include a treatment arm for treating depression and then reassessing desire for death.

The intention of Rosenfeld et al.[118] was to create a research tool for assessing the degree of desire for death, rather than a clinical tool to determine or predict who may or may not request assistance in dying. The scale was not aimed at determining whether such a request might be "appropriate." Their data suggested that while high scores on the SAHD may correspond to a substantial desire for hastened death, this desire may be largely influenced by depression, as evidenced by the significant correlations with the Desire for Death Rating Scale, as well as the BDI and HAM-D. Clearly, this important tool, which reliably assesses patients' attitudes, could be used in further studies.

Research Methodologies and Areas for Future Research

In reviewing the research conducted in HIV palliative care, a number of urgent issues present themselves. There is a critical need for properly conducted randomized, double-blinded, placebo-controlled trials to show efficacy for interventions in major areas such as the treatment of pain, fatigue, dementia, and depression. Too many of the interventions offered to patients are based on small case series, non-evidence-based clinician preferences, or research conducted with other medically ill populations and not specific to HIV/AIDS. Much of the research into symptomatic therapies for HIV/AIDS predates the introduction of HAART.

A critical review of the literature concerning major psychiatric syndromes and HIV/AIDS must include a recognition of the massive impact of the introduction of protease inhibitors on those living with HIV and AIDS. Rabkin and Ferrando[120] point out that researchers need to consider that the introduction of these drugs poses new research and policy issues. They suggest that research be conducted into the development of strategies to enhance medication adherence and into psychological restructuring of lives and expectations in the event of clinical benefit. They suggest that research will need to develop strategies with which to manage the distress associated with clinical failure. They further recommend studying the effect of restored health on the appraisal of HIV risk behaviors and assessment of the effect on neurocognitive functioning, as well as further research into psychotropic drugs and protease inhibitor drug interactions. They conclude that there will need to be behavioral research to inform provision of those considered difficult to treat, specifically those with severe and persistent mental illness.[98]

There is enormous need for research in the psychiatric care of AIDS patients. A huge majority of outpatients studied reported symptoms suggestive of psychological distress and possibly psychiatric illness, including worry (85%), feeling sad (81%), feeling nervous (68%), and difficulty concentrating (64%).[4] There is also a need for psychiatric research concerning later-stage AIDS patients, including those with dementia, particularly those in the palliative care setting. Accurate diagnosis and treatment of psychiatric disorders could substantially improve quality of life for this population.[121] Research from the cancer literature illustrates this principle. Breitbart and colleagues[80] discovered that 30% of hospitalized patients with cancer who express suicidal ideation had an unrecognized, untreated delirium. Given the complexity of the HAART regimens as well as the incidence of HIV dementia, the complexity of the psychiatric psychopharmacological management of late-stage illness would be well served by some empirical research in this population of patients.

Hope of increasingly effective treatments for HIV is offered by HAART, yet clinicians and patients alike are becoming increasingly aware of treatment side effects and toxicities which make for poor quality of life for some AIDS patients. Palliative care clinicians have a great deal to offer patients at earlier stages of living with HIV/AIDS in the spectrum of "supportive care" throughout the early, middle, and late stages of illness and in managing long-term survival.

To address each of the areas in this chapter in turn, pain remains a central issue in AIDS, with 76% of patients reporting it.[4] There is an urgent need for randomized controlled trials for treatments aimed at HAART-induced peripheral neuropathies to assess the efficacy of new anticonvulsants of all types. This issue is highly prevalent and will affect large numbers of patients who are on long-term HAART. Palliative care physicians could assist in breaking down barriers to effective pain control simply by educating primary medical care providers about the administration of opioids without the stigma of addiction or abuse, which research has illustrated is not the problem that clinicians or the public fear.

Breitbart and colleagues[77] have provided a landmark study in delirium, which should have impact in clinical practice and decrease the use of benzodiazepines, which worsen cognitive impairment in hospitalized delirious patients. Further studies into novel antipsychotics are needed to improve treatment of delirium. Encouraging drug manufacturers to develop parenteral forms of novel antipsychotics would also be useful in the palliative care setting.

Dementia and its behavioral manifestations are a key area in which randomized controlled trials would clarify useful treatment, both in combating the viral load and in controlling behavioral symptoms of dementia. Depression is likewise an area where clinical trials would be helpful in assessing the efficacy of newer antidepressants, including the SSRIs, serotonin and norepinephrine specific reuptake inhibitors and antidepressants with dopaminergic effects. The psychopharmacological concentration of these drugs combined with HAART is largely unstudied at this time.

Finally, there is still room for good phenomenological and epidemiological studies which address the fundamental psychological responses of large groups of patients as they struggle to maintain hope in the face of great uncertainty and great advances in the treatment of HIV/AIDS.

References

1. Pallela F, Delaney K, Moorman A, et al. Declining morbidity and mortality among patients with advanced human immunodeficiency virus infection. N Engl J Med 1998; 338:853–860.
2. Center for Disease Control and Prevention. HIV/AIDS Surveillance Report. Atlanta: CDC, 1998.
3. Breitbart W. Pain in AIDS. In: Jensen J, Turner JA, Wiesenfeld-Hallin Z, eds. Proceedings of the 8th World Congress on Pain. Progress in Pain Research and Management, vol 8. Seattle: IASP Press, 1997:63–100.
4. Vogl D, Rosenfeld B, Breitbart W, et al. Symptom prevalence, characteristics and distress in AIDS outpatients. J Pain Symp Manage 1999; 18:253–262.
5. Breitbart W. Pain in AIDS: an overview. Pain Rev 1998; 5:247–272.
6. Breitbart W, Rosenfeld B, Passik S, et al. The undertreatment of pain in ambulatory AIDS patients. Pain 1996; 65:239–245.
7. Breitbart W, McDonald MV, Rosenfeld B, et al. Pain in ambulatory AIDS patients. 1: Pain characteristics and medical correlates. Pain 1996; 68:315–321.
8. Larue F, Fontaine A, Colleau S. Underestimation and undertreatment of pain in HIV disease: multicentre study. BMJ 1997; 314:23–28.
9. Hewitt D, McDonald M, Portenoy R, et al. Pain syndromes and etiologies in ambulatory AIDS patients. Pain 1996; 70:117–123.
10. Jacox A, Carr D, Payne R, et al. Clinical Practice Guideline Number 9: Management of Cancer Pain. AHCPR Publication 94-0592. Rockville MD: US Department of Health and Human Services, Public Health Service, Agency for Health Care Policy and Research, 1994:139–141.
11. Kimball LR, McCormic WC. The pharmacologic management of pain and discomfort in persons with AIDS near the end of life: use of opioid analgesia in the hospice setting. J Pain Symptom Manage 1996; 11:88–94.

12. Kaplan R, Conant M, Cundiff D, et al. Sustained-release morphine sulfate in the management of pain associated with acquired immune deficiency syndrome. J Pain Symptom Manage 1996; 12:150–160.

13. Lefkowitz M, Newshan G. An evaluation of the use of duragesic for chronic pain in patients with AIDS. In: Proceedings of the 16th Annual Scientific Meeting of the American Pain Society, Oct 23–26, 1997:A-71. Abstract Nr. 684.

14. Breitbart W, Passik S, MacDonald M, et al. Patient-related barriers to pain management in ambulatory AIDS patients. Pain 1998; 76:9–16.

15. Caraceni A, Zecca E, Martini C, et al. Gabapentin as adjuvant to opioid analgesia for neuropathic cancer pain. J Pain Symptom Manage 1999; 17:441–445.

16. Hewitt D, McDonald M, Portenoy R, et al. Pain syndromes and etiologies in ambulatory AIDS patients. Pain 1996; 70:117–123.

17. Portenoy RK. Adjuvant analgesics in pain management. In: Doyle D, Hanks GWC, MacDonald N, eds. Oxford Textbook of Palliative Medicine, 2d ed. New York: Oxford University Press, 1998:361–390.

18. Hewitt D, Portenoy R. Adjuvant drugs for neuropathic cancer pain. In: Bruera E, Portenoy R, eds. Topics in Palliative Care, vol 2. New York: Oxford University Press, 1998:41–62.

19. Watson CP, Chipman M, Reed K, et al. Amitriptyline versus maprotiline in post-herpetic neuralgia: a randomized double-blind, cross-over trial. Pain 1992; 48: 29–36.

20. Max MB, Culnane M, Schafer SC, et al. Amitriptyline relieves diabetic neuropathy pain in patients with normal and depressed mood. Neurology 1987; 37:589–596.

21. Sindrup SH, Gram LF, Broen K, et al. The selective serotonin reuptake inhibitor paroxetine is effective in the treatment of diabetic neuropathy symptoms. Pain 1990; 42:135–144.

22. von Moltke L, Greenblatt D, Grasssi J, et al. Protease inhibitor as inhibitors of human cytochromes P450: high risk associated with ritonavir. J Clin Pharmacol 1998; 38: 106–111.

23. Ackerman Z, Levy M. Hypersensitivity reactions to drugs in acquired immunodeficiency syndrome. Postgrad Med J 1987; 63:55–56.

24. Backonja M, Beydoun A, Edwards K, et al. Gapabentin for the symptomatic treatment of painful neuropathy in patients with diabetes mellitus: a randomized controlled trial. JAMA 1998; 280:1831–1836.

25. Rowbotham M, Harden N, Stacey B, et al. Gabapentin for the treatment of postherpetic neuralgia: a randomized controlled trial. JAMA 1998; 280:1837–1842.

26. Harati Y, Gooch C, Swenson M, et al. Double-blind randomized trial of tramadol for the treatment of the pain of diabetic neuropathy. Neurology 1998; 50:1842–1846.

27. Lantz M, Buchalter E, Giambanco V. Serotonin syndrome following the administration of tramadol with paroxetine. Int J Geriatr Psychiatry 1998; 13:343–345.

28. Mason B, Blackburn K. Possible serotonin syndrome associated with tramadol and sertraline coadministration. Ann Pharmacother 1997; 31:175–177.

29. Simpson D, Dorfman D, Olney R, et al. Peptide T in the treatment of painful distal neuropathy associated with AIDS: results of a placebo-controlled trial. The Pep-tide T Neuropathy Study Group. Neurology 1996; 47:1254–1259.

30. Kieburtz K, Simpson D, Yiannoutsos C. A randomized trial of amitriptyline and mexiletine for painful neuropathy in HIV infection. AIDS Clinical Trial Group 242 Protocol Team. Neurology 1998; 51:1682–1688.

31. Breitbart W, Rosenfeld B, Kaim M. Clinician's perceptions of barriers to pain management in AIDS. J Pain Symptom Manage 1999; 18:203–212.

32. Cleeland CS, Gonin R, Hatfield AK, et al. Pain and its treatments in outpatients with metastatic cancer: the Eastern Cooperative Group's Outpatient Study. N Engl J Med 1994; 330:592–596.

33. Rosenfeld B, Breitbart W, McDonald MV, et al. Pain in ambulatory AIDS patients. II: Impact of pain on psychological functioning and quality of life. Pain 1996; 68: 323–328.

34. Ferrando S, Evans S, Goggin K, et al. Fatigue in HIV illness: relationship to depression, physical limitations and disability. Psychosom Med 1998; 60:759–764.

35. Darko DF, McCutchen JA, Kripke DF, et al. Fatigue, sleep disturbance, disability and indices of progression of HIV infection. Am J Psychiatry 1992; 149:514–520.

36. Breitbart W, McDonald MV, Rosenfeld B, et al. Fatigue in ambulatory AIDS patients. J Pain Symptom Manage 1998; 15:159–167.

37. Cella D, Peterman A, Passik S, et al. Progress toward guidelines for the management of fatigue. Oncology 1998; 12:369–377.

38. Revicki DA, Brown RE, Henry DH, et al. Recombinant human erythropoietin and health-related quality of life in AIDS patients with anemia. J Acquir Immune Defic Syndr 1994; 7:474–484.

39. Rabkin JG, Rabkin R, Wagner G. Testosterone replacement therapy in HIV patients. Gen Hosp Psychiatry 1995; 17:37–42.

40. Miller RG, Carson PJ, Moussavi RS, et al. Fatigue and myalgia in AIDS patients. Neurology 1991; 41:1603–1607.

41. Hellerstein MK, Kahn J, Mudie H, et al. Current approaches to the treatment of human immunodeficiency virus–associated weight loss: pathophysiologic considerations and emerging management strategies. Semin Oncol 1990; 17:17–33.

42. Breitbart W, DiBiase L. Current perspectives on pain in AIDS, Part 2. Oncology 2002; 16:964–972.

43. Holmes VF, Fernandez F, Levy JK. Psychostimulant response in AIDS-related complex patients. J Clin Psychiatry 1989; 50:1–8.

44. Krupp LB, Coyle PK, Cross AH, et al. Amelioration of fatigue with pemoline in patients with multiple sclerosis. Ann Neurol 1989; 26:155–156.

45. Bruera E, Chadwick S, Brennels C, et al. Methylphenidate associated with narcotics for the treatment of cancer pain. Cancer Treat Rep 1987; 71:67–70.

46. Weinshenker BG, Penman M, Bass B, et al. A double-blind, randomized crossover trial of pemoline in fatigue associated with multiple sclerosis. Neurology 1992; 42:1468–1471.

47. Fernandez F, Adams F, Levy J, et al. Cognitive impairment due to AIDS related complex and its response to psychostimulants. Psychosomatics 1988; 29:38–46.

48. Breitbart W, Rosenfeld B, Kaim M, et al. A randomized, double-blind placebo-controlled trial of psychostimulants for the treatment of fatigue in ambulatory patients with HIV disease. Arch Intern Med 2001; 161:411–420.

49. Piper BF, Lindsey AM, Dodd MJ, et al. The development of an instrument to measure the subjective dimension of fatigue. In: Funk SG, Tornquist EM, Champagne MT, et al., eds. Key Aspects of Comfort: Management of Pain, Fatigue, and Nausea. New York: Springer, 1989:199–208.

50. Ferrando S, Evans S, Goggin K, et al. Fatigue in HIV illness: relationship to depression, physical limitations, and disability. J Psychosom Med 1998; 60:759–764.

51. Perry SW. Organic mental disorders caused by HIV: update on early diagnosis and treatment. Am J Psychiatry 1990; 147:696–710.
52. Rabins PV, Folstein MD. Delirium and dementia: diagnostic criteria and fatality rates. Br J Psychiatry 1982; 140:149–153.
53. Lipowski ZJ. Delirium (acute confusional states). JAMA 1987; 258:1789–1792.
54. Derogatis LR, Morrow GR, Fetting J, et al. The prevalence of psychiatric disorders among cancer patients. JAMA 1983; 249:751–757.
55. Fleishman S, Lesko LM. Delirium and dementia. In: Holland J, Rowlands JH, eds. Handbook of Psychooncology. New York: Oxford University Press, 1989:342–355.
56. Francis J, Martin D, Kapor WN. A prospective study of delirium in hospitalized elderly. JAMA 1990; 263:1097–1101.
57. Treisman GJ, Angelino AF, Hutton HE. Psychiatric issues in the management of patients with HIV infection. JAMA 2001; 286:2857–2864.
58. Perry SW. Organic mental disorders caused by HIV: update on early diagnosis and treatment. Am J Psychiatry 1990; 147:696–710.
59. Bruera E, Miller MJ, McCallion J, et al. Cognitive failure in patients with terminal cancer: a prospective study. J Pain Symptom Manage 1992; 7:192–195.
60. Fainsinger RL, MacEachern T, Bruera E, et al. Symptom control during the last week of life in a palliative care unit. J Palliat Care 1991; 7:5–11.
61. Wise MG, Brandt GT. Delirium. In: Yudofsky SC, Hale RE, eds. Textbook of Neuro-psychiatry, 2d ed. Washington DC: American Psychiatric Association Press, 1992: 89–105.
62. American Psychiatric Association. Diagnostic and Statistical Manual of Mental Disorders. Washington DC: American Psychiatric Association Press, 1994:124–133.
63. Breitbart W, Sparrow B. Management of delirium in the terminally ill. Prog Palliat Care 1998; 6:107–114.
64. American Psychiatric Association. American Psychiatric Association Practice Guidelines for the Treatment of Patients with Delirium. Am J Psychiatry 1999; 156 (Suppl):1–18.
65. Smith M, Breitbart W, Platt M. A critique of instruments and methods to detect, diagnose, and rate delirium. J Pain Symptom Manage 1995; 10:35–77.
66. Breitbart W, Rosenfeld B, Roth A, et al. The Memorial Delirium Assessment Scale. J Pain Symptom Manage 1997; 13:128–137.
67. Cohen BM, Lipinski JF. Treatment of acute psychosis with non-neuroleptic agents. Psychosomatics 1986; 27(Suppl):7–14.
68. Salzman C, Green AI, Rodriguez-Villa F, et al. Benzodiazepines combined with neuroleptics for management of severe disruptive behavior. Psychosomatics 1986; 27 (Suppl):28–32.
69. Rosen HS. Double-blind comparison of haloperidol and thioridazine in geriatric outpatients. J Clin Psychiatry 1979; 40:17–20.
70. Smith GR, Taylor CW, Linkous P. Haloperidol versus thioridazine for treatment of psychogeriatric patients: a double-blind clinical trial. Psychosomatics 1974; 15: 134–138.
71. Tsuang MM, Lu LM, Stotsky BA, et al. Haloperidol versus thioridazine for hospitalized psychogeriatric patients: double blind study. J Am Geriatr Soc 1971; 9: 593–600.
72. Kirven LE, Montero EF. Comparison of thioridazine and diazepam for the control of nonpsychotic symptoms associated with senility: double-blind study. J Am Geriatr Soc 1973; 12:546–551.

73. Thomas H, Schwartz E, Petrilli R. Droperidol versus haloperidol for chemical restraint of agitated and combative patients. Ann Emerg Med 1992; 21:407–413.
74. Thompson WL, Johnson AD, Maddrey WL, et al. Diazepam and paraldehyde for treatment of severe delirium tremens. Ann Intern Med 1975; 82:175–180.
75. Massie MJ, Holland J, Glass E. Delirium in terminally ill cancer patients. Am J Psychiatry 1983; 140:1048–1050.
76. Fernandez F, Levy JK, Mansell PWA. Management of delirium in terminally ill AIDS patients. Int J Psychiatry Med 1989; 19:165–172.
77. Breitbart W, Marotta R, Platt MM, et al. A double-blind trial of haloperidol, chlorpromazine, and lorazepam in the treatment of delirium in hospitalized AIDS patients. Am J Psychiatry 1996; 153:231–237.
78. Sipahimalani A, Masand PS. Use of risperidone in delirium: case reports. Am Clin Psychiatry 1997; 9:105–107.
79. Sipahimalani A, Sime R, Masand P. Treatment of delirium with risperidone. Int J Geriatr Psychopharmacol 1997; 1:24–26.
80. Breitbart W, Chochinov H, Passik S. Psychiatric aspects of palliative care. In: Doyle D, Hanks G, MacDonald N, eds. Oxford Textbook of Palliative Medicine, 2d ed. New York: Oxford University Press, 1988:933–954.
81. Ventafridda V, Ripamonti C, DeConno F, et al. Symptom prevalence and control during cancer patients' last days of life. J Palliat Care 1990; 6:7–11.
82. Fainsinger R, MacEachern T, Hanson J, et al. Symptom control during the last week of life in a palliative care unit. J Palliat Care 1991; 7:5–11.
83. Bottomley DM, Handks GW. Subcutaneous midazolam infusion in palliative care. J Pain Symptom Manage 1990; 5:259–261.
84. Moyle J. The use of propofol in palliative medicine. J Pain Symptom Manage 1995; 10:643–646.
85. Grant I, Marcotte T, Heaton, R. Neurocognitive implications of HIV disease. Psychol Sci 1999; 10:191–195.
86. Aweeka F, Jayewardene A, Staprans S, et al. Failure to detect nelfinavir in the cerebrospinal fluid of HIV-1 infected patients with and without AIDS dementia complex. J AIDS 1999; 20:39–43.
87. Chang L, Ernst T, Leonido-Yee M, et al. Highly active antiretroviral therapy reverses brain metabolite abnormalities in mild HIV dementia. Neurology 1999; 53:782–789.
88. Melton S, Kirkwood C, Ghaemi S. Pharmacotherapy of HIV dementia. Ann Pharmacother 1997; 31:457–453.
89. Sidtis J, Gatsonis C, Price R, et al. Zidovudine treatment of the AIDS dementia complex: results of a placebo-controlled trial. Ann Neurol 1993; 33:343–349.
90. Porgegies P, Enting R, deGans J, et al. Presentation and course of AIDS dementia complex: 10 years of followup in Amsterdam, the Netherlands. AIDS 1993; 7:669–675.
91. Melton S, Kirkwood C, Ghaemi S. Pharmacotherapy of HIV dementia. Ann Pharmacother 1997; 31:457–453.
92. Fernandez F, Levy J. Adjuvant treatment of HIV dementia with psychostimulants. In: Ostrow D, et al., eds. Behavioral Aspects of AIDS. New York: Plenum Press, 1990.
93. Catalan J. Psychosocial and neuropsychiatric aspects of HIV infection: review of their extent and implications for psychiatry. J Psychosom Res 1988; 32:237–248.

94. Rabkin J, Ferrando S, Jacobsberg L, et al. Prevalence of axis I disorders in an AIDS cohort: a cross-sectional, controlled study. Compr Psychiatry 1997; 38:146–154.

95. Elliot A, Uldall K, Bergam K, et al. Randomized, placebo-controlled trial of paroxetine versus imipramine in depressed HIV-positive outpatients. Am J Psychiatry 1998; 155:367–372.

96. Ferrando S, Goldman J, Charness W. Selective serotonin reuptake inhibitor treatment of depression in symptomatic HIV infection and AIDS. Gen Hosp Psychiatry 1997; 19:89–97.

97. Elliot A, Russo J, Bergam K, et al. Antidepressant efficacy in HIV-seropositive outpatients with major depressive disorder: an open trial of nefazodone. J Clin Psychiatry 1999; 60:226–231.

98. Wagner G, Rabkin J, Rabkin R. A comparative analysis of standard and alternative antidepressants in the treatment of human immunodeficiency virus patients. Compr Psychiatry 1996; 37:402–408.

99. Wagner G, Rabkin J, Rabkin R. Dextroamphetamine as a treatment for depression and low energy in AIDS patients: a pilot study. J Psychosom Res 1997; 42:407–411.

100. Atkinson J, Grant I, Kennedy C, et al. Prevalence of psychiatric disorders among men infected with human immunodeficiency virus. Arch Gen Psychiatry 1998; 45:859–864.

101. Rabkin J, Rabkin R, Remien R, et al. Stability of mood despite HIV illness progression in a group of homosexual men. Am J Psychiatry 1997; 154:231–238.

102. Maj M, Janssen R, Starace F, et al. WHO neuropsychiatric AIDS study, cross-sectional phase I, study design and psychiatric findings. Arch Gen Psychiatry 1994; 51:39–49.

103. Catania J, Turner H, Choi K, et al. Coping with death anxiety: help seeking and social support among gay men with various HIV diagnoses. AIDS 1992; 6:999–1005.

104. Sewell DD. Schizophrenia and HIV. Schizophr Bull 1996; 22:465–473.

105. Sewell DD, Jeste DV, McAdams JL, et al. Neuroleptic treatment of HIV-associated psychosis. HNRC Group. Neuropsychopharmacology 1994; 10:223–229.

106. Kotler D, Grunfeld C. Pathophysiology and treatment of AIDS-wasting syndrome. In: Volberding P, Jacobson M, eds. AIDS Clinical Review 1992. New York: Marcel Dekker, 1996:229–276.

107. Van Roenn J, Armstrong D, Kotler D, et al. Megestrol acetate in patients with AIDS-related cachexia. Ann Intern Med 1994; 121:393–399.

108. Beal J, Olson R, Laubenstein L, et al. Dronabinol as a treatment for anorexia associated with weight loss in patients with AIDS. J Pain Symptom Manage 1995; 10:89–97.

109. Bucher G, Berger D, Fields-Garner C, et al. A prospective study on the safety and effect of nandrolone decanoate in HIV-positive patients. XIth International AIDS Conference, Vancouver, B.C., Canada. July 7–12, 1996. Abstract nr. Mo.B.423.

110. Corcoran C, Grinspoon S. Diagnosis and treatment of endocrine disorders in the HIV-infected patient. J In Assoc Physicians AIDS Care 1998; 4:10–14.

111. Laudat A, Blum L, Guechot J, et al. Changes in systemic gonadal and adrenal steroid in asymptomatic immunodeficiency virus–infected men: relationship with the CD4 cell counts. Eur J Endocrinol 1995; 133:418–424.

112. Berger D, Murahainen N, Wittert H, et al. Hypogonadism and wasting in the era of HAART in HIV-infected patients. XIIth World AIDS Conference, Geneva, Switzerland. June 28–July 3, 1998. Abstract nr. 32174.

113. Wagner G, Rabkin J. Testosterone therapy for clinical symptoms of hypogonadism in eugonadal men with AIDS. Int J STD AIDS 1998; 9:41–44.

114. Coodley, GO, Coodley, MK. A trial of testosterone therapy for HIV-associated weight loss. AIDS 1997; 1347–1352.

115. Martinez E, Gatell J. Metabolic abnormalities and body fat redistribution in HIV-1 infected patients: the lipodystrophy syndrome. Curr Opin Infect Dis 1999; 12: 13–19.

116. Carr A, Samaras K, Chishold D, et al. Pathogenesis of HIV-1 protease inhibitor–associated peripheral lipodystrophy, hyperlipidaemia, and insulin resistance. Lancet 1998; 35:1881–1883.

117. Breitbart W, Rosenfeld B, Passik S. Interest in physician-assisted suicide among ambulatory HIV-infected patients. Am J Psychiatry 1996; 153:238–242.

118. Rosenfeld B, Breitbart W, Stein K, et al. Measuring desire for death among patients with HIV/AIDS: the Schedule of Attitudes towards Hastened Death. Am J Psychiatry 1999; 156:94–100.

119. Chochinov H, Wilson K, Enns M, et al. Desire for death in the terminally ill. Am J Psychiatry 1995; 152:1185–1191.

120. Rabkin J, Ferrando J. A "second life" agenda: psychiatric research issues raised by protease inhibitor treatments or people with the human immunodeficiency virus or the acquired immunodeficiency syndrome. Arch Gen Psychiatry 1997; 54: 1049–1053.

121. Breitbart W. Psychiatric disorders in patients with progressive medical disease: the importance of diagnosis. In: Portenoy R, Bruera E, eds. Topics in Palliative Care, vol 3. Oxford: Oxford University Press, 1998:165–173.

Index

Page numbers followed by *f* and *t* indicate figures and tables, respectively